"In the present conjuncture, authoritarianism has spread across the world and fascism is looming. How can we understand the appeal of these destructive trends and begin to oppose them? In this inspiring Reader, Alasdair Cannon and Tom Fielder provide some essential texts bringing psychoanalysis to bear on these questions. Their own Introduction and Conclusion draws this material together into a powerful new account of the dynamics of fascism (the 'fascist state of fantasy') that sets the agenda for political and psychoanalytic resistance. This is an essential text for a deeply troubling world."

Stephen Frosh, *Emeritus Professor, Birkbeck, University of London, UK*

"Against the backdrop of contemporary political culture, Alasdair Cannon and Tom Fielder's excellent Reader provides an important contribution to the field of psychopolitics at a time when authoritarian leaders, far-right populism, and processes of radicalisation are widespread. The book brings together significant texts drawing on a range of perspectives and traditions, past and present, addressing the interweaving of conscious and unconscious forces that underlie the pull of fascism and how to resist it. The authors' substantial introduction and conclusion reflect critically on the essays in this volume, providing original insights into fascism as a 'multi-dimensional psychosocial phenomenon' shaped by 'fascist states of fantasy.' This is urgent work: as forces associated with fascism reassert themselves across the political landscape, the task of understanding and countering their psychic hold has rarely felt more pressing, and this book offers vital resources for that task."

Candida Yates, *Emerita Professor, Bournemouth University, UK*

"This is not simply a book about fascism; it is a profound exploration of the vulnerabilities of the human mind, the fragility of democratic life, and the psychic conditions that render cruelty, exclusion, and dehumanization imaginable. At a moment when authoritarian fantasies are once again gaining political traction, this volume demonstrates that understanding these processes is not merely an intellectual exercise—it is itself an act of ethical and political resistance.

Bringing together an outstanding group of psychoanalytic thinkers, this collection shows with remarkable clarity that fascism cannot be understood solely as a historical or political phenomenon. It must also be approached as a recurring psychic formation that emerges wherever fear, humiliation, omnipotence, and the longing for certainty eclipse the capacity to tolerate difference and uncertainty.

Essential reading for psychoanalysts, psychologists, psychiatrists, political theorists, historians, and all those concerned with the psychological foundations of contemporary democracy, this volume will become an indispensable resource for scholars, clinicians, and engaged readers alike. It stands as a major contribution to the growing dialogue between psychoanalysis, critical social thought, and political theory, and will undoubtedly serve as a landmark reference for years to come."

Fanny Guglielmucci, *Professor, Roma Tre University, Italy*

"This work is a huge contribution towards psychoanalytic thinking in relation to fascism. It is a gift to the psychoanalytic community who continue to make efforts in understanding human destructiveness and what can repair our human relationships in times of polarisation.

It gathers seminal works on psychoanalysis and fascism together in one place and is carefully curated drawing on the principles of free association so that it can create space for new insights to be made. It is a timely and important contribution and has been crafted with much care, attention and thoughtfulness."

Dr Anna Harvey, *The Tavistock and Portman NHS Foundation Trust, UK*

"This ambitious collection accomplishes a difficult task. Alasdair Cannon and Tom Fielder have brought together a stellar team of scholars, philosophers and psychoanalysts. Each author has already published their contribution during different post-war decades. The achievement of this collection is that the book chapters read as though these have been written recently.

Being timely, the volume interweaves its thinking about fascism by presenting its social, political and psychical dimensions without reduction or conflation. As a 'psychosocial' study, it is indeed 'multi-dimensional' (to quote the Editors' Introduction). The 'group ego' and the 'mass psychology of fascism' are familiar phrases. Yet these meet our understanding of how fascisms deal with what they find unbearable. Is there a 'fascist mindset?' Stock terms from psychoanalysis return: the 'paranoid-schizoid position,' 'narcissism,' 'mourning and melancholia.' These can all be re-theorized and investigated as 'states of fantasy' (to use Jacqueline Rose's term). Masculinity can be conceptualised less as a gendered term and more as an intolerable experience of separation: it is superficially solved only by joining an in-group of like-minded fascists who cannot bear internal differences. What is regarded as truth invites delirium.

Cannon and Fielder present the concept of 'ante-fascism' as occupying those sovereign states in which 'fascism has not fully arrived' while it lurks with a 'ghostly' presence. To use Freud's phrase 'terminable and interminable,' fascism may persist, may come to an end or do both. *Psychoanalysis and Fascism* should be read by psychoanalysts, academics, politicians and citizens. It is not a self-help book. Rather, it is an intellectual guide for survival in a period when even thinking about fascism is under assault.'

Dr. Catherine Lord, *University of Amsterdam, Netherlands*

"This is a very exciting collection of papers that address psychoanalytic thinking on fascism. While fascism has historical and economic components, the psychological reasons for why people participate in this project of hate when it is so costly, are important to know. But the gripe I have with psychoanalysis is that it has kept these ideas in the inner academic circles. I hope what this book leads to is reading circles, awareness projects, street plays and other mediums to help people understand their mind and how it could become fascist—and how the release with violence is only temporary. I have faith that if taken in the right spirit, this book could help us come up with ways to combat polarization."

Sadaf Arafati, *Guftagu Counselling and Psychotherapy Services*

"The editors of *Psychoanalysis and Fascism* provide an excellent selection of essays, and an indispensable map for exploring dark times. The book contains a thoughtful editorial introduction, a varied selection of perspectives by illustrious writers, on history, psyche and politics, and an urgent conclusion. This collection has implications for the study of the twentieth-century past, the new millennium, and our possible futures. It deserves to become required reading for all those who are grappling now with the dire and enduring attractions of fascism."

Daniel Pick, Professor Emeritus, Birkbeck College, training analyst, British Psychoanalytical Society, and author of *The Pursuit of the Nazi Mind and Brainwashed*

Psychoanalysis and Fascism

Psychoanalysis and Fascism: A Reader brings together some of the most significant papers papers from a century-long history of psychoanalytic writings on fascism.

Alasdair Cannon and Tom Fielder situate key work by authors including Wilhelm Reich, Christopher Bollas, Jacqueline Rose, Otto F. Kernberg, and Theodor W. Adorno in the context of fascism's return as a locus of renewed political anxiety and scholarly debate. Organised into five parts—The Fascist State of Mind, Mass Psychology, Masculinity and Perversion, Psychosocial Approaches, and an Afterword—and featuring an extensive Introduction and Conclusion by the Editors, the book includes a diverse and comprehensive view of the major contributions to the field, from its inception to the present day.

Psychoanalysis and Fascism: A Reader will be a valuable resource for scholars and students of psychoanalytic studies, critical theory, cultural studies, political studies and political psychology, and for psychoanalytic and group analytic practitioners seeking a psychosocial perspective on the proliferation of rage and terror in today's world of systemic breakdown.

Alasdair Cannon is a British-Australian writer and independent researcher based in London. He is the author of *Infinite Discontent: Writings on the Allure of Fascism* (eidolon ink, 2024) and holds an MA in Psychoanalytic Studies from Birkbeck, University of London.

Tom Fielder, PhD, is an Associate Lecturer at the Centre for Psychosocial Research, Birkbeck, University of London, and a member of the Executive Board of the Association for Psychosocial Studies.

Psychoanalysis and Fascism

A Reader

Edited by Alasdair Cannon
and Tom Fielder

Routledge
Taylor & Francis Group
LONDON AND NEW YORK

Designed cover image: Spaarnestad Photo Thousands of 'Blackshirts' listen to Mussolini's speech in the old Colosseum in Rome, Italy 1926.

First published 2027
by Routledge
4 Park Square, Milton Park, Abingdon, Oxon OX14 4RN

and by Routledge
605 Third Avenue, New York, NY 10158

Routledge is an imprint of the Taylor & Francis Group, an informa business

British Library Cataloguing-in-Publication Data
A catalogue record for this book is available from the British Library

ISBN: 978-1-041-24638-1 (hbk)
ISBN: 978-1-041-24637-4 (pbk)
ISBN: 978-1-003-74287-6 (ebk)

DOI: 10.4324/9781003742876

Typeset in Times New Roman
by SPi Technologies India Pvt Ltd (Straive)

Contents

Contributors

Theodor W. Adorno (1903–1969) was a leading member of the Frankfurt School. His critical theory examined authoritarianism, ideology, and the psychodynamics of fascist propaganda. Notable works include *The Authoritarian Personality* (with Else Frenkel-Brunswik, Daniel Levinson, and Nevitt Sanford), *Dialectic of Enlightenment* (with Max Horkheimer), *Negative Dialectics*, and *Minima Moralia*.

Christopher Bollas is a British psychoanalyst and writer who has been in psychoanalytical practice for over 50 years. A former Professor of English at the University of Massachusetts and Professor of Psychoanalysis at the University of Rome, he is the author of more than 25 books.

Michael J. Diamond is an American psychoanalyst and clinical psychologist. Author of five books, he is a Fellow of the International Psychoanalytic Association, the American Psychological Association, and the American Academy of Clinical Psychology.

Stephen Frosh is Emeritus Professor in the Department of Psychosocial Studies at Birkbeck, University of London, UK, and a Founding Member of the Association of Psychosocial Studies. He is the author of over 20 books on psychosocial studies and psychoanalysis.

Sue Grand is faculty and supervisor at the NYU Postdoctoral Program in Psychotherapy and Psychoanalysis. She is the author and co-editor of multiple books on psychoanalytic theory and works in private practice in NYC and in New Jersey.

Otto F. Kernberg is Past President of the International Psychoanalytic Association, and Training and Supervising Analyst of the Columbia University Center for Psychoanalytic Training and Research. The author of 12 books and co-author of 11 others, he has received numerous awards for his excellence in psychiatry

Noëlle C. McAfee is Professor of Philosophy at Emory University and holds a secondary appointment as Professor of Psychiatry and Behavioural

Sciences. She is the author of over 80 articles and 5 books, including *Fear of Breakdown: Politics and Psychoanalysis* (Columbia, 2019).

Wilhelm Reich (1897–1957) was a leading psychoanalyst and deputy director of Freud's Psychoanalytic Polyclinic in Vienna. A pioneer of body-oriented psychotherapy, he authored influential works including *Character Analysis* and *The Mass Psychology of Fascism*. He fled Nazi Germany in 1933 and emigrated to the United States in 1939.

Jacqueline Rose is Professor of Humanities at Birkbeck, University of London, and Co-Director of the Birkbeck Institute for the Humanities and of the London Critical Theory Summer School. She is internationally known for her writing on feminism, psychoanalysis, literature and the politics and ideology of Israel-Palestine.

Jill Salberg is faculty at the NYU Postdoctoral Program in Psychoanalysis, where she teaches and writes on topics including the relationship of psychoanalytic free association to democratic free speech. She also completed psychoanalytic training at the Institute for the Psychoanalytic Study of Subjectivity, and is in independent practice in Greenwich Village, NY, and in Highland Park, NJ.

Alberto Toscano is Adjunct Professor within the School of Communication at Simon Fraser University in Burnaby, British Columbia. He is the author of *Fanaticism* (Verso, 2017) and *Late Fascism* (Verso, 2023).

Christina Wieland is Visiting Fellow at the Department of Psycho-Social and Psychoanalytic Studies, University of Essex, and a psychoanalyst in private practice. She is the author of two books, including *The Fascist State of Mind and the Manufacturing of Masculinity: A Psychoanalytic Approach* (Routledge, 2014).

Introduction

Psychoanalysis and Fascism

Alasdair Cannon and Tom Fielder

We live in a paranoid state of alarm and planetary dread, bewildered and beset by a staggering concatenation of economic, environmental, technological, political and geopolitical crises. It is the era of polycrisis, in which wildly disparate shocks intersect so that the whole is much more dangerous, and much more difficult to conceptually 'contain', than the sum of its parts. Yet even as we blindly advance into the brave new world of the twenty-first century, peering over the ends of history towards dramatic tipping points, we regress into the horrors of the past. Never entirely transcended, the history of the twentieth century weighs like a compulsive nightmare on the critical imagination, simultaneously clarifying and repugnant. Almost everywhere we look, strongmen are on the march, recklessly propagating new forms of right-wing nationalism in the guise of restoring a forsaken identity, and a lost or stolen sense of collective security and greatness. Has the plague returned? The invisible worm released into the deepening night? Are we witnessing the resurgence of fascism in liberal societies? We awake from this dream—which is not a dream—with pounding hearts, short of breath as we search the landscape for reasons to confirm or contest our fears. Alert to the risks of misrecognition and moral panic, we seek to apprehend the political trajectory of the destructiveness that has resurfaced in our societies by asking each other and ourselves if we are in the early stages of a new 'fascism'.

In the USA, the second Trump administration has galvanised these fears and insistently provoked this debate. Proclaiming a new "GOLDEN AGE" (The White House, 2026), perhaps only insofar as "gold is a sign or symbol for faeces" (Freud, [1911] 2024, p. 186), Trumpism has attracted comment from a range of politicians and prominent scholars, including Ruth Ben-Ghiat, Judith Butler, Naomi Klein, Robert Reich, Avi Shlaim, Timothy Snyder, Alberto Toscano and Slavoj Žižek. Each Democratic presidential candidate from the last decade—Clinton, Biden, and Harris—has now called Trump a fascist (Bowman, 2024; Clinton, 2024; Williams and Waldenberg, 2024). And as ICE spends $38 billion on converting warehouses across the US into detention and deportation centres (Jones, 2026), US imperialism threatens old allies (Canada,

DOI: 10.4324/9781003742876-1

Greenland) and enemies (Iran, Cuba) alike, Trump issues orders decreeing that the state will recognise only "two sexes" (The White House, 2025), and senior figures in Trump's administration claim he has "plenary authority" to deploy federalised National Guard troops against US citizens (Chidi, 2025), speculation about the US government's incipient fascism hardly seems unwarranted.

But even as they invoke the haunting spectre of fascism, critical scholars qualify its (re)appearance with various epithets: late fascism, liberal fascism, American fascism, ante-fascism, end-times fascism, failed fascism. Others more robustly reject implicit or explicit equivalences with the 1930s, warning that such critical hyperbole diminishes the urgency of self-scrutiny on the Left, and elides more careful consideration of Trump's actual appeal to voters. Historian of fascism Roger Griffin insists that the word has a specific, technical meaning which we must not dilute: "You can be a total xenophobic racist male chauvinist bastard, and still not be a fascist" (Matthews, 2020). There may be more historically appropriate terms to describe the current global conjuncture instead of "fascism", such as "neoliberalism" (Brown, 2019), "necropolitics" (Mbembe, 2019), and "technofeudalism" or "neofeudalism" (Varoufakis, 2024; Dean, 2025). Given the complexity and ideological diversity of contemporary far-right movements, it may be best to adopt or create an entirely new terminology to describe the reactionary, authoritarian class that now reaches from Silicon Valley to the White House. Or perhaps, given that this disparate group embraces old and new ideas from the Dark Enlightenment, tech-bro transhumanist eschatology, incel ideology, White nationalism, Christian theocracy, neo-Nazism, and free-market fundamentalism, alongside MAGA's opportunistic, illiberal politics and narrative of national rebirth, it may be most accurate to say that "fascism" comprises and brings into focus only one aspect of a novel, syncretic, chaotically improvised and ongoing (re)organisation of ideology and power in the early twenty-first century.

From Trump's ruthless, intoxicated assault on immigrant populations in the USA and his illegal attacks on Iran and Venezuela, to Putin's grinding imperialism in Ukraine and Netanyahu's genocidal war in Gaza—via Farage, Modi, Milei, Orbán, Duterte, Bolsonaro, Le Pen and Meloni—reflection on the meaning of 'fascism' has become a pressing political concern. A foundational object within critical theory, generations of writers and readers have turned to the history and conceptual articulation of fascist politics to locate an incipient logic of destruction within liberal democratic societies, ideally before this logic has had the chance to fully disclose itself. This history of writing about the connection between liberalism and fascism invites us to clarify our moral and ideological orientation in certain ways, shifting gears in our dialectical engagements with the crises of contemporary capitalism. And as we seek to orient ourselves to the present conjuncture, with its bewildering brew of sadistic performative politics, racism, and irrationality at the collective level, the return of fascism deserves a much wider discussion within psychoanalytic studies, not least because psychoanalysis has been so integral to the theorisation of fascistic psychopolitics. In this reader, we have collected some of the most generative writings in the history of psychoanalytic studies of fascism, to ask: what can psychoanalysis contribute to our understanding of fascism and to contemporary anti-fascist critique?

Diagnosis, Resistance, Suppression, & Collaboration: A Century of Psychoanalysis and Fascism

The sheer scale and dynamism of violent destructiveness around the world today confronts the critical imagination with the limits of its powers, pointing beyond materialist analysis and folk-psychological frameworks towards an unconscious zone of intrigue and irrationality which has been filled with fresh, concrete life by the latest generation of tyrannical agitators and nativist 'rabble-rousers'. Even scholars such as Adam Tooze (2025), who remain more cautious about directly calling Trump a fascist, recognise that the fascisms of Mussolini's Italy, or Nazi Germany, had a psychological dimension which cannot be so easily confined to the historical circumstances of the 1930s. There are fascisms, to borrow from Freud, both "terminable" and "interminable" (Freud, [1937] 2024). Or, as Michel Foucault (in Deleuze and Guattari, 1983, p. xii) observed in his famous preface to the English translation of *Anti-Oedipus*: fascism can also be considered as a permanent potential "in our heads and in our everyday behavior". The murderous and death-driven, suicidal and millenarian idealism of historic fascisms have inspired significant volumes of psychoanalytic writing. For almost a century now, psychoanalysis has tried to reckon with the worst of what the mind is really capable *en masse*.

Historians of psychoanalysis have frequently observed the "chronological simultaneity of origin" between fascism and psychoanalysis (Forrester, 2009, p. 272). Fascism emerged in Italy in the wake of the First World War, and although psychoanalysis had already been substantially formed by 1914, it only became "a movement with a major cultural resonance" as John Forrester (2009, p. 271) notes, "whose ripples from a certain moment onwards extended very widely and with no coordinated control through the arts and sciences, in the same historical moment". While the development of Freud's thought after 1914 had its own theoretical and clinical rationale, it was also clearly propelled and even inspired by the deterioration of European society and the rise of new forms of political barbarism within "the great world-dominating nations of white races" (Freud, [1915] 2024, p. 276). Freud responded to the famous "loss of authority" which simultaneously provoked and precipitated artistic and literary modernism by positing something "radically unmasterable" about human subjectivity (Rose, 2021, p. 203). Drawing on his experience with shell-shocked soldiers, Freud introduced the death drive to psychoanalysis in 1920, the year the Nazi Party was formed in Germany. Observing the compulsive tendency of such patients to "repeat… unwanted situations and painful emotions", Freud ([1920] 2024, p. 21) laments that "no lesson has been learnt from the old experience of these activities having led... only to unpleasure". He then published *Group Psychology and the Analysis of the Ego* in 1921, the year before Mussolini's March on Rome, critically engaging Gustave Le Bon's (1895) earlier work on the psychological character of the "group mind"—a text which was also influential for Mussolini (Freud, [1921] 2024, pp. 69–77; see Paxton, 2004, pp. 32–33).

In this decisive period of the early twentieth century, Freud's psychoanalysis and Mussolini's fascism revealed and manifested the unconscious of the European liberal tradition, rupturing the image of the self as forged in the mirror of reason, and exposing the myths of progress and Enlightenment as interminably conflicted and precarious. In diametrically opposing ways, their respective movements showed that the empires of civilization had never finally triumphed over barbarism, because they continued to draw their power from a barbaric or repressed "primitive" otherness at their core. In the development of the mind, as Freud ([1915] 2024, pp. 284–285) observed, every earlier, "primitive" stage persists alongside the later, "civilized" stage which has emerged from it, in the form of a "special capacity" for involution and regression.[1] But while psychoanalysts such as Freud theorised and remembered this repressed material in order to release their patients from demonic repetition, fascists repeated it as a contemporary experience of return. For Federico Finchelstein (2009), Freud understood fascism in exactly these terms. When he was asked to dedicate a copy of *Why War?*—his 1933 response to a letter from Albert Einstein—to Mussolini, Freud cryptically referred to Il Duce as the "*Kultur Heros*". In so doing, Finchelstein argues that Freud posited a subtle form of identification between Mussolini and Prometheus—for Freud, an ambivalent symbol of heroic "modernity" and resurgent primitivism that together brought "unmediated violence, death and destruction" (2009, p. 113).

Just as Freud's investigation of the neuroses revealed tormenting inner conflicts simultaneously produced and repressed by society—and thereby rendered impossible to resolve—so psychoanalytic approaches to fascism promised to expose the unrequited yearnings and "undeniable... hypocrisy" (Freud, [1915] 2024, p. 283) within liberal selves and their societies, which were continuing to ferment political catastrophe at home and abroad. In Finchelstein's (2009) account of Mussolini's "fascist unconscious", Freud's theory describes an intrapsychic analogue to what Aimé Césaire and Hannah Arendt would later describe as the "boomerang effect" of European imperialism: the return to Europe of forms of domination and technologies of violence previously projected outward onto colonial populations. The violence historically exercised by European powers against colonial subjects returns homeward in fascism, now directed against racialized enemies located within the body politic. In this sense, fascism appears structurally analogous to Freud's account of melancholia: aligned with a punitive ego ideal against a debased ego, fascist states "direct against [themselves] the hostility" that represents their "original reaction to objects in the external world" (Freud, [1917] 2024, p. 225). Where the melancholic ego denigrates itself as a hated object, the fascist state redeploys against its own society the terroristic violence already practised and refined at the imperial frontier.

"Psychoanalysis, in its encounter with fascism", writes Finchelstein, "became a form of anti-fascism". Against Mussolini's idealisation of war and radical violence, Freud forwarded a psychoanalytic anti-fascism based on pacifism, critical irony, the deflation of myth, and recognition of the unconscious (Finchelstein, 2009, pp. 99–100). In another essential paper which we have not been able to include in this reader, Daniel Pick (2009) warns against underestimating the role of Freudian thought in the wider struggle against fascism between the 1920s and 1950s. Although scholars have tended to diminish the extent of Freud's own political resistance to fascism, diverse psychological theories derived from psychoanalysis in fact suffused anti-fascist commentaries in both the interwar and immediate post-war periods. Pick emphasises Allied investigations of the "Nazi mind" led by Henry Dicks and others during the Second World War, alongside interventions from a range of eminent psychoanalysts: Anna Freud, Karl Menninger, Wilfred Bion, Edward Glover, John Rickman, Ernest Jones, Roger Money-Kyrle, Erich Fromm, John Bowlby, Erik Erikson, Ernst Simmel, Walter Langer, Bruno Bettelheim, Edith Jacobson, Franz Alexander, and Ernst Kris (Pick, 2009, p. 140; cf. Pick, 2012). "We might debate the quality of each of these contributions", as Pick observes, "but suffice to say that there was a shared endeavour to understand both the psycho-social conditions in which the extreme right flourished and the unconscious factors that made Fascism attractive to so many" (2009, p. 140).

The most famous of these early psychoanalytic writings was Wilhelm Reich's *The Mass Psychology of Fascism* ([1942] 1970). In his 1942 preface to the third edition of the book—originally published in 1933—Reich helpfully insists on the "general and international" nature of fascism as "the organized political expression of the structure of the average man's character" in what he calls "our authoritarian machine civilization and its mechanistic-mystical conception of life". Charged with the perverse sadism of "race ideology", fascism in its pure form, Reich claims, "is the sum total of all the irrational reactions of the average human character" (Reich, [1942] 1970, p. xiv). In this reader, we have included the second chapter of Reich's seminal text, in which he investigates the mass psychological structure of the middle class and the role of "authoritarian family ideology" in rendering the "average man" vulnerable to demagogy. Emphasising the central role of desire in fascism, Reich's work would eventually be enormously influential on Deleuze and Guattari's schizoanalytic theory of the "non-fascist life" ([1972] 1983). In turn, Deleuze and Guattari's work would inform Klaus Theweleit's *Male Fantasies* ([1977] 1987; [1978] 1989), a seminal psychoanalytic study of the German Freikorps men of the 1920s that combined pre-Oedipal psychoanalytic ideas from Michael Balint and Margaret Mahler with an outspoken feminist standpoint (see [1977] 1987, pp. 204–215). Theweleit's study was a surprise bestseller in Germany upon its release, much like Alexander and Margarete Mitscherlich's *The Inability to Mourn* (1967) had been a decade before. A rare example of psychoanalytic writing that had a powerful political impact in its time—selling 100,000 copies in the original edition—the Mitscherlichs called for a collective reckoning with the Nazi past via hundreds of case histories and an original "socio-psychological analysis" of the Third Reich. "World-redeeming dreams of ancient greatness", as they so evocatively write, "arise in peoples in whom the sense of having been left behind by history evokes feelings of impotence and rage" (Mitscherlich and Mitscherlich, 1984, p. 12). Such dreams, as the success of these texts by Theweleit and the Mitscherlichs demonstrated, left subsequent generations in Germany with a terrible thirst for psychoanalytic insight.

Approaching fascism by way of Freud's theories on narcissism and mass psychology, and brilliantly elucidating Freud's anticipation of the 1930s, Theodor Adorno developed another early and important contribution to the psychoanalysis of fascism. In his essay on "Freudian Theory and the Pattern of Fascist Propaganda" (Chapter 4 of this reader), Adorno refers to "the externalization of the super-ego" and its "replacement through a 'group ego'" as "one of the most decisive observations about the fascist personality" and "exactly what happens to fascist personalities" (note 7, p.89). "They fail to develop an independent autonomous conscience", Adorno continues, "and substitute for it an identification with collective authority which is irrational as Freud described it, heteronomous, rigidly oppressive, largely alien to the individuals' own thinking and, therefore, easily exchangeable in spite of its structural rigidity" (note 7, p. 89). Adorno even refers to the speeches of "American fascist demagogues who never appeal to their prospective followers' own conscience but incessantly invoke external, conventional and stereotyped values" (note 7, p. 89). Drawing on Adorno's essay, and his preceding study of "the authoritarian personality", alongside the psychoanalytic contributions afforded by Klein, Jones and Bion, Pick (2009, pp. 152–153) emphasises Freud's introduction of the superego as the crucial concept for psychoanalytical investigations of the Nazi mind, even suggesting that the encounter between psychoanalysis and fascism in the twentieth century was defined in essential respects by the application of this theory of a sadistic and vengeful, inner "moral" authority to the formation of fascist collectives (cf. Ffytche, 2016). In *The Ego and the Id* ([1923] 2024), published in the same year as Hitler's abortive putsch in Munich, Freud ([1923] 2024, p. 47) resonantly observes that, in melancholia, this superego is embroiled within "a pure culture of the death drive"—a formulation one could adopt with minimal modification to describe Hitler's Nazi government. After the Anschluss in 1938, Freud was forced to flee Vienna, arriving in London together with his wife Martha and their daughter Anna, in June 1938. Freud's sisters Rosa, Marie, Adolfine and Pauline could not leave Austria, and were deported to concentration camps in 1942, where they either died of internal injuries or were murdered in the gas chambers.

As a diagnostic tool that can reveal the disavowed fears and desires that underwrite the deadly allure of fascism, psychoanalysis has a long history of mutual antagonism with fascist movements. Freud's texts were among the first targets of the book burnings at the outset of the Nazi regime, signalling the Third Reich's compulsive hostility towards the "Jewish science" of Freud and his followers. To the Nazis, as Stephen Frosh (2005, p. 74) explains, "psychoanalysis was a prime example of the corrosive nature of Jewish thought, its degenerate capacity to poison the sources of idealism and feeling for race and nation… sucking the life blood out of the Aryan nations and using it to feed the growth of Jewish corruption." Its Jewish origins and its focus on sexuality, combined with its critical and ironic perspective on German society, and the links with socialism shared among so many of its adherents, "all added up to compelling evidence", as Frosh writes, "of its perniciousness, and made it a prime candidate for persecution" (2005, p. 74). Numerous European-Jewish psychoanalysts, including Freud, were forced to flee from Germany and Austria in the 1930s, seeking refuge in the USA and England, as well as Palestine, the Netherlands and elsewhere in Europe. Some analysts were directly murdered by the Nazis: Karl Landauer, co-founder of the Frankfurt Institute of Psychoanalysis, was arrested in the Netherlands and deported to Bergen-Belsen with his wife and eldest daughter, where he died of starvation in January 1945, while Dr. John F. Rittmeister was arrested in September 1942 and executed in May 1943 for taking part in the resistance activities of the 'Red Chapel' or 'Red Orchestra' anti-fascist organisation. Others still were detained and imprisoned: Bruno Bettelheim's influential paper, "Individual and Mass Behaviour in Extreme Situations", had its basis in the author's first-hand observations during his year "at Dachau and at Buchenwald" (Bettelheim, 1943, p. 417).

However, more widely across the psychoanalytic movement in Germany, and under substantial pressure from the Nazi authorities, there was also a discomfiting history of "appeasement" among many practitioners, especially at the notorious Göring Institute in Berlin (Cocks, 1997; Frosh, 2005). The non-Jewish analysts Felix Boehm and Carl Müller-Braunschweig negotiated with the Nazis in 1933, overseeing the Aryanisation of psychoanalysis in the Third Reich, under the leadership of Hermann Göring's cousin, Matthias. Müller-Braunschweig penned a notorious "Memorandum" on psychoanalysis for the Nazis in 1933, in which he adopted the language of "mastery" so resonant with fascism, even claiming that psychoanalysis "works to remodel incapable weaklings into people who can cope with life… those indifferent to the totality of life into those willing to serve the whole" (Brecht et al., 1985, p. 116). Both Boehm and Müller-Braunschweig survived the war, the latter going on to head the new post-war psychoanalytic organisation in West Germany. It was not, in fact, until the IPA Hamburg Congress of 1985 that the full scope of this history of collaboration with Nazism finally emerged into institutional consciousness, through a remarkable exhibition on German psychoanalysis before and after 1933, the result of a series of historical "recoveries" and the searching efforts of a new generation of German analysts (Frosh, 2005, p. 3; see also

Brecht et al., 1985; Chasseguet-Smirgel, 1987; Cocks, 1997; Goggin and Goggin, 2001). Infamously, Carl Jung's relationship to the Third Reich exposed a notorious tendency towards anti-Semitism in his thought, although he later modified and even reversed his initial tacit support for Nazism (Pick, 2009, p. 139; cf. Samuels, 1992a, 1992b; Cocks, 1997; Shamdasani, 2003). But for Stephen Frosh (2012), there are still real questions for contemporary psychoanalysis regarding its ability to work through the past, including specifically the history and ongoing existence of anti-Semitism within its institutional body (see also Frosh, 2005, 2019, 2023).

Psychoanalysis and Fascism: A Reader

Beginning with Freud's seminal reflections on mass psychology and incipient fascism in interwar Europe, and the subsequent contributions of Wilhelm Reich and the 'political Freudians' of the 1930s and 1940s like Fenichel, Simmel, and Loewenstein (Zolkos, 2022), the archive of psychoanalytic studies on fascism now reaches back almost a century, branching through the critical theories of Erich Fromm, Theodor Adorno, Gilles Deleuze, and Félix Guattari, as well as the varied psychoanalytic traditions of Klein, Winnicott, Bowlby, Bion, Lacan, Kristeva, Volkan, and Benjamin. For decades, a range of influential scholars have used psychoanalysis to reflect on fascism as both a political 'state of mind' and as a pathological mass movement, ambiguously positioned between psychic life and the social order. Today, this discontinuous seam of psychoanalytic engagement with far-right politics, episodically triggered by political dread and "regression", includes works produced by some of the field's most eminent researchers—Jessica Benjamin, Jacqueline Rose, Christopher Bollas, Janine Chasseguet-Smirgel, Stephen Frosh, and Slavoj Žižek—and continues to attract exciting contributions from younger researchers in psychoanalysis and psychosocial studies.

But despite this abundant and ongoing history of psychoanalytic interest, the archive of psychoanalytic studies in fascism remains somewhat limited, disorganised, and incoherent. In general, there is a Eurocentric bias to the study of fascism within psychoanalysis and critical scholarship more broadly, with its characteristic emphases on Italy, Germany, and the contemporary USA, which we would like to signal and to contest in this reader (see "Directions for Future Research and Further Readings"). Major contributions in the field from earlier decades have also been neglected by later writers who themselves authored seminal contributions. Chasseguet-Smirgel's paper (1990), for example, does not cite Theweleit, Adorno, or Reich, despite obvious overlaps in their arguments. The same is true of Bollas's paper (1991), which makes only a passing reference to Reich. The Marxist-Lacanian theory of fascism Žižek developed in the 1990s and 2000s has also been largely ignored by later psychoanalytic theorists: Toscano and Frosh are the only authors in this reader (see Chapters 10 and 11) who discuss his work (e.g. Žižek, 2006). Though contemporary writers generally take more care to recognise and build upon the contributions of their forebears (see, e.g., Diamond, Chapter 2 of this reader), it seems that psychoanalytic theorists of fascism have often been inclined to set out alone against the enemy, theorising and resisting fascism as if preceding works did not exist—a fact, perhaps, that itself calls for psychoanalysis.

Similarly, and in a perplexing refusal of the interdisciplinary approach often deployed within psychoanalytic studies of social phenomena, psychoanalytic writers frequently ignore the political elements of fascism. Encountering the psychoanalytic archive on fascism, one wonders if the famous slipperiness of fascism as a concept confuses psychoanalysis. One anonymous reviewer of this volume referred to the pervasive "all in the mind" orientation of psychoanalytical researchers. There is indeed a notable tendency to reduce fascism, with its complex socioeconomic, political, and historical dimensions, to a generic and pathological extremist "state of mind". Christopher Bollas's landmark paper (Chapter 1 of this reader) refers to Stalin's Russia, the French Revolution, and Bakunin's revolutionary anarchism alongside Hitler's Germany and Mussolini's Italy in the development of his immensely influential notion of the "fascist state of mind" (pp. 79–83). Michael Diamond similarly conflates contemporary forms of anti-colonial resistance with instances of state terrorism as examples of the same reductively psychologistic phenomenon: "fascistic-friendly leanings", he writes, appeared "among extremists in both the pro-Israeli and pro-Palestinian enclaves" after Hamas's October 7th attack (this reader, note 9, p. 54). Both authors are undoubtedly correct to claim that the governments, movements, and thinkers they mention display similar kinds of psychic extremism. But labelling all these movements as "fascist" occludes the very real political, ideological, structural, historical, and material differences between them—distinctions that, as psychoanalysts know, will inevitably reflect and generate acute variations in the political fantasies of the people whose psychic lives they hope to describe.[2] The idea of a 'state of mind' itself also sits uneasily within psychoanalysis, which more characteristically asserts the mobility of the mind against the identity of any particular 'state', and in the conclusion to this reader we propose fascist "states of fantasy" as an alternative rubric, with reference to Jacqueline Rose's (1996) pivotal account of the intersection between psyche and politics.

Notwithstanding its limitations, the remarkable extant archive of psychoanalytic work contained in this reader and beyond presents a powerful resource for continued transgenerational creativity, suggesting new pathways for the further development of its ideas and analyses in the diverse and rapidly changing circumstances of global humanity—at a time when the question of fascism has become urgent once again. The papers we have been able to include in this volume sample almost a century of psychoanalytic writing about fascism. Wilhelm Reich's pioneering work on Nazi psychology from 1933 sits alongside cutting-edge papers on US fascism by Sue Grand and Jill Salberg published in late 2025. The major works by Christopher Bollas and Theodor Adorno referred to above join more recent pieces from some of the foremost living scholars of psychoanalysis like Stephen Frosh, Jacqueline Rose, and Otto Kernberg. The reader also includes pieces by Christina Wieland, Noëlle McAfee, Alberto Toscano, and Michael Diamond, scholars whose particular contributions to the field are essential to its future. Most of these contributions were authored relatively recently, with as many as nine of the reader's twelve papers published within the last decade. This is in part a reflection of the contemporary productivity of anti-fascist critique: inspired by the recent upsurge in authoritarian and populist right-wing politics, especially in the USA, many psychoanalytical theorists have returned to the topic of fascism to understand the imaginary, symbolic, and affective underpinnings of contemporary political ideologies and movements. (Perhaps inevitably, Trumpism therefore looms large among the most recent papers, although Trump himself is not always explicitly mentioned.) Despite its diversity, the literature appears to be approaching a kind of consensus on the psychopolitics of fascism, at least to the extent that narcissistic, schizoid, psychotic, and perverse phenomena are central to the most recent psychoanalytic explanations of fascist politics.

Each chapter in this reader begins with a short paragraph that explains the reasons for its inclusion. In these segments, the reader will find a brief statement of the significance or value of each paper as a distinctive contribution to the field. However, the papers chosen for this reader should not be read as anything like an official "canon" for psychoanalytic studies of fascism. Our original pitch for the reader, in fact, only included four of the papers it now contains. Most of these original papers were excluded because the licensing fees were prohibitively expensive (a fact Marxist scholars of fascism, for whom fascism is related to the defence of capitalist private property rights, will inevitably find ironic); those finally included were either the property of our publisher, Routledge, or of other publishers and copyright holders who were generous enough to grant us reprint permissions *gratis* or at a steep discount. The inclusion of a relatively large number of recent papers is partly a consequence of these factors; had it been possible, it is likely that we would have included additional, earlier works in this reader by authors like Klaus Theweleit, Janine Chasseguet-Smirgel, and Alexander and Margarete Mitscherlich. Works by these and other authors—including Freud himself—are instead included on the list of "Further Readings" at the end of this book. With this in mind, we have included each paper because of our sense of its generativity for future psychoanalytic thinking and writing on fascism, sometimes as a representative instance of a particular author's oeuvre. Each paper, we think, has the capacity to inspire new thought in a variety of useful directions. Taken together, we believe the contributions collected in this reader have the power to catalyse excellent new work in the field as a whole (see "Directions for Future Research and Further Readings").

The papers in this reader are organised in a deliberately loose and associational, rather than linear or evolutionary fashion. Though they are grouped with other papers that share similar themes—gender, for example, or group psychology—there is significant overlap between papers throughout the book. Crucially, we decided not to sequence the pieces chronologically. To do so, we felt, would generate a false impression of an oedipal, authoritarian structure of influence and descent in psychoanalytic studies of fascism, beginning with Freud, and moving through Reich and Adorno up to the present day, as though each of these authors were participants in a coherent and sequential project of developing anti-fascist critique. Instead, the papers are sequenced to encourage free association between papers past and present, and to rupture any fantasy of psychoanalytic mastery. This, we hope, will help readers to generate their own creative and unexpected connections between papers, and to theorise fascism anew in the present moment, drawing upon historical and contemporary experience from diverse global contexts in the process of collectively and independently grappling with fascism's uncanny return. Indeed, we wish for readers to experience a kind of Freudian *Nachträglichkeit* in their encounters with our reader, with the perspectives presented in later papers retroactively adjusting their understanding of earlier texts (and earlier historical moments), or vice versa.

This mode of thinking and reading, inspired by the psychoanalytic praxis of free association, is itself anti-fascist, in an albeit limited sense. The selected papers in this reader suggest that the fascist "state of fantasy" elicits transgressive enjoyment while simultaneously restricting mental life to a set of fixed ideas. "For Freud," writes Finchelstein, "the fascist leader thinks in terms of circular images" (2009, p. 99). "The similarity of the utterances of various agitators… is so great", as Adorno observes in this reader, "that it suffices in principle to analyse the statements of one of them in order to know them all." "Moreover," he continues, "the speeches themselves are so monotonous that one meets with endless repetitions as soon as one is acquainted with the very limited number of stock devices. As a matter of fact, constant reiteration and scarcity of ideas are indispensable ingredients of the entire technique" (p. 72). Fascist subjectivity involves a kind of cyclonic rage, where all signifiers furiously circle a still centre of hypercathected ideas: nation, race, masculinity, purity, wholeness, rebirth. Fascism, for this reason, functions as a paradoxically destructive and mobile *edification* of the self, issuing a phantasmatic psychological security to the ego even as it undermines the actual material and relational basis of personal and collective life. Fascist desire flows only in its rigidity, its violent simplifications of psyche and society obeying the strict inner logic issued by the superego. The continuous displacements and reconfigurations of fantasy, thought, and meaning produced by a mind in free association are therefore necessary (if insufficient) features of any "non-fascist life", whatever else those lives might otherwise entail (Foucault in Deleuze and Guattari, 1983, p. xii).

And what more can psychoanalysis say about the "non-fascist life"? The psychoanalytic studies of fascism collected in this reader generally emphasise description and diagnosis over *resistance*, as such. Nevertheless, they each forward their own visions of anti-fascist ethics, whether implicitly or explicitly. Within these texts the reader will find overt criticisms of the ideals and norms typical of fascism—racism, misogyny, patriarchy, nationalism, ableism, violence, and so on. But behind and beyond the critical delineation of these stereotyped structures of signification and power lurks a more visceral apprehension of fascism as a potential forever latent within ourselves and our societies, which—as kin to the death drive—can never be finally localised, identified, or contained in a particular form of personal or political consciousness, but incessantly manifests itself in newly destructive ways, eliding the mastery of critique. Within psychoanalysis, anti-fascist criticality requires an active and continued encounter with the unconscious—with those deathly urges, ideas, and fantasies that we cannot consciously avow or consistently countenance—and a refusal to take flight into consoling illusions of personal safety or immunity. We are all ensnared in the allure of fascism, just as we are all ensnared in the global economic system. But if it is in the unconscious, as Rose (1996, p. 10) writes, "that you most profoundly submit to the law, the unconscious is also, according to psychoanalysis, the place where all your other and better ideas can be found". While fascism gives new life to the worst aspects of the unconscious mind, cathecting the corrupt and degraded law (of the leader or Führer) with murderous, sadistic violence, the unconscious also preserves a capacity for fierce resistance, creativity, and survival, in which we might ultimately discover something stronger and more truthful than the fascist state and its spiralling (self-)destructiveness.

Rather than licensing complacently concretised diagnostic norms, an anti-fascist psychoanalysis demands an acute awareness of historical context, and a creative refusal of any reliance on clichés, tropes, or settled forms of thought. No two fascist movements are ever identical: fascist desires can only ever garb themselves in the signs and symbols of a particular period and place. As is the case in the encounter between analyst and patient in the psychoanalytic clinic, it is never enough to rely on established perspectives, codified theories, and accepted approaches when we try to comprehend and resist fascism, although these may be immensely influential. Animated by the insistent, conflictual forces of desire and destructiveness, and expressed through the memories and signifiers of a specific moment in time, fascism must be treated like a psychoanalytic symptom. The generic strategies and goals of treatment may inform an overall approach, but in a live encounter with fascism, the psychoanalytic process of working-through is achievable only if we are able to sufficiently respond to the idiosyncrasies and singularity of the symptom's active presentation. As the psychoanalyst does for the patient, anti-fascists must actively listen to fascist political actors and their audiences to locate the real sources of malaise, and creatively respond to the odious expression of hatred, resentment, anger, and destructiveness as a symptomatic knot or ghostliness in the political field. Against fascism, we need empathy—an empathy that can bear the unbearable about ourselves, our histories and our social structures; an empathy that hurts.

Alongside the continued rise in the terrifying threat posed by far-right political actors, there remains fierce debate today about the status of fascism in the contemporary world. We hope that this reader will show that psychoanalysis remains an invaluable and varied resource for the present and future of anti-fascist writing, complementing structural critique with a challenging and highly sophisticated—as well as self-critical—perspective on the 'mass psychology' of the 'fascism in us all' (Reich [1946] 1970; Foucault in Deleuze and Guattari, 1983, p. xii).

Notes

1 The role of references to the "primitive" mind within psychoanalysis has been forcefully criticised by postcolonial scholars such as Ranjana Khanna (2003). Freud ([1915] 2024, p. 283), however, was also at least signalling the "undeniable… hypocrisy" of liberal civilization.
2 Bollas counterposes the "fascist state of mind" against the "democratic" mind (Bollas, 2011, p. 81). Diamond also states that "fascism is antithetical to liberal democracy in that differences, including the narcissism of minor differences (Freud 1921, 1930), are turned into hated, demonized oppositions to be eradicated." By doing so, both Bollas and Diamond impliedly conflate liberal democratic politics and "states of mind" with sanity. Yet the forms of psychic extremism they describe as fascistic can be found amongst adherents of liberal democratic politics: note, for example, the dehumanising perspectives on the Israeli state's genocide of the Palestinian people adopted by mainstream Democrats like Joe Biden or Kamala Harris, both of whom characterised Trump as a "fascist" during the 2024 election cycle (see Bowman, 2024; Williams and Waldenberg, 2024).

References

Bettelheim, B. (1943) 'Individual and Mass Behavior in Extreme Situations', *The Journal of Abnormal and Social Psychology*, 38(4): 417–452.

Bowman, E. (2024) *Harris Called Trump a 'Fascist.' Experts Debate What Fascism Is — And Isn't*. Available at: https://www.npr.org/2024/10/29/nx-s1-5164488/harris-trump-fascist-explained (Accessed: 23/02/2026).

Bollas, C. (2011[1992]) *The Fascist state of mind*. The Christopher Bollas Reader. London: Routledge.

Brecht, K., Friedrich, V., Hermanns, L., Kaminer, I. and Juelich, D. (eds) (1985) *'Here Life Goes On in a Most Peculiar Way': Psychoanalysis before and after 1933*. London, Goethe Institut.

Brown, W. (2019) *In the Ruins of Neoliberalism: The Rise of Antidemocratic Politics in the West*. New York, Columbia University Press.

Chasseguet-Smirgel, J. (1987) 'Time's White Hair We Ruffle'. Reflections on the Hamburg Congress. *International Review of Psychoanalysis* 14:433–444.

Chasseguet-Smirgel, J. (1990) Reflections of a Psychoanalyst Upon the Nazi Biocracy and Genocide. *International Review of Psycho-Analysis*, 17(2):167–176. https://psycnet.apa.org/record/1990-28120-001

Chidi, G. (2025) *Stephen Miller said Trump has 'Plenary Authority'. What does that Mean?* Available at: https://www.theguardian.com/us-news/2025/oct/09/what-does-plenary-authority-mean-stephen-miller-trump (Accessed: 05/03/2026).

Clinton, H. (2024) 'Trump's rhetoric has become blatantly fascist.' October 14th, 2024. Available at: https://x.com/HillaryClinton/status/1845830956252275096?lang=en (Accessed: 05/03/2026).

Cocks, G. (1997) *Psychotherapy in the Third Reich.* Oxford, Oxford University Press (second edition).

Dean, J. (2025) *Capital's Grave: Neofeudalism and the New Class Struggle.* London, Verso.

Deleuze, G., & Guattari, F. (1983) *Anti-Oedipus: Capitalism and Schizophrenia.* Minneapolis, MN, University of Minnesota Press.

Ffytche, M. (2016) 'The Superego as Social Critique: Frankfurt School Psychoanalysis and the Fall of the Bourgeois Order', in D. Pick & M. Ffytche (Eds.), *Psychoanalysis in the Age of Totalitarianism* (pp. 55–70). London, Routledge.

Finchelstein, F. (2009) 'Fascism Becomes Desire: On Freud, Mussolini and Transnational Politics', in J. Damousi & M. B. Plotkin (eds.) *The Transnational Unconscious: Essays in the History of Psychoanalysis and Transnationalism*: 99–123.

Forrester, J. (2009) 'Afterword: Psychoanalysis, Fascism, Fundamentalism And Atheism', *Psychoanalysis and History* 11(2): 271–278.

Freud, S. [1911] (2024) 'Dreams in Folklore', in M. Solms (ed.) *The Revised Standard Edition of the Complete Psychological Works of Sigmund Freud, Volume XII.* Lanham, MD, Rowman & Littlefield: 179–204.

Freud, S. [1915] (2024) 'Thoughts for the Times on War and Death', in M. Solms (ed.) *The Revised Standard Edition of the Complete Psychological Works of Sigmund Freud, Volume XIV.* Lanham, MD, Rowman & Littlefield: 275–306.

Freud, S. [1917] (2024) 'Mourning and Melancholia', in M. Solms (ed.) *The Revised Standard Edition of the Complete Psychological Works of Sigmund Freud, Volume XIV.* Lanham, MD, Rowman & Littlefield: 217–238.

Freud, S. [1920] (2024) 'Beyond the Pleasure Principle', in M. Solms (ed.) *The Revised Standard Edition of the Complete Psychological Works of Sigmund Freud, Volume XVIII.* Lanham, MD, Rowman & Littlefield: 7–66.

Freud, S. [1921] (2024) 'Group Psychology and the Analysis of the Ego', in M. Solms (ed.) *The Revised Standard Edition of the Complete Psychological Works of Sigmund Freud, Volume XVIII.* Lanham, MD, Rowman & Littlefield: 67–138.

Freud, S. [1923] (2024) 'The Ego and the Id', in M. Solms (ed.) *The Revised Standard Edition of the Complete Psychological Works of Sigmund Freud, Volume XIX.* Lanham, MD, Rowman & Littlefield: 10–62.

Freud, S. [1927] (2024) 'The Future of an Illusion', in M. Solms (ed.) *The Revised Standard Edition of the Complete Psychological Works of Sigmund Freud, Volume XXI.* Lanham, MD, Rowman & Littlefield: 5–58.

Freud, S. [1937] (2024) 'Analysis Terminable and Interminable', in M. Solms (ed.) *The Revised Standard Edition of the Complete Psychological Works of Sigmund Freud, Volume XXIII.* Lanham, MD, Rowman & Littlefield: 209–254.

Frosh, S. (2005) *Hate and the "Jewish Science".* New York, Palgrave Macmillan.

Frosh, S. (2012) 'The Re-enactment of Denial', in Gülerce, A. (eds) *Re(con)figuring Psychoanalysis.* Palgrave Macmillan, London.

Frosh, S. (2019) *Those Who Come After: Postmemory, Acknowledgement and Forgiveness.* London, Palgrave Macmillan.

Frosh, S. (2023) *Antisemitism and Racism: Ethical Challenges for Psychoanalysis.* London, Bloomsbury Publishing.

Goggin, J. and Goggin, E. (2001) *Death of a 'Jewish Science': Psychoanalysis in the Third Reich.* West Lafayette, Purdue University Press.

Jones, R. P. (2026) *ICE to Spend $38.3 Billion on Detention Centers across US, Document Shows.* Available at: https://www.reuters.com/world/us/ice-spend-383-billion-detention-centers-across-us-document-shows-2026-02-13/ (Accessed: 05/03/2026)

Khanna, R. (2003) *Dark Continents: Psychoanalysis and Colonialism*. Durham, NC, Duke University Press.
Le Bon, G. (1895) *Psychologie des foules*. Paris, Félix Alcan.
Matthews, D. (2020) *Is Trump a Fascist? 8 Experts Weigh In*. Available at: https://www.vox.com/policy-and-politics/21521958/what-is-fascism-signs-donald-trump (Accessed: 05/03/2026).
Mbembe, A. (2019) *Necropolitics*. Durham, NC, Duke University Press.
Mitscherlich, A., & Mitscherlich, M. (1984) *The Inability to Mourn: Principles of Collective Behavior*. Grove Press, New York, NY.
Paxton, R. O. (2004) *The Anatomy of Fascism*. New York, Alfred A. Knopf.
Pick, D. (2009) 'In Pursuit of the Nazi Mind?' The Deployment of Psychoanalysis in the Allied Struggle Against Germany', *Psychoanalysis and History*, 11(2): 137–157. https://doi.org/10.3366/e1460823509000373
Pick, D. (2012) *The Pursuit of the Nazi Mind: Hitler, Hess, and the Analysts*. Oxford: Oxford University Press.
Reich, W. [1946] (1970) *The Mass Psychology of Fascism*. New York, Farrar, Strauss and Giroux.
Rose, J. (1996) *States of Fantasy*. Oxford, Clarendon Press.
Rose, J. (2021) *On Violence and on Violence Against Women*. London: Faber & Faber.
Samuels, A. (1992a) 'National Psychology, National Socialism, and Analytical Psychology: Reflections on Jung and Anti-Semitism. Part I', *Journal of Analytical Psychology* 37: 3–28.
Samuels, A. (1992b) 'National Psychology, National Socialism, and Analytical Psychology: Reflections on Jung and Anti-Semitism. Part II', *Journal of Analytical Psychology* 37: 127–148.
Shamdasani, S. (2003) *Jung and the Making of Modern Psychology: The Dream of a Science*. Cambridge, Cambridge University Press.
The White House (2025) *Defending Women from Gender Ideology Extremism and Restoring Biological Truth to the Federal Government*. Available at: https://www.whitehouse.gov/presidential-actions/2025/01/defending-women-from-gender-ideology-extremism-and-restoring-biological-truth-to-the-federal-government/ (Accessed: 27/03/2026).
The White House (2026) *The White House*. Available at: https://www.whitehouse.gov/ (Accessed: 04/03/2026).
Theweleit, K. [1977] (1987) *Male Fantasies, Volume 1: Women, Floods, Bodies, History*. Minneapolis: University of Minnesota Press.
Theweleit, K. [1978] (1989) *Male Fantasies, Volume 2: Male Bodies: Psychoanalyzing the White Terror*. Minneapolis: University of Minneapolis Press.
Tooze, A. (2025, May 6). 'Chartbook 380 Trump's Futurism: Elon's Rockets and Fewer Dolls for "Baby Girl" - Part I', *Adam Tooze Substack*. Available at: https://adamtooze.substack.com/p/chartbook-380-trumps-futurism-elons
Toscano, A. (2020) 'Capitalism without Capitalism. Fascism According to Žižek', *Res Pública*, 23(3). Available at: https://doi.org/10.5209/rpub.71030 (Accessed: 05/03/2026).
Varoufakis, Y. (2024) *Technofeudalism: What Killed Capitalism*. London, Vintage.
Williams, M., & Waldenberg, S. (2024) *Biden Believes Trump is a Fascist, White House Says*. Available at: https://edition.cnn.com/2024/10/23/politics/biden-trump-fascism (Accessed: 26/02/2026).
Žižek, S. (2006) 'The Fetish of the Party', in R. Butler & S. Stephens (eds.) *The Universal Exception*. London, Continuum.
Zolkos, M. (2022) 'The Phantasmatic Core of Fascism: Psychoanalytic Theories of Antisemitism and Group Aggression Amongst the "Political Freudians"', *Redescriptions*, 25(1): 49–64. Available at: https://doi.org/10.33134/rds.367 (Accessed 28/02/2026).

Part I

The Fascist State of Mind

Chapter 1

The Fascist State of Mind

Christopher Bollas

Reasons for Inclusion

Bollas' paper is a modern classic within psychoanalytic studies of fascism. Working in a post-Freudian register that draws on Klein, Fairbairn, and Winnicott, Bollas presents an elegant account of how anxieties and needs that generate a drive towards psychic certainty create a 'vicious cycle' in the subject, whose catastrophic endpoint is a mind evacuated of complexity and prepared for murder. The essay is an important contribution to our understanding of the genesis of genocidal psychic states and the processes of radicalization. However, its focus on the psychic dimension of fascism as a 'state of mind' has been criticized for its lack of sociological sensitivity, which has arguably exerted a problematic influence on the field, and needs to be read in relation to a more structural register—such as provided in Žižek's analysis of fascism.

***

'Our program is simple,' wrote Benito Mussolini in 1932. 'They ask us for programs, but there are already too many. It is not programs that are wanting for the salvation of Italy but men and willpower' (1983, p. 185). 'What is Fascism?' asked Gramsci some ten years before Mussolini's spartan statement. 'It is the attempt to resolve the problems of production and exchange with machine-gun fire and pistol shots' (1983, p. 82).

Fascism seemed to simplify the ideological, theological, and cultural confusions that emerged from the failure of the Enlightenment view of man to comprehend human existence. It was, argues Fritz Stern, a 'conservative revolution' constituting 'the ideological attack on modernity, on the complex of ideas and institutions that characterize our liberal, secular, and industrial civilization' (1974, p. xvi). Where the Enlightenment had partly emphasized the integrity of individual man, twentieth-century Fascism extolled the virtue of the state, an organic creation driven by the militant will of the masses, a sharp contrast indeed to the federal republic encumbered by checks and balances dividing power so that the people remained individually free to speak their minds in a pluralistic society.

While Freud reconsidered the dark side of man's self, this id never was free as a virtuous agent of the innate will of man. It became part of an internal

DOI: 10.4324/9781003742876-3

federation of complex checks and balances, of ego working with superego against id, or id with superego in compromise negotiations with the ego. Freud rethought man and maintained some considerable belief in the power of reason to influence the id, and even if his theory of the death instinct accounts for the possibility of a mass negation of life, he remained a Bismarckian with a sense of real politics: life was to be an endless series of compromise solutions between the parts of the self. At the end of a Freudian life it is possible to be a Montaigne, rendered far too wise by the mayorial negotiations of existence to characterize ontology as a 'pursuit of happiness,' but nonetheless continuously respectful of the individual skills of man to negotiate a good enough life.

Like many Europeans of his time, Freud deferred recognition of a deeply troubling factor in human culture, an element which preoccupies us now with its haunting relevance: the related issues of terror and genocide. In February 1915 the Ottoman government decreed that its Armenian population would lose the privileges of the ordinary civilian, and immediately the slaughter began. In that year 800,000 Armenians were massacred, and although the *entente* nations (Britain, France, Russia) protested to the Ottoman government and Arnold Toynbee collected a volume of essays testifying to the atrocities against the Armenians, this was to be a massacre that could not be inscribed in the symbolic orders of Western thought; references to it were scarce indeed. There is no mention in Freud's work of the elimination of 75 percent of the Armenian population. Nor indeed does he make more than a single reference to the pogroms that preceded it in European history.

Although the genocide against the Jewish population in Nazi Germany—the Holocaust—seems an irreplaceable icon to evil in the twentieth-century mind, we may wonder if its ironic function (the Jew now used once again to serve as a point of projection) is to serve as a continued mental negation of the continuation of genocide. We seem to know this, as citizens of the Western world do try not to eliminate from their thoughts the re-emergence in Cambodia of the Khmer Rouge which put to death millions of people. 'Never forget,' the cry of the Holocaust victim, seems a tellingly apt injunction: we seem all too able to forget.

'Terror is the realization of the law of movement: its chief aim is to make it possible,' writes Hannah Arendt, 'for the force of nature or of history to race freely through mankind unhindered by any spontaneous human actions.' Is genocide, the mass implementation of terror, social license to remake the world according to one's vision? 'Those who are not of my species are not my fellow men … a noble is not one of my species: he is a wolf and I shoot' (O'Sullivan, 1983, p. 49). So spoke a French revolutionary. And from 3 executions a week in 1793 to 32 a week in early 1794, the revolutionaries executed, on average, 196 people a week in the summer of 1794.

But a noble is not man but wolf, so is this the destruction of a lowly creature? In genocide a person is killed for who he is, not for what he does, which prompts Kuper to pose an uncomfortable question: as there is a 'thoroughgoing dehumanization of the bourgeoisie' in the Communist manifesto, is it possible to see this intellectual act as a precondition for Stalin's elimination of such bourgeois elements in his death camps (1981, p. 95)? In other words, is this famous act of Marxist objectification, the vilification of the bourgeoisie to which thousands of intellects since that time have paid lip service, the 'warrant' for killing some 20 million human beings in the years between 1919 and 1939 (1981, p. 59)?

In the *perestroika* world created by Mikhail Gorbachev it now seems not only possible but equally essential to think not only about what we have done but about who we are, or what we are, when we license genocide. As a psychoanalyst I turn my attention to that frame of mind which is the warrant for the extermination of human beings. I term it the Fascist state of mind, knowing that in some respects this is historiographically incorrect, as Fascism was a particular movement in world history with highly unique features to it, but I justify this license by playing on the double meaning of the word 'state.' There was a Fascist state. The coming into being of that state and its political theory can tell us quite a lot about another state: the state of mind that authorized a Fascist theory. Furthermore, like it or not, 'Fascist' is now a metaphor in our world for a particular kind of person, and I wish to reserve this ironic scapegoating of the Fascist from the convenient movement of its personification of evil, as, like Wilhelm Reich and Hannah Arendt, I shall argue that there is a Fascist in each of us and that there is indeed a highly identifiable psychic profile for this personal state.

Noel O'Sullivan, a political theorist and author of a fine study of Fascism, dismisses the psychoanalytical literature on Fascism as 'dangerously complacent … since it merely explains Fascism away by pushing it out of sight into a psychiatric ward.' He disagrees with Martin Wangh's view (O'Sullivan, 1983, p. 247) that the idealization of Hitler relieved homosexual tensions through submission to the leader, and objects to this and other analytical studies of Nazi pathology as failing to 'explain why other nations whose children were left fatherless in the First World War did not produce successful Führers and Nazi-type mass movements.' Psychoanalytic studies, he continues, 'explain everything, and therefore tell us nothing'; they assume that any sane person would be a liberal, and 'once this hidden postulate is granted, it naturally follows that those who dislike parliamentary institutions, respond to nationalistic appeals, and show a taste for heroism and self-sacrifice, are the victims of some psychological disorder.' The psychoanalytic argument, O'Sullivan concludes, ultimately claims that Fascists are the insane, and liberals and psychoanalysts are the sane (1983, p. 27).

Some analytic studies of the Nazi movement may have suggested that there was an illness peculiar to the Germans, and if such a disorder is regarded as an idiosynchrome of culture and history, then I would join O'Sullivan in regarding such psychoanalytical positions as worryingly simplistic. It is my understanding of a prominent feature of psychoanalysis that the pathology found in the Fascist movement is inside each of us, and that one aim of a training analysis is to provide the analyst-to-be with the evidence of neurotic and psychotic processes within the ordinary self. Indeed I shall argue that it is possible to be both a liberal believing in a parliamentary world and yet capable of developing a Fascist frame of mind. I thus find no contradiction between a belief that a world of checks and balances mitigates genocide and the view that as the Fascist state of mind is ordinary, it can indeed subvert the democratic mind.

There is a view now fairly common in psychoanalysis that the subject is composed of varied parts of the self. These parts are the ordinary functioning parts of the mind (i.e., the workings of the mind according to Freud, Klein, Fairbairn, and Winnicott) and the differing selves and objects represented in this internal world. It is rather like a parliamentary order with instincts, memories, needs, anxieties, and object responses finding representatives in the psyche for mental processing. When under the pressure of some particularly intense drive (such as greed), or force (such as envy), or anxiety (such as the fear of mutilation), this internal world can indeed lose its parliamentary function and evolve into a less representative internal order, particularly as differing parts of the self are projected out into other objects, leaving the mind denuded of its representative constituents.

To see the mind's move to Fascism, we need to consider just how this democratic order is changed. How does one become Fascist? Eric Brenman suggests that 'the practice of cruelty' is a 'singular narrow-mindedness of purpose' that when 'put into operation … has the function of squeezing out humanity and preventing human understanding from modifying the cruelty' (1988, p. 256). In object relations terms, humanity is presumably represented or representable by the presence of different capacities of the self (such as empathy, forgiveness, and reparation) which had been squeezed out of the self.

Kleinian psychoanalysts frequently refer in their literature to the 'killing off' of those parts of the self, thereby emphasizing the factor of murder as an ordinary feature of intrapsychic life. Rosenfeld, for example, describes an aggressive aspect of the narcissistic self state achieved by 'killing their loving dependent self and identifying themselves almost entirely with the destructive narcissistic parts of the self which provides them with a sense of superiority and self admiration' (1987, p. 248). Compare this psychoanalytic observation to the terrorist credo of Mikhail Bakunin's *Revolutionary Catechism* written in 1869.

> All the tender feelings of family life, of friendship, love, gratitude, and even honor must be stifled in the revolutionary by a single cold passion for the revolutionary cause.
>
> (1869, p. 67)

Bakunin's statement is a conscious articulation of what the revolutionary must do to achieve his cold passion, and perhaps because he knows (has made conscious) what must be squeezed out, we can feel the horror and sadness of this psychic movement. Rosenfeld, however, addresses the unconscious equivalent of this process, and in a passage strikingly relevant to our subsequent considerations of political genocide, he likens destructive narcissism to the work of a gang:

> The destructive narcissism of these patients appears often highly organized, as if one were dealing with a powerful gang dominated by a leader, who controls all the members of the gang to see that they support one another in making the criminal destructive work more effective and powerful.
>
> (1987, p. 249)

The death camps of Buchenwald and Dachau come to mind, the training ground for the SS, a gang dominated by a hierarchy of Hitler clones who watched each other commit atrocities in order to ensure that no one in the gang stepped outside the ethos of terror. There could be no internal opposition to the gang's operation of the death camps, organized by their 'death work' (Pontalis, 1974, p. 184). 'Terror becomes total when it becomes independent of all opposition,' says Arendt. 'It rules supreme when nobody any longer stands in its way' (1986, p. 464). Other psychoanalysts (e.g., Kovel and Federn) have addressed certain mental mechanisms that are useful to an understanding of the Fascist state of mind.

It is incumbent to very briefly outline the extraordinary study by Robert J. Lifton, who believes the key to understanding how Nazi doctors committed acts of genocide yet remained ordinary family men lies in the psychology of doubling: 'the division of the self into two functioning wholes, so that a part self acts as an entire self' (1986, p. 418). Such doubling may be ordinary—for example, when a surgeon needs to be his ordinary doctor self in order to perform operations. Nazi doctors escaped the sense of guilt arising from their evil actions by transferring the guilt from the ordinary to the 'Auschwitz self.' Nonetheless, argues Lifton, the Auschwitz self must become psychically numb to commit atrocities, something partly achieved by refusing to name the act of killing, finding instead many alternative words.

Lifton brilliantly illustrates the link between these Nazi doctors' sense of being inside the atmosphere of death and their increased omnipotence and mechanization of self as they transcended the death feeling. German genocide, argues Lifton, emerged from the sense of death that followed on from the First World War, a war that left Germans with a 'profound experience of failed regeneration' (1986, p. 468). A sense of collective illness pervaded the country, leading to a 'vision of total cure' (1986, p. 470) which the charismatic Hitler provided. The cure that becomes genocide, according to Lifton, must be total, invincible, transcendental. The victim of genocide is designated a disease that could contaminate the self and must therefore be eliminated, sponsoring a 'genocidal necessity' that is a 'fierce purification procedure' (1986, p. 482).

The Fascist State of Mind

Whatever the factors that sponsor any specific social act of genocide, the core element in the Fascist state of mind (in the individual or the group) is the presence of an ideology that maintains its certainty through the operation of specific mental mechanisms aimed at eliminating all opposition. But the presence of ideology (either political, theological, or psychological) is hardly unusual; indeed it is quite ordinary. The core of the Fascist state of mind—its substructure, let us say—is the ordinary presence of ideology, or what we might call belief or conviction. Arendt finds the seeds of totalitarianism in ideology because ideologies 'claim … total explanation,' divorce themselves from all experience 'from which they cannot learn anything new,' insisting therefore on the powerful possession of a secret truth that explains all phenomena, and operates from a logic which orders facts to support the ideological axiom (1986, pp. 470–71).

Thus something almost banal in its ordinariness—namely, our cohering of life into ideologies or theories—is the seed of the Fascist state of mind when such ideology must (for whatever reason) become total.

To achieve such totality, the mind (or group) can entertain no doubt. Doubt, uncertainty, self-interrogation, are equivalent to weakness and must be expelled from the mind to maintain ideological certainty.

This is accompanied, in my view, by a special act of *binding* as doubts and counter views are expelled, and the mind ceases to be complex, achieving a simplicity held together initially by bindings around the signs of the ideology. Political slogans, ideological maxims, oaths, material icons (such as the flag), fill the gap previously occupied by the polysemousness of the symbolic order. When the mind had previously entertained in its democratic order the parts of the self and the representatives of the outside world, it was participant in a multifaceted movement of many ideas linked to the symbolic, the imaginary, and the real—Lacan's terms. Specifically, words, as signifiers, were always free in the democratic order to link to any other words, in that famous Lacanian slide of the signifiers which expressed the true freedom of the unconscious (this Other) to represent itself. But when representational freedom is foreclosed, signifiers lack this freedom, as ideology freezes up the symbolic order, words becoming signs of positions in the ideological structure. When Michael Dukakis tried to introduce complex issues in the American presidential campaign of 1988, George Bush made the word 'liberal' a sign of weakness visited upon the certain mind by doubt and complexity. To supplement his destruction of the symbolic order Bush made the American flag the sign of the difference between Dukakis and himself; sadly, it signified the end of discourse and the presence of an emergent Fascist frame of mind.

As the empty binding of the order of signs constitutes an act of de-semiosis, it enables the mind to function in a highly simplified way, cushioned initially by the success of such binding.

O'Sullivan believes there is a 'marshall sense' to Fascism, which I shall define here as a binding of mental forces to create a sense capable of murder. In a way the elimination of the symbolic, of polysemousness is the first murder committed by this order, as the symbolic is the true subversion of ideology. The slide of signifiers will always dissipate a bound meaning and subvert any act of solidarity, a fact which Freud showed so very simply in his numerous demonstrations of how the parapraxis subverts the position of the conscious subject.

Aware of the pathological functions of certainty, Freud wrote in *The Future of an Illusion*:

> An enquiry which proceeds like a monologue, without interruption, is not altogether free from danger. One is too easily tempted into pushing aside thoughts which threaten to break into it, and in exchange, one is left with a feeling of uncertainty which in the end one tries to keep down by over-decisiveness.
>
> (1927, p. 21)

Ideological certainty, then, in spite of its binding of the self through simplification and the exile of other views, is threatened by the sudden breakthrough of the pushed-aside thoughts, which now must be dynamically ordered by an overdecisiveness.

This will work for some time, perhaps for a long time. Stuart Hampshire claims that the Nazi movement created 'a dizzying sense in German minds that all things are possible and that nothing is forbidden ... and that there is an infinite moral space now open for natural violence and domination' (1989, p. 69). The psychoanalyst Janine Chasseguet-Smirgel sees this infinite moral space as the pervert's accomplishment eliminating (at first Oedipal) opposition to desire and gaining objects without opposition. Hampshire argues that the violence inherent in the Nazi moral space has left 'a great vacancy ... a moral void' (1989, p. 69), which psychoanalysts such as Chasseguet-Smirgel, Khan, and Stoller, who study the perversions, would agree lies at the now empty heart of the pervert.

The moral void created by the simplifying violence of an ideology that brooks no true opposition is also an essential consequence of this stage in the evolution of the Fascist state of mind. For although the binding of signs and the power of certainty dull the subject into complacency, the moral void created by the destruction of opposition begins to make its presence felt. At this point the subject must find a victim to contain that void, and now a state of mind becomes an act of violence. On the verge of its own moral vacuum, the mind splits off this dead core self and projects it into a victim henceforth identified with the moral void. To accomplish this transfer, the Fascist mind transforms a human other into a disposable nonentity, a bizarre mirror transference of what has already occurred in the Fascist's self experience.

As contact with the moral void is lost through projective identification into a victim, and the victim now exterminated, the profoundly destructive processes involved are further denied by a form of delusional narcissism which is constructed out of the annihilation of negative hallucination, an idealization of self accomplished by the negation of any alternative (and thus enviable or persecutory) self or environment. As the negation of the qualities of the other are destroyed via the annihilation of the other, a delusional grandiosity forms in the Fascistically stated mind.

It is at this point that the process of annihilation is idealized in order to supply the Fascist mind with the qualities essential to delusional narcissism. Mental contents are now regarded as contaminates, and the Fascist mind idealizes the process of purging itself of what it has contained. The cleansing of the self suggests the possible birth of a new, forever empty self to be born with no contact with others, with no past (which is severed), and with a future entirely of its own creation.

The foregoing mental processes can be seen, in some respects, in Nietzsche's semi-autobiographical *Ecce Homo*. At a time when he suffered from continuous episodes of vomiting, traveling about Europe he became preoccupied with 'the question of nutriment,' by which he meant not only literally what one ate but also what sort of national culture one took into oneself. He proclaimed, for example, that 'the German spirit is an indigestion' while extolling the virtues of Italian culture and life (1908, p. 52).

Ecce Homo is, by any account, a deeply anguished text, full of contradictions, which, if they evoke our interest and compassion, are nonetheless remarkable actions of split consciousness. 'I am by nature warlike,' he proclaims (1908, p. 47); yet elsewhere he claims: 'no trace of struggle can be discovered in my life ... I look out upon my future as upon a smooth sea ... ruffled by no desire' (1908, p. 65). Perhaps this is a sea of vomit, accomplished through a continuous warlike spirit that leaves him feeling serene.

I refer to Nietzsche because at times he defines quite precisely the unconscious idealization of the self as an empty, and therefore pure, container. 'I possess a perfectly uncanny sensitivity of the instinct for cleanliness,' he writes, adding that this instinct has given him a sense of smell for the unclean 'innermost parts, the "entrails," of every soul' which are the cause of his 'disgust.' No doubt in such moments he would have to vomit up these noxious internal objects in order to maintain his sense of inner purity: 'As has always been customary with me an extreme cleanliness in relation to me is a presupposition of my existence, I perish under unclean conditions' (1908, p. 48).

Such a state of mind extols the virtue of being pure, uncontaminated because nothing is taken into the self, the psyche living from its sense of antiseptic accomplishment by maintaining purity in its own right, achieved by the continuous oral evacuation of the noxious. We can find this phenomenon, however, in ordinary life, whether it be spoken by those who attempt to claim the position of pure Christianity, pure objectivity, pure science, or, dare I say, pure analysis!

The greater the annihilation of the opposition, the more delusionally narcissistic the Fascist mind must become, a psyche now empty of ideas other than those performing a pure sign function—to bind the state of mind—a mind that idealizes itself as a cleaning process. It is not difficult to see, then, why the Fascist did not share the Marxist's belief in a logical history, but supported a movement that idealized struggle (or riddance) in its own right. As Mussolini wrote:

> War alone brings up to their highest tension all human energies and puts the stamp of nobility upon the peoples who have the courage to meet it. Fascism carries this anti-pacifist struggle into the lives of individuals. It is education for combat ... war is to man what maternity is to the woman. I do not believe in perpetual peace; not only do I not believe in it but I find it depressing and a negation of all the fundamental virtues of man.
>
> (1983, p. 185)

But this so-called struggle is, in fact, no combat at all. How far we are indeed from that 'noble' warfare found in the chivalric code of the *Song of Roland* when the virtue of one's opponents ennobled the act of physical battle. What is this male maternity to which Mussolini refers? Is it not the death camps, where the living are brought to a container, stripped of their culture, their loved ones, their adult characters, and turned into bizarre fetuses eventually to be killed in this deadly womb?

Some who opposed Fascism, such as Giovanni Zibordi, were able to diagnose the Fascist need to be at war. In 1922, in 'Towards a Definition of Fascism,' he wrote that after the First World War 'the officers sympathize with Fascism because it represents a prolongation of the state of war internally, and of a possibility of war externally' (1983, p. 89). Psychoanalytically considered, this permanent war is actually against struggle, against the conflicts brought on by continued engagement with opposition views. The idealization of war and of the warrior is a call to a state of mind that rids itself of opposition by permanent violence.

Cotta suggests that there is a 'circuit of de-personalization' conducted by the person who submits to domination by passing on to another victim his own circumstance. 'Violence has its origins and triumphs within the circuit of depersonalization thus actuated, which ultimately leads to a dispossession of oneself' (1985, p. 63).

This loss of self seems to me to be that loss of humanity to which Brenman referred, and which leaves in its place an idolized skeleton, a figure (leader, ideology, or state) revered for its militant capacity, in the end an idealization of the capacity to murder the self.

Thus the concentration camp, a metaphor of the psychic process of Fascism, is the place where, as the humane parts of the self are dehumanized and then exterminated, the death work is idealized in the death workers who cleanse the body politic of the undesirables. As Susan Sontag argues (1976), when illness is used as a metaphor for the opposition, then the act of elimination is viewed only as a necessary surgical intervention. Reference to the opposition as a disease or cancer that must be removed from society (and mind) is a frequent feature of the Fascist mental state, leading eventually to an idealization of the anti-human. Writing of the mobile killing units of the SS, Leo Kuper muses that 'the "ideal" seems to have been that of the dispassionate, efficient killer, engaged in systematic slaughter, in the service of a higher cause' (1981, p. 122). 'Higher' here is a metaphor of that grandiosity that achieves nobility by rising above the human: Kuper quotes from an address by the chief of the SS to his top commanders in October 1943:

> Most of you know what it means when 100 corpses lie there, or when 500 corpses lie there, or when 1,000 corpses lie there. To have gone through this and—apart from a few exceptions caused by human weakness—to have remained decent, that has made us great.
>
> (1981, p. 122)

Intellectual Genocide

'Genocide' is a word coined by the jurist Raphael Lemkin in 1944, from the Greek *genos* (tribal race) and the Latin *cide* (killing). Lemkin found a word that linked up with 'tyrannicide' and 'homicide' and thus inscribed itself in the symbolic order, enabling us finally to think about this crime.

The process that leads to a Fascist state (of mind, group, or nation) is unremarkable, and evidence of its emergence is easy to detect. I intend to list the features of what I shall term *intellectual genocide*, to name the mental processes precursor to, and eventually part of, the genocidal act. I do so, as will be clear toward the end of the chapter, not only out of interest in this problem but because I think identification of ordinary genocide (the genocide of everyday life) may lead us toward self scrutiny and confrontation of others when we see that an individual or a group has taken on this form of representation of the other. Because it is so ordinary, it is easily identifiable but, equally, because of its unremarkable status, it is also capable of emergence into mass murder.

I start by differentiating between committive genocide, identifying its visible traits, and omittive genocide, which is an act of omission.

Committive Genocide

Distortion. In the early stages of a possible move to a Fascist state of mind, the subject subtly distorts the view of the opponent, rendering it less intelligent or credible than hitherto. This is an ordinary part of debate, but in the extreme manifests itself as slander.

Decontextualization. A point of view held by the opposition is taken out of its proper context, which recontextualized would make the content more credible. This is an ordinary part of debate and the victim of decontextualization will naturally struggle to fill the gaps created by this rhetorical violence. The extreme of this act is the removal of a victim from his tribe, home (i.e., context), isolated for purposes of persecution.

Denigration. The belittling of an opponent's view combines distortion and decontextualization, rendering the opponent's views ridiculous. This is a door through which affects (of scorn and belittlement) move and displace ideation as the machinery of conflict with the opposition.

Caricature. This is the move from the denigration of the opponent's views to cartooning of the individual who presumably holds the views. Again, it is part of ordinary rhetoric to caricature the opposition's view and yet it is a transfer from the view held to the holder of the view. It therefore represents a significant step in the identification of a person or group with ascribed undesirable qualities.

Character assassination. This refers to the attempt to eliminate the opposition by discrediting the personal character of the holder of a view. An unacceptable form of debate, it is an ordinary part of discourse, usually referred to as 'gossip.' This perfectly harmless act of character assassination ('Oh, I do love gossip! Tell me all about it!') which discredits an opponent by conveying fictions or facts in a nonjudicial place—notably where the victim cannot speak for himself—can eliminate a person from the scene of consideration.

Change of name. Again, this is sometimes an acceptable part of debate but with obviously more disturbing manifestations ('kikes' for Jews, 'gooks' for Vietnamese) that form part of the act of elimination of the proper name, precursor to the elimination of the person himself (from the scene of consideration or from life itself). It is ordinary ('You know, what's his name. Thingy'), sometimes acceptable, if tiresome (when a person's name is consciously distorted for humorous purposes), and may be an unconscious parapraxis when the name is unknowingly altered.

Categorization as aggregation. These terms, used by Kuper, are useful to define the moment when the individual is transferred to a mass in which he loses his identity. It may be ordinary: 'Oh, but of course she is Freudian.' It may be permissible, if dicey: 'Well, of course she is ill' or 'Well, he is a psychopath.' Or it may be an extreme act of lumping together: 'He's a Jew.'

Omittive Genocide

Absence of reference. This is an act of omission, when the life, work, or culture of an individual or group is intentionally not referred to. Again, this is an ordinary feature of life: one group may get rid of the contributions of another group by never referring to them, or a writer such as Solzhenitsyn may be removed from bookshelves, or in the extreme there are no references to crimes against humanity.

When a person or a group addresses the opposition in the terms outlined above, alarms should ring in the witnesses to such action, who may respond by not engaging in vicious gossip or by directly confronting an individual who distorts, decontextualizes, denigrates, or caricatures the holder of different views. Such confrontation aims to arrest, at the very least, intellectual genocide. It is ordinary. Yet even in its purely rhetorical expression it can be extremely destructive. If an individual or group, previously participant in discourse, is a ceaseless object of intellectual genocide, then the recipients will show the effects. Some will simply leave the scene, no longer partaking in the group—a kind of voluntary exile in the face of persecution. Some may be pushed to express extreme views, victims of a violent innocence who appear to have gone over the edge. Others may somatize the conflict: a heart attack, we know, is often the outcome of extreme duress in one's place of work. Others may attempt to form alliances with the persecutor in an effort to gain some form of protection against their own potential destruction.

My point here is to raise intellectual genocide within our consciousness as a crime against humanity. Since it is ordinary, we can do something about it in the simple Freudian way of talking about it in the here and now and therefore partly divesting the act of its potential by addressing it.

The Vicious Circle

We could say that until Lemkin created a word for mass murder, 'genocide' managed to elude the signifier and thus escaped its representation in a symbolic order. To this list of obstacles I wish to add a few more.

One of the most perplexing features of the success of intellectual genocide is that its most gifted practitioners not only seem to achieve places of prominence by viciously attacking others; indeed they also seem to become objects of endearment to those who otherwise—one would have thought—would be horrified by such behavior. I recall a right-wing political figure in my hometown in Southern California, a person who vilified the opposition, spread vicious gossip, and damaged many, many people. Yet he was almost loved as a kind of cute monster. I also recall, only a few miles down the road, another person known for his viciousness who was finding himself the object of endearment: Richard Nixon. And though we knew of Stalin's monstrosity we still turned him into good old Uncle Joe.

The puzzle is why we 'love' these monstrous monsters rather than oppose them. Why are they allowed to climb so far up the ladder of success, sometimes to a place of leadership where they continue to eliminate the opposition in vicious ways? Perhaps they represent us. Perhaps we fear to challenge such an individual. There must be some truth to that, but I also think we observe an interpersonal sleight of hand in which the monster person is 'the impossible loved object' because love here exonerates the subject from responsible opposition: 'I wish I could stand up to Mary, but you know she's just impossible and

I'm afraid I love the old monster.' Presumably confrontation of the monster must be reserved for those who don't love the monster, and yet almost everyone gives the same shrug of the shoulder: 'How can Mary be challenged? She is Mary and her very monstrous qualities, darn it, are what we kind of love about her.' In some ways this seems to me to be the interpersonal equivalent of creating a type of joke. Aggression—the anger or outrage evoked by such a person's behavior—is turned into humor: Mary becomes the basis of our laughter about the atrocious. But such an obstacle to confronting viciousness in a person, and in some cases the practice of intellectual genocide, is no laughing matter and deserves our continuing study. I consider this further through a personal vignette.

I attended high school in Orange County, California, during the 1950s, and for a limited period of time it became compulsory for the students to attend Christian anti-Communist crusades in—of all appropriate places—Disneyland, and usually with a visiting speaker, who now and then was Ronald Reagan. I particularly admired one of my history teachers, who struck me as an intelligent and very decent man. Yet in the weeks approaching such events and most intensively at the crusade itself, he became rabid in his hate of the liberal conspiracy that was plotting to overthrow the U.S. government.

I had not known his politics until then and I recall being shocked at the utter transformation in his character whenever contemporary politics entered his mind. I think most of us were bewildered by him and by what I would now term a local psychotic state. But what we did is of interest: we turned this aspect of his behavior into a joke. He became our loved madman, and occasionally one or another of the group would 'push his button' and send him across the boundary from the sane to the insane part of his personality.

Discussing the vicious behavior of a person, people will often say, 'But you know, she really is quite a lovely and kind person' or 'Well, you know, removed from her pulpit she is really quite a different person.' And this is true. But it is not the point. In fact, this opposes the point: humanity (the good parts of the self) is now used to excuse the destructive side of the self. The joke, as always, now borders on the perverse. The humane now authorizes the inhumane as Mary's viciousness is loved, in the economical exchange between the Fascistic and the non-Fascistic parts of her personality.

Even if we accept that compliance with a Mary is in the interests of vicarious support of one's own viciousness, which will always be partly true, the act of dissociative acceptance (the 'how Mary is really privately a nice person' story) colludes with the function of genocide. In this case, however, it is the witness who, by tacitly accepting Mary's viciousness, accepts the eradication of the humane as a joke: the world will then be full of monstrous Mary stories, tales of her beastliness.

When we excuse the destructive behavior of anyone by citing their humanity, we commit a crime against the function of humanity. When we distance ourselves from collusive responsibility for the destructive effects of the vicious person by turning them into a joke of sorts, we pervert the truth. It is this corruption in the citing of humanity that perverts truth and that constitutes essential contextual support for any vicious person's successful establishment of the Fascistic parts of themselves in the successful movement of the social group to its own Fascism.

The noncollusive witness to that personality change that occurs when the person crosses over from the sane to the insane parts of the self, is initially shocked by this transference. We all know how stunning it is, when discussing an issue with someone, to witness the person's vicious espousal of a doctrine that derives part of its energy from the intellectual annihilation of the other. We may be speechless. Such a rupture also occasions a sense of dissociation: we feel immediately separated out from the conversant's insanity. And following this dissociation, part of us will feel deadened by the eruption, as now it is clear to us that the other is subject to an internal Fascistic process. In a way our response is our victimage. It is in feeling shocked, dissociated, and deadened that we share elements in common with those who are more severely traumatized by socially operant Fascism.

We may also share responsive qualities in common with a collusive witness, whereby we may try to recover from this trauma by reminding ourselves how, in so many other ways, this person is not only sane but likable. In this respect we use our humanity and its link to the humane parts of the other to recuperate from the trauma, but, as suggested, the irony of this is that it ultimately excuses, and finally supports, the destruction of humanity. Often we feel a certain dread as we sense our responsibility to those who are the objects of this person's intellectual genocide. We must say something that at the very least marks our opposition to the Fascistic state of mind.

When we exonerate a vicious person's actions by citing elements of their humanity, I think we create a perversion in logic itself—in thinking—that is part of what we may consider the vicious circle. It is of interest that from the seventeenth century the word 'vicious' was used to describe a fault in logic, when a conclusion was realized by false means of reasoning. Webster's third definition of the vicious circle cites this fault in logic: 'an argument which is invalid because its conclusion rests upon a premise which itself depends on the conclusion.' The argument that Mary is really a good human being, in spite of her nefarious actions, because she is at the same time a human being, is a circular argument, a flawed logic that perverts the truth because it comes round full circle. Indeed, I use the word 'vicious' to describe the person in a Fascist state of mind not only because this word signifies one who is 'full of faults,' which seems an apt description of one carrying moral voids determined by massive evacuations, but because we may also speak of a particular process—the vicious circle—which is definitionally affiliated with the vicious person, that suits my analysis of such a person as involved in a particular mental process.

A vicious circle is also defined as 'a situation in which the solution of one problem gives rise to another, but the solution of this, or of other problems rising out of it, brings back the first, often with greater involvement.' Another definition states: 'a situation in which one disease or disorder results in another which in turn aggravates the first.' It is exactly this type of process which, in my view, takes place in the Fascist state of mind: whatever the anxiety or need that sponsors the drive to certainty, which becomes the dynamic in the Fascist construction, the outcome is to empty the mind of all opposition (on the actual stage of world politics, to kill the opposition), a process that ironically undermines the vicious person. It does this by creating a moral void which further increases the underlying uncertainty which set the mind on its pathological track to certainty in the first place.

It is a procedure which Nietzsche regards as a virtue: 'the doctrine of "eternal recurrence," that is to say of the unconditional and endlessly repeated *circular course* [italics mine] of all things' (1908, p. 81). The cycle of purification through violent expulsion leaves a void which Nietzsche tries to fill with a notion of tranquillity derived from the liquefaction of opposition: 'I swim and bathe and splash continually as it were in water, in any kind of perfectly transparent and glittering element' (1908, p. 48), which is possible until he meets up with any human element which fills him with a sense of disgust (1908, p. 48). To the extent to which Nietzsche portrays early on the process of thought subsequently peculiar to the Nazi movement, we can see how the Fascist sea of inner tranquillity is mirrored by those horrid seas of internment camps that contain the Fascist's vomit: the place that purifies them because it contains the indigestible opposition.

For a person incarcerated in the concentration camp, it is hard to find any vestige of the humane that could possibly offer resistance to the Fascist state. In *The Informed Heart* (1960), Bruno Bettelheim tells us that humane gestures expressed by one detainee to another were punished by death. One eventually could not help the other. Nor indeed could the subject express any of his feelings about the treatment meted out to the other and to oneself. Expression of feeling led to further torture and sometimes to extinction. Thus, those qualities we value so highly as expressions of humanity—helping others in need and expressing our feelings and views—were eliminated. In that situation, incarcerated in Buchenwald, Bettelheim knew that to lose one's humanity was to risk personal madness. How could he remain sane? He discovered that it was through an ironic act sponsored by his extreme state: he would observe the SS, study them, consider at an intellectual remove what was taking place. 'If I should try to sum up in one sentence what my main problem was during the whole time I spent in the camps,' he writes, 'it would be: to protect my inner self in such a way that if, by any good fortune, I could regain liberty, I would be approximately the same person I was when deprived of liberty' (1960, p. 126). He had to accept, therefore, a split in his personality between the private world of his own thoughts—which ultimately were unreachable by the SS—and 'the rest of the personality that would have to submit and adjust for survival' (1960, p. 127). This is an extreme state of victimage in which the subject can only retain his humanity by preserving his sanity, which he accomplishes by accepting a split of sorts in his personality. It is interesting that thought and memory, the capacity to perceive reality, to think it, and remember it, become the core of potential recovery to a humane future.

We can see, then, why any person or group which has suffered a genocide must reach a point in the process of recuperation when remembering what actually happened is crucial. It is not only an action aimed at objectifying the crimes committed against the self, but, as Bettelheim hints, to recuperate from one's own destruction of the humane parts of the self in the interests of survival. As the victim seeks his own safety and deserts his fellow man, there will be an enormous loss of self respect. Only through further self analysis and self expression can the victim recuperate that love of himself that is an ordinary part of the generative narcissistic structure of human relations. I suggest, therefore, that the ultimate human response to genocide is self preservation: following physical liberation from the terms of aggression, this curiously inhuman side of the preservation of one's humanity (the will to survive) will move toward its abandoned humanities first by memory, then by speech, and finally by true grief. There is a triumph, here, of the seemingly inhuman (our Darwinian move) that is curiously more humane than the collusive acts of humanizing the monstrous parts of the self.

If a person, group, institution, or country truly wishes to recover from the traumas of intellectual or physical genocide, then it will have to remember the crimes it has committed. The act of remembering is the antecedent to forgiveness (of self and others) and instrumental to the reparative rehumanization of the group. This painful process is often bypassed by denials ('it is water under the bridge') aimed to thwart recollection, and by transfers to the next generation, which is somehow meant to naturalistically displace the crimes of the older generation and absolve that generation from its collective responsibility. And, as we know, a new generation, though seemingly possessed of its own displacing vision of the future, is highly liable to inherit the sins of the fathers.

References

Arendt, H. (1986) *The Origins of Totalitarianism*. London, Deutsch.

Bakunin, M. (1869) *Revolutionary Catechism*. New York, Knopf.

Bettelheim, B. (1960) *The Informed Heart*. London, Penguin.

Brenman, E. (1988) 'Cruelty and narrow-mindedness', in E. Spillius (ed.) *Melanie Klein Today*, Vol. 1. London, Routledge, pp. 256–270.

Cotta, S. (1985) *Why Violence?* Gainesville, FL, University of Florida.

Freud, S. (1927) 'The Future of an Illusion', in J. Strachey, A. Freud, A. Strachey, & A. Tyson (eds.) *The Standard Edition of the Complete Psychological Works of Sigmund Freud, Volume XXI (1927–1931): The Future of an Illusion, Civilization and its Discontents and Other Works*. London, Hogarth Press, pp. 3–56.

Hampshire, S. (1989) *Innocence and Experience*. London, Allen Lane.

Kuper, L. (1981) *Genocide*. London, Penguin.

Lifton, R. J. (1986) *The Nazi Doctors*. New York, Basic Books.

Mussolini, B. (1983) 'Dottrina del fascismo', in *Encyclopaedia Britannica, Vol. 7*. Chicago, University of Chicago Press, pp. 182–188.
Nietzsche, F. (1908) *Ecce Homo*. London, Penguin.
O'Sullivan, N. (1983) *Fascism*. London, Dent.
Pontalis, J.-B. (1974) 'Dream as object', *International Review of Psychoanalysis*, 1, pp. 125–133.
Rosenfeld, H. (1987) *Impasse and Interpretation*. London, Tavistock.
Sontag, S. (1976) *Illness as Metaphor*. New York, Farrar Strauss.
Stern, F. (1974) *The Politics of Cultural Despair*. Berkeley, CA, University of California Press.
Zibordi, G. (1983) 'Towards a definition of fascism', in D. Beetham (ed.) *Marxists in Face of Fascism*. Manchester, Manchester University Press, pp. 88–96.

Chapter 2

Toward Eradicating the Unbearable

The Dangerous Allure of Fascistic States of Mind

Michael J. Diamond

Reasons for Inclusion

Diamond's article is one of the best contemporary papers on psychoanalysis and fascism. Drawing on a range of past psychoanalytic scholarship on fascism, and taking care to define fascism precisely (though not unproblematically) at the outset of his argument, Diamond makes a highly convincing case that fascism is rooted in fears of annihilation provoked by times of crisis, and the violent narcissism and paranoid-schizoid defences enacted in response. Importantly, Diamond also considers (again, not unproblematically) contemporary political events and figures including Orbán, Putin, Trump, Modi, and Netanyahu, clarifying the psychopolitical dimensions of their far-right politics and their relation to fascism. We were concerned by his use of the fascist "state of mind" to insinuate a psychic equivalence between "pro-Israeli" and "pro-Palestinian enclaves" (see below, p. 54, n. 9), which may be read in the context of ongoing debates within psychoanalytic institutions across the USA. Notwithstanding this qualification, Diamond's paper is exemplary for its contemporary focus, the highly convincing theory of fascism it presents, and for recognising the archive of psychoanalytic studies of fascism while avoiding some of the major pitfalls of those works.

***

Introduction

Nearly one-half century ago, Václav Havel (1979) addressed the seductive power of fascistic movements in declaring, "Individuals need not believe all these mystifications, but they must behave as though they did … They must *live within a lie* … For by this very fact, individuals confirm the system, fulfil the system, make the system, *are* the system" (p. 31, original italics). Today, we are living in troubling times characterized by ethno-nationalistic, autocratic populist movements "drawn toward endless mobilization of destructiveness" (Loewenstein 2024a, pp. 8–9). To address the allure of fascism, and because conscious reasoning alone is inadequate to rein in the destructive forces that provide relief from unbearable mental states, I will consider the unconscious

DOI: 10.4324/9781003742876-4

fantasies, impulses, and the accompanying dynamics of fascistic states of mind within all of us. In addition, I will explore how these states of mind can move from the individual psyche to fuel rising autocratic, proto-fascistic group movements worldwide.

Although psychoanalysis is uniquely situated to understand fascistic, more destructive states of mind, caution is nonetheless called for when applying the psychoanalytic understanding of individual minds to larger sociopolitical groupings, so as not to fall into the trap of overgeneralizing from the individual to the collective. Nonetheless, as Segal (2006) advocated, as analysts treating patients, we must not confuse analytic neutrality with our responsibilities as citizens that demand that we not allow ourselves to be neutered. This is especially true given that, as we can so clearly observe, we cannot escape fascism; fascistic states of mind reside within each of us and particularly so in the context of the worldwide rise in tendencies toward nationalism.

Unfortunately, the ubiquity of such states of mind, under certain circumstances, can be harnessed by agitating demagogues who operate as *prophets of deceit* (Löwenthal and Guterman, 1949), offering seductively appealing leadership to susceptible groups and individuals. In this context, primitive, regressive group processes may easily result in authoritarian and/or fascistic, cult-like movements. I will particularize this by describing the unconscious dynamics of fascistic mental states that can be tied to destructively narcissistic identifications and to the Freudian notion of the death drive. I will then extend our understanding by exploring how fascistic states of mind can progress from the individual, primarily unconscious psyche to a large, regressed group mind. Finally, I will offer some thoughts on how we might recognize and hopefully contain the seductive allure of fascistic states.

A Note on Democracy Within the American Polity

Implicitly aware of the allure that fascistic states of mind hold not only for the individual but for collective movements at the extremes of both the right and left wings of the political spectrum, the framers of the US Constitution recognized—as have many scholars over the past two and a half centuries—that modern democracies in which pluralism is called for are always accompanied by a fascistic-friendly underbelly that must be guarded against. As the iconic folk rock classic "Me and Bobby McGee" (Kristofferson and Foster, 1969) ironically suggests, "Freedom is just another word for nothin' left to lose." Accordingly, the American democratic ideal of freedom can be misunderstood if it promises an escape from loss, uncertainty, meaninglessness, and responsibility, especially as applied to the acceptance of differences and its accompanying tensions.

America's experiment in representative democracy was founded on an inherent tension between the elected ruling class of elites and the ordinary common people or populace exercising their voting rights. Ideally, such a democratic system (known as republicanism) requires the two sectors of the polity to work in tandem in pursuing truth together while bearing its inherent *uncertainty*, especially through the acceptance of loss of an election. Most significantly, a functioning democracy helps in containing both individual and societal unconscious fears and impulses while framing the polity's ability to adapt to changing social/historical reality. Consequently, democracy's fluid, messy, dynamic, and creative character requires protection of the inherent dialectical tension, uncertainty, and commitment to truth. Yet as we know from our psychoanalytic work and our own life experiences, truth, loss, conflict, and uncertainty—all so-called *facts of life* (Money-Kyrle, 1968)—can be extremely difficult to bear.

Inevitably, rather than becoming a veneer for an increasingly authoritarian agenda (as we see, for instance, in Viktor Mihaly Orban's *illiberal* form of democracy), liberal democracy's survival requires that its participants reckon with grief, guilt, and truth. This entails relinquishing omnipotent leanings, if only to manage the losing of elections and the grieving of formerly valued policies and respected leaders. In this respect, Joseph Goebbels, the Nazi party's chief propagandist, correctly asserted that in the face of extreme nationalistic trends, "the big joke on democracy is that it gives its mortal enemies the tools to its own destruction" (Goebbels, quoted in Gopnik, 2024, p. 76).

The theme of the seeds of such a threat to American democracy being sown by mobilizing internal fascistic tendencies was explored by the seminal 20th-century historian Richard Hofstadter (1965). He emphasized the paranoid character within the American polity, in which there is a particular affinity for bad, rather than good, causes. He suggested that, typically, a central preoccupation of the grievance-based, nationalistic, and paranoid style is the fear of a plot designed to perpetrate fiendish acts that aim to destroy an idealized and treasured way of life.

As I have discussed in other writings (Diamond, 2022, 2023), these plots are evident throughout the history of the United States and are typically described in apocalyptic terms. Such conspiratorial thinking is evident in purported attempts to undermine and destroy a way of life; and it often appeals to fundamentalist beliefs, including, for example, beliefs having a Christian theme in which there is a spiritual wrestling match between absolute good and absolute evil. This can lead to the creation of a prophetic cult of a Manichean psychology that eschews compromise, so that the only acceptable outcome is complete victory over a clearly delineated, malicious enemy. When ensnared within this conspiratorial bubble, the constructed enemy represents a projection of idealized and unacceptable aspects of the self and is viewed as possessing an especially effective source of power, while it is also conceived as "sinister, ubiquitous, cruel, sensual, luxury-loving" (Hofstadter, 1965, pp. 32–33).

Authoritarianism and its more destructively virulent cousin fascism do not occur in a vacuum; instead, environmental and societal conditions giving rise to existential, annihilating forms of anxiety—the most primordial dangers to the psyche—set the stage for its appearance (Diamond, 2022). Moreover, authoritarian and proto-fascist populist movements are more likely to gain ground in the context of significant social progress, increasing multiculturalism and plurality, societal and personal trauma, environmental threat, rapid technological changes, and the failure within liberal democracies to sufficiently address real social and economic problems, including massive inequities in income, privilege, and other aspects of society; border control; climate change; and economic mismanagement (Diamond, 2022). These social determinants add to mounting identity/ status instability and existential anxieties in the form of what social scientists term as *normative and dominant group status threats* that jeopardize a sense of sameness, identity, and a way of life. Because democratic systems are held together by a common belief in democracy itself, one that serves to transform more unconscious fears of extinction as Christina Wieland (2024) adeptly argues, democracy begins to collapse when such social meaning signified by the trust placed in democratic government is under severe threat. As a consequence, fascistic states can rise to the fore by providing new meaning while averting more primary annihilation terrors.[1]

Under these social conditions, skillful propagandists and fiery demagogues use agitating tactics marked by fraudulent indoctrination to harness unconscious fears and phantasies within regressed groups. Promoting illusionary solutions, proto-fascist leaders utilize fear-mongering to generate submission and idealization, resulting in the disposition to follow (Bohleber, 2024). Consequently, a symbiosis with the leader is formed in which destructive impulses are managed largely through paranoid processes characterized by highly demonized forms of splitting, disavowal, and projective identification (Löwenthal and Guterman, 1949; Money-Kyrle, 1937, 1941). As I will elaborate, fascistic states characterized by violent, sadistic impulses to exterminate the demonized out-group or *other(s)* are mobilized through such proto-fascist leadership. Here, imaginary enemies or dangers carried within are transformed into something very real. In short, a vicious spiral of effective hate serves to preserve the group's existence (Money-Kyrle, 1941).

Before diving more deeply into what is meant by a *fascistic state of mind* and its allure—and given that terms such as *authoritarianism* and *fascism* are repeatedly used without a definitional consensus—it is useful to consider next what is meant by fascism, how it might be distinguished from authoritarianism, and how either or both may be evident in today's autocratic regimes.

Defining and Differentiating Fascism from Other Forms of Authoritarianism

Fascism today is a very loosely used term that is often conflated with and rather crudely distinguished from authoritarianism, illiberal democracy, autocracy, totalitarianism, and tyranny. Somewhat undefinable due to its emotional charge and force, fascism—much like sexuality, pornography, love, and war—is something we tend to recognize when we see it but may have trouble explicating. For instance, Umberto Eco (1995) called fascism a *fuzzy totalitarianism* with a timeless quality. Nonetheless, it is helpful to define how it is being used and how it might be differentiated from other forms of authoritarianism, either in individual states of mind or in larger group movements.

In its political countenance, *authoritarianism* can be described as a form of government that favors strong central power; it is characterized by large-scale weakening of the rule of law, of separation of powers, and of democratic voting. In the democratic polity, the executive branch overrides the other governing branches. In an individual, the *authoritarian personality*, associated with the F-scale developed by Adorno and his colleagues (Adorno et al., 1950), indicated a disposition for extreme rigidity and intolerance for ambiguity and differences (Gandesha, 2019). Today, this is best understood as an *authoritarian dynamic* (Stenner, 2005; Stenner and Haidt, 2018) in which obedience and conformity are favored over freedom, plurality, and differences.

Rather than constituting an individual character trait, authoritarian thinking is activated on a broader scale when social conditions are perceived as existentially threatening, which is typically triggered by fear and threats in a climate where political plurality is rejected; consequently, forced obedience and conformity are favored over freedom, diversity, and differences.[2]

In contrast, *fascism* is an extreme form of authoritarian ultranationalism, ultra-institutionalism, and/or ultra-tribalism characterized by dictatorial power, severe societal regimentation, and forcible, violent suppression of opposition. While the word *fascism* is ubiquitous in contemporary discourse, its roots lie in the ancient Roman past. The word stems from the Latin *fascis* (plural: *fasces*), referring to a bundle of wooden rods bound together with a leather cord surrounding an axe, an object that signifies the power of high Roman officials to enforce order through fear of the rods. The emblem of the fasces became a symbol for political power of dictators and kings who were allowed to inflict multiple beatings and executions, including "flogging and decapitation" (Brennan, 2022, p. 14). In the early twentieth century, it became the emblem and source of the name of Mussolini's National Fascist Party (PNF); and at the beginning of the 2000s, several American, white-supremacist groups incorporated the fasces into their logos to reflect "unity by means of authority" (2022, p. 14). Though a long-dormant signifier, today it is again being put to use by extremist movements that presume the right to impose one's will on others through the use of force.

Fascism is especially perilous because it is organized around intolerance and the destruction of "the individuality of others" (Prince, 2023, p. 733).[3] Located at the extreme of the authoritarian spectrum, fascism is distinguished by a *violently destructive force*. As a reaction to uncertainty, when conditions are suitable, it is not an ideology per se (though it may purport to be one); instead, it can be described as "a bolus of rage, anger, resentment, victimization, and grievance…in search of an ideology" (2023, p. 73). This reliance on an emotionally charged passion coalesces by attacking the perception of reality, while creating its own delusional reality that disguises its destructiveness with a "perverted idealism" (2023, p. 81). It brings perversity together with destructive narcissism in *omnipotent object relations* (Rosenfeld, 1984a, 1984b, 1987), while phantasy remains unchecked by perception, and the mind—operating within a psychotic register—becomes dominated by Mafia-like states that exterminate oppositional states of mind (Rosenfeld, 1971).[4]

Much like authoritarianism, totalitarianism, and tyranny, fascism is antithetical to liberal democracy in that differences, including the *narcissism of minor differences* (Freud, 1921, 1930), are turned into hated, demonized oppositions to be eradicated. Still, a simple opposition between democracy and authoritarianism or fascism cannot be posited since there are benevolent dictators, just as there are malevolent democratic leaders (Hinshelwood, 2025). Moreover, democracy is not so much about individual freedoms, but rather about collective decision-making; consequently, who is designated as the leader in communal decisions is vital (Hinshelwood, 2023). In fascistic groups, even those arising in democratic settings, splitting is a major factor in creating an identity, and "alienable others are powerful" (2023, p. 113) in ensuring the group's solidarity by means of an *us-against-them* dynamic.

Parenthetically, we might ask how a nationalistic movement or country can move from being a populist-fueled, anti-democratic autocracy to a fullblown fascistic state. As Argentine historian Federico Finchelstein (2024) proposes, fascism at the state level can be distinguished from autocratic, proto-fascistic regimes by utilizing all five of the following methods: *political violence*; *repetitive propaganda*; *widespread dissemination of misinformation*; *xenophobia* (including, especially, *an intense anti-immigrant stance*); and the *leader's adoption of dictatorial powers*. In Trump's America, and despite his cult-like following, democracy's guardrails continue to hold, tenuously, with respect to the MAGA movement's dictatorial powers, seemingly leaving Trump merely a "wannabe fascist"[5] (Finchelstein, 2024, p. 2).

To reiterate, fascism is an intrinsic state of mind that stems from the core of man's instincts (Musil, 1976). Considered an omnipotently based, narcissistically organized mental quality or structure, it becomes pathological during conditions of upheaval and insecurity (Prince, 2023). Reich (1933) went further in considering it the organized political expression of the average man's character structure. Bollas (1992) observes that this state is present "in each of us," noting that it kills off the democratic parts of the mind in order to become "the warrant for the *extermination* of human beings" (1992, p. 196, italics added). As I will subsequently elaborate, such annihilation or extinction is idealized since the fascist mental state "extols the virtue of being pure" (1992, p. 204), purging itself of what had previously been contained but now seems contaminated.

This is evident today in Trump's use of Hitlerian propaganda and disinformation tactics in which the opposition—which he designates as radical leftists, socialists, Democrats, immigrants, the "fake press," and/ or the "deep state," among other pejoratively used terms—becomes a cancer, virus, or toxin, a "vermin...poisoning our blood" that must be totally eliminated. Whether present in the individual or in the group, this mind-state operates to maintain certitude by expelling doubt, uncertainty, and critical self-reflection through whatever means necessary to annihilate all opposition (Bollas, 1992; Figlio, 2006; Prince, 2023).[6]

Next, I will consider the unconscious dynamics of fascistic states of mind in order to further our understanding of its perverse allure.

A Brief Overview of the Dynamics of Fascistic States of Mind

At the manifest level, fascistic states are characterized by an absolutism marked by the erasure of critical thinking (Figlio, 2006; Loewenstein, 2024a). From a Kleinian perspective, this primitive form of black-and-white thinking resides in the paranoid-schizoid position, in which there are simple binaries between the *good* (us) and the *bad* (them). Originating from the deeply unconscious dread of falling apart, disintegrating, or not existing—described as *annihilation anxiety* that begins in the mother-infant experience—the primary and largely unconscious dread of annihilation and/or of the agony of disintegration requires, for both an individual and the group psyche, transformation through healthy containment, typically through *maternal reverie* (Bion, 1962b). However, when such transformative containment (or holding) is lacking, it becomes psychically urgent to create a *bad* object outside the self, which averts the unthinkable internal anxieties of *going to pieces* or *falling forever* (Winnicott, 1962; see also Wieland, 2024).

Once the fascistic mind begins to take hold to protect the self from unbearable anxieties of extinction, phantasies and impulses of forever ridding the self of the bad object predominate.[7] Particularly when one feels helpless and impotent, omnipotent phantasies characterized by unlimited power serve as a vital defense against a desperate internal situation (Feldman, 2022). Weakness, vulnerability, and need are averted, pain and frustration are disavowed, and magical certitude prevails, often in the countenance of identification with an idealized superior being.

When existentially threatening conditions are suitable, forceful efforts are more likely to be undertaken to eliminate uncertainty, insecurity, and ambivalence. Consequently, collectively shared unconscious fantasies tend to be triggered in which the identified-with group or nation becomes an "imagined community" through a narcissistic mirroring that revels in "ideal-narcissistic states of purity and homogeneity" (Bohleber, 2024, p. 1). As evident in the U.S. today, far-right populist ideologies become particularly attractive when large groups are under the sway of a "narcissistic longing for a homogeneous society" (2024, p. 1).[8] Such rigidly held, demonizing forms of splitting, forceful projection, fantasized purification, and identification are evident among those rooted in the Trumpian world, as well as in many virulent anti-Trumpists. Notably, these processes are seen among extremist segments within both the right and left wings of the political spectrum, presumably mobilized to ward off more unconscious terrors.

True believers (Hoffer, 1951) who inhabit radical fundamentalism reflect a form of group thinking—more aptly termed *non-thinking*, in which uncertainty is eradicated—that can easily lead to a Manichean psychology in which the righteous in-group alone personifies the *good* that must extinguish the *bad*, with the latter embodied by the out-group. Such absolute states of mind entail a common psychotic core of massive projective identification, fostering the illusion of inner purity and certitude with a paranoid dread of impurity and badness. This badness is seen as producing an excessive force that must be cleansed in order for one to remain enthralled by one's own righteous goodness. Hence, grandiose, psychotic idealization ferments as the ego and ego-ideal merge to create manic elation (Figlio, 2006). The connection between collective narcissism and violence is evident in the production of action-oriented forces, or "mobilizing passions," that collapse thinking into violent behavior capable of wiping out internal and external enemies, "without legal or moral limits" (Paxton, 2004, pp. 218–219).[9]

Such passionate, hypnotic-like submission to a fascistic propagandist, not dissimilar to the hate-fueled self-pity and manic elation that may be seen at Trump's MAGA rallies, was aptly described by Money-Kyrle (1941) after attending a 1932 rally for Hitler just before the latter came into power. In Money-Kyrle's words, Hitler…

> …was preceded by Goebbels, and both orators said the same things in the same order. The repetition did not bore the audience, but … seemed only to increase the emotional effect. It was not easy to keep one's balance; for if one was unable to identify oneself with the crowd and share its intense emotions, one almost inevitably personified it as a sinister and rather terrifying super-individual. …The people seemed gradually to lose their individuality and to become fused into a not very intelligent but immensely powerful monster, which was not quite sane and therefore capable of anything … for it was under the complete control of the figure on the rostrum … [who] evoked or changed its passions as easily as if they had been the notes of some gigantic organ. … The monster seemed to indulge in an orgy of self-pity … [that] gave place to hate; and the monster seemed on the point of becoming homicidal … [and] intoxicated by the belief in its own omnipotence.
>
> (1941, pp. 165–166)

As noted by Reich (1933) and observed more recently by Bollas (1992) and Loewenstein (2023, 2024a, 2024b), fascism as a state of mind—both within the individual psyche and in fascistic political regimes—remains an unavoidable part of the human condition, one in which there is an enemy, a *bad* object outside the self, to be eliminated. Moreover, as with any paranoid pursuit, there is typically something in the out-group's or opposing mind-state's differences that seems threatening to the competing in-group or mental state. Within the in-group, individuals narcissistically identify with and establish strong emotional bonds with each other (Freud, 1920); consequently, when the in-group is threatened by mixing with the impure, outgroup other, then fears, resentments, and sources of envy become routes to unleashing violence promoted by fascist-leaning leadership.

As a mass phenomenon of organized irrationality under suitable existentially threatening conditions, authoritarian temptations prevail, and an authoritarian bargain is often made. That is, an autocratic, protofascist leader partners with a religious institution or nationalistic mythology that legitimizes the hypermasculine, strongman leader's lack of morality in order to exterminate the threat posed by the demonized, bad object (Ben-Ghiat, 2020). We see this, for example, in Trump's alliance with Christian nationalists and in Putin's allegiance to Russian orthodoxy.[10]

In considering some of the tactics and characteristics of autocratic, nationalistic, and populist proto-fascists, from Orban and Putin to Trump, Modi, and Netanyahu, we see that the fascist playbook entails ongoing attacks on truth and reality, as the decline of critical thinking and of listening to differing viewpoints is orchestrated and perpetuated. In this sociopolitical surround, the courage to disagree and speak freely is wiped out, and personalist rule is widely diffused through the leadership of authoritarian, hypermasculine strongmen who seek to co-opt and destroy democracy for power and personal gain (Ben-Ghiat, 2020; Loewenstein, 2024a; Wieland, 2015).

The Fascistic Leader in the Fascistic Mind

Malignant, narcissistic, paranoid, and psychopathic leaders infect vast numbers of people by stimulating fascistic states, especially under conditions of societal or personal trauma. Through the stimulation of these fascistic states of mind that dominate individual and group psyches, critical thinking is largely immobilized (Kernberg, 2020[11]). Utilizing both agitating and soothing tactics that access unconscious, archaic fears of ego annihilation and extinction, as well as redemptive rebirth and omnipotent phantasies, such leaders create a form of mass hypnosis in which personal autonomy and responsibility are abdicated. In identifying with a powerful and seemingly omnipotent leader, the group can evade painful truths, conflictual tensions, and reality itself. Large-group regressions are promoted in which basic assumptions and archaic psychic processes flourish, and manic elation accompanies the promise of salvation offered by a savior, a godlike Messiah (Bion, 1961; see also Money-Kyrle, 1941), or a secular pope (Wieland, 2024).

Consequently, a personality cult emerges to take over the group mind, now obtaining considerable pleasure in expressing hatred of the demonized other. Mob violence can easily erupt when individuals who feel helpless and impotent avert a desperate internal situation by delegating their own inner violence to the state, while also managing their annihilation anxieties through splitting and dissociation, fragmentation, violent projection, and disavowal. As the reality principle recedes and the group mind becomes coopted by the pleasure-unpleasure principle, wishes to cross boundaries, break norms, act on violent impulses, and relieve guilt and shame can lead to devastating destruction.

Authoritarian and fascist movements easily take hold when malignantly narcissistic demagogues and autocrats skillfully agitate to deceive, thereby serving as perverse containers for the nonthinking group mind (Diamond, 2023; Zienert-Eilts, 2020). As a result, fascist groups obtain considerable pleasure in expressing hatred of their demonized other, who through massive projective forces comes to represent desperate needs for achieving power through violence. Moreover, there is perversely pleasurable relief from the removal of repression in the permission to destroy or kill the hated object (Money-Kyrle, 1937), which is a "kind of cure for the ordinary neurosis of peace" (Bell, 2022, p. 681). Crossing boundaries, breaking norms, sanctioning violent and sadistic impulses, and relieving guilt and shame states may ultimately lead to devastation enacted by pathologically contained, regressed, proto-fascist groups (Diamond, 2022, 2023).[12]

Next, to better understand the allure of such fascistic states, I will introduce another key facet in the dynamics of the fascistic mind: namely, the role played by the death drive and its relationship to destructive narcissism.

The Role of the Death Drive and Destructive Narcissism in Promoting the Fascistic Mind

To reiterate, a central characteristic of fascism is its attacks on thinking, as well as on linking and binding—attacks that impede functioning in accordance with the reality principle and the symbolic register. Because external reality serves as an obstruction to omnipotence, it is hated, which in Bionian terms results in *attacks on linking* (Bion, 1961). From a Kleinian perspective, within each individual's and group's fascistic mental structure, there is an omnipotent, extremely violent force that is called upon when primordial annihilation fears are not transformed, and so, instead, the psyche "hates anything felt as an *obstruction... to anything ... not itself*" (Bell, 2015, p. 415, italics added).

Bion (1962a) used the term *–K* or "false links" to describe this malignant form of destructive negation or hatred of "any new development, as if ... *a rival to be destroyed*" (1962a, p. 82, italics added). When frustrations are too difficult to bear, and when rational, critical thinking is scorned, agitating tactics aim to obliterate reality by destroying knowledge and creating omnipotent solutions, with the result that the usual thinking processes are crippled and learning from experience is thwarted (Bion, 1962a).

Consequently, part of fascism's allure is that by extinguishing the bad other, whether it be a person, group, or mental function, the intoxicating illusion is created of *never having to lose*, let alone to *die*, thereby averting annihilation fears while avoiding the tensions, grief, and guilt of the depressive position. In terms of more deeply held, unconscious fantasies, the fascistic, destructively narcissistic state of mind retains the sense of omnipotence as his or her "majesty the baby" (Freud, 1914, p. 91), while avoiding having to compete in the oedipal realm, escaping from grief, and sidestepping the need to bear the tensions and guilt of the depressive position.[13] This forceful and fundamentally destructive state of mind is understood as the *negative* or as *death narcissism* that contrasts with *life narcissism* (Green 1999, 2001, 2023), which will be further discussed in what follows.

Accordingly, the ubiquitous *wish to flee death* is a key facet of fascism's allure. Primordial, omnipotent unconscious phantasy wishes of escaping death require that bodily and self-identity annihilation anxieties are defended against by means of splitting processes and projection outward into a demonized other—one who deserves being extinguished as the *dead* other. In this respect, the excessive use of projective processes by fascistic movements aims to gain the omnipotent power to escape death itself, even if it means destroying millions of others to do so. *Kill or be killed* becomes the prevailing ethic, and the appeal of fascism becomes preferable to reckoning with unthinkable, yet still unconscious, terrors. Perhaps something in human beings actually welcomes the level of violence seen in war, given that, as Bell (2022) argues, the psyche is "a soil that is so hospitable to the seeds of destruction … [that violence can] rapidly germinate with little obstruction" (2022, p. 675).

The death drive, or Thanatos—championed by Freud (1920, 1930, 1933), Klein (1933, 1946), and seminal French analysts (e.g., Lacan, 1966; and Green 1999, 2001, 2023)—remains a controversial concept. Nonetheless, both the forceful magnetism of phantasies underlying human destructiveness and the eternal appeal of murderous destruction, which manifests in fascist regimes, is evident throughout world history and in discussions of disturbed psychic processes.[14] In this respect, the human longing for violence and destructiveness is an aspect of the death drive's effort to eradicate threats posed by difference, conflict, and thinking itself. Indeed, "the apparent caesura between man and animal is somewhat illusory" (Bell, 2022, p. 678), something that Adorno (1951) seemed to detect when he described the inscrutable ruthlessness of the mob psychology among fascist crowds, noting that "if they would stop to reason … the whole performance would fall to pieces and they would be left in panic" (1951, p. 137).[15] Indeed, the limits of rational thinking and the relevance of unconscious forces become more apparent when violent power and destructiveness harken us back to Freud's (1930) linkage of the death drive to destructive omnipotence characterized by the pleasure of destructiveness for its own sake.

We might ask how the conceptual basis for the death drive is useful in understanding fascism. I find it valuable to consider three vectors of the death drive that seem applicable to fascism's allure.[16] First, Freud's (1933) *nirvana principle* of striving "to reduce life to its original condition of inanimate matter" (1933, p. 211) represents the lure toward *nothingness*, *quietude*, or *zero*—a nirvana-like mindlessness that, in restoring the previous non-life state, opposes thought, complexity, and life (or Eros) itself. In relieving the psyche of tensions, the drive is aimed toward the pleasure derived from negating all desires through mindlessness (Bell, 2015).

The second vector is Klein's (1933, 1946, 1958) pure pleasure in destructiveness as an expression of primary envy, which Bion (1962a) subsequently stressed in malignant attacks on linking or binding that falsifies and obliterates reality. This pull toward *manifest destructive violence* undoes connections, unbinds, breaks linkages, disinvests, and destroys objects; this paralyzes or annihilates the libidinal aspect of the life instinct (Haas and Topfer, 2024; see also Green, 1999). Klein (1933, 1946, 1958), situating its focus largely in her clinical work, understood the drive or instinct to reflect a persistent, unconscious, violent, and sadistic phantasy inscribed in the infant's mind, from which annihilation anxieties originate (and likewise fuel it). As an expression of primary envy, there is a pure pleasure in destruction, including destruction of thinking itself (Bion, 1962a). Consequently, congruent with most analytic thinkers, both Klein and Bion posit that the heart of the ubiquitous human struggle lies in the lifelong conflict between love and destructiveness.[17]

The third vector, especially relevant in balancing constructive and destructive forces, has been articulated in slightly different ways by Lacan (1966) and subsequently more precisely by Green (1999, 2001, 2023). In the Lacanian perspective, the constructive life force is embedded within a destructiveness expressed in the willingness to sacrifice life itself in pursuit of ecstasy or *jouissance*. Lacan considers the painful arousal of libidinal gratification as taking a form inherent within all drives, so that this symbolic destruction of the psyche related to *jouissance* reflects a "desperate affirmation of life" (1966, p. 263). Other analysts have addressed such destructiveness as demonstrating an "unrelenting life-in-excess-of life" (Ackerman et al., 2023, p. 680).

Following Lacan's contribution, Green (1999, 2001, 2023) furthered this intertwining of the life and death drives by positing a *death narcissism*, mentioned earlier, which is fueled by a wish for the omnipotence of immortality and timelessness that aims to escape life by glorifying the libidinal gratification of psychic death. In short, Green noted the pleasurable allure of the *negative* derived from abolishing all desires and returning to the nothingness of non-existence.[18]

Thanatos and the Mob

The death drive, directed toward undoing the bonds of love and hate, produces an overall deadening of the self and its objects, which can manifest in both self- and other destructiveness. Within the body politic, the death drive cultivates the very forces that would destroy it. This is exemplified in the fundamentalist Christian, evangelical, nationalistic belief manifest in sectors of Trumpism that welcome the coming of Armageddon, idealized as the will of God and a prelude to nothingness as the gateway to eternal bliss (Segal, 1987).

As Freud (1930) observed, natural aggression and hatred must be suppressed in order that we may live in civilization. Nonetheless, hatred does not simply disappear and can easily become manifest through group dynamics that foment violent action. Consequently, part of fascism's appeal resides in the fact that it allows sadistic desires to be fulfilled, and it permits guilt and shame to be absolved; furthermore, the seduction of the fascist mind is enhanced by the leader's use of a form of mass hypnosis.

Mob violence can easily arise when there is a conjunction between the narcissistically fueled destructive disposition within an individual or group and the presence of destabilizing social/environmental conditions (Money-Kyrle, 1934, 1937). Culture and civilization itself require the binding of the drives, particularly Eros and Thanatos, in order for disruptions to be tolerated and to enable individuals to think sufficiently with others (Green, 2023). The internal and external come into relation with one another in ways that Freud (1930) suggested when he described how individuals delegate their own internal violence to the state, especially under conditions of societal or personal trauma, as well as existential fears. Arguably, social trauma marked by the loss of meaning leads to massive group regression (Wieland, 2024), whereas the accompanying existential annihilation anxieties foster primitive defenses and phantasies of returning to a safe, conflict-free womb (Diamond 2022, 2023). Moreover, such large regressed groups tend to become aggregated through massification processes in which basic assumptions and archaic psychic processes flourish, and, as I've noted, manic elation accompanies the promise of salvation.

Next I will elaborate on the interminability of fascistic states in the unconscious mind.

The Timeless Allure of Fascistic States of Mind

To understand the allure of fascism in political groupings as well as in the individual mind, it is important to underscore that, rather than longing for freedom, humans often seek to be led and brought together with others to make meaning out of dread (Bion, 1961) and to be enveloped by something bigger and stronger (Musil, 1976; Reich, 1933; see also Bion, 1961; Freud, 1921). As Erich Fromm (1941) persuasively argues, relief is sought by *escaping from freedom* through surrendering to dictators of all kinds, relinquishing individual liberty, and transforming oneself into a cog in a much larger machine. To surrender to a powerful leader, and to regard them as a god or Messiah, is "an enormous relief from anxiety and inner conflict" (Money-Kyrle, 1941, p. 173). In particular, when social conditions evoke primordial, annihilating anxieties, relief in varied forms of surrender, ranging from conformity and idealization to authoritarianism and destructiveness, aids in evading what is most terrifying of all, namely, disintegrating and dying.[19]

Nonetheless, especially in democracies, we often frame our rhetoric and create our governing structures as though the deepest roots of human desire revolve around *being free*. But we should not overlook the innate, entrenched desire *to obey* and *to be dominated by a savior* in order to attain relief and to satisfy basic drives, including that of destructiveness, as well as the absolution of guilt and shame. The overarching wish to be cared for while de-repressing less civilized aspects of human nature helps us understand why fascism is an ever-present unconscious accompaniment to democratic ideals.

In examining fascist groupings and their relationship to group members' individual minds, Herbert Rosenfeld's (1971, 1984a, 1984b, 1987) incisive work is especially clarifying in addressing the malignant, psychotic part of the mind that functions as a kind of Mafia boss, an internal Führer, or a gang leader who promises welcome relief from uncertainty, meaninglessness, guilt, pain, and the confusion born of complexity (see, e.g., Diamond, 2023, 2024; Loewenstein, 2023, 2024a; Zienert-Eilts, 2024). Rosenfeld (1971, 1987) characterizes this internal psychic organization, namely, the *bad* or *mad* parts of the self or group culture, as idealizing omnipotence and cruelty; its thrust is largely against a dependence on loving, libidinal objects, including the dependent self, and on *sane* object relations.

In this malignant psychic realm dominated by destructive narcissism, a so-called Mafia gang seduces, stands above, and overpowers the healthy part of the personality.[20] Consequently, both within the individual and within the group mind, an internal Hitler, Stalin, or Mussolini stands ready to autocratically take hold of the plurality of psychic states and exterminate whatever seems most terrifying within. As every psychoanalytic clinician knows, taming the ruthless internal object or the obliterating inner madness—largely superego-driven—in order for the patient to regain control of his or her mind is part and parcel of the psychoanalyst's daily bread.

Applying his understanding of primitive states more directly to the political sphere, Rosenfeld (1984a, 1984b, 1987) posited that extremist, totalitarian systems, such as national socialism in Nazi Germany, promote delusional states in which the destructive narcissism of a Mafia-gang structure comes to dominate an entire population. Fascism ensues when the group's leader or Fuhrer is primarily "sadistic, omnipotent, completely lacking compassion, and demanding an absolute obedience from all parts of the [group's] self" (Rosenfeld, 1984b, pp. 159–160). Much like those under the sway of malignant narcissism, the fascist group functions in accordance with an ego-destructive, severe-superego-fueled, and rigidly organized structure that, as the bearer of authority and moral guidance, is not easily modified. Because destructive power is idealized, an omnipotent structure emerges that cannot be questioned (Rosenfeld, 1987).

Viewing its forcefulness in accordance with the death drive, Bion (1962a) posited that destructive idealization is "an envious assertion of moral superiority without any morals...[and a] stripping of all good ... that in turn degenerates into nullity" (1962a, p. 97). When this formation is outsourced to the collective group psyche, there is often a symbiotic relationship between the minds of autocratic, fascistic leaders and their followers, which provides a sense of belonging and cohesion, a sanctioning of grievances, and an erasure of differences, competitions, and tensions within the group (Kernberg, 2020; Volkan, 2020).

Though it is not possible to more fully explicate here the shift from the individual to the group mind, I have elaborated elsewhere the ways in which regressed large groups can begin to deal with primitive anxieties and fantasies in more psychotic ways (Diamond, 2022, 2023, 2024). This dynamic can easily lead to the creation and dominance of proto-fascistic defensive systems—ranging from authoritarianism to radical fascism—in which splitting, projection, and disavowal reign supreme, and violent action itself can ward off dissolution fears. For example the autocratic and perverse leader of the regressed group, such as Trump with his zealous MAGA followers who are faithful to his personality cult, is likely not the *shaper* of the group but is more accurately described as the narcissistically idealized executive of the group's latent spirit (Beland, 2024), the one who provides the group with a strong affective bond and, as the supreme, omnipotent leader, protects it from feared annihilation (Loewenstein, 2024b).

Arguably, this sort of pathological, fascistic organization can be described as a poorly contained psychological field, which German analyst Karin Zienert-Eilts (2020; 2024; see also Diamond, 2023) thinks of as a negative or *perverse container* that distorts and perverts reality while providing a delusional libidinal structure.[21] Perversion is evident in the twisting of good and evil, the idealized admiration of disruption and chaos, and the legitimization as well as dissociation of violent, destructive impulses (Zienert-Eilts, 2024). This malignant and hate-filled state then provides relief from the inherent tensions of living with differences and the unbearable anxieties of annihilation and death. In its destructive group dynamic, this perverse container serves to defend against anxiety caused by diversity and the inherent frustrations and losses that accompany a democracy (Diamond, 2023).

Next, I consider the operation of these processes in the large-group MAGA movement characterized by autocratic and proto-fascistic collective mental states, currently dominating the polity in the United States.

Perverted Containment and the Role of Fascistic States in Trump's America

These group dynamics are most evident in what I've described as the cult of Trumpism (Diamond, 2022, 2023), in which Trump and his enablers serve as the perverted container that abolishes the individuality of diverse group members. These members range from Main Street workers and rural laborers to tech bros, neo-Nazi thugs, and Wall Street power brokers. Rather than containing by detoxifying and transforming the mad, psychotic elements within the larger group—specifically, via *alpha functioning*—this malignant brand of containment fuels destructive processes. For instance, destruction itself was perversely idealized in the January 6, 2021, insurrection at the U.S. Capitol. Moreover, a reciprocal fascistic form of destructiveness often arises in which the impulse to eradicate the putative evil residing in MAGA members is apparent among virulent anti-Trumpists. Such eradicating forms of sadism aim to abolish anything other than the group's self, which Ron Britton (2021) describes as a "xenocidal" mental state in which there is a love of destroying and even killing (2021, p. 92).[22]

Within the Trumpian world, Trump appears in the same paranoid/schizoid mode as the larger group—speaking the same language, executing the group's spirit, and sharing "hatred of the 'establishment mother'" (Zienert-Eilts, 2020, p. 980). In this symbiosis between the leader and his followers, the other or out-group is projectively identified with the group members' hateful imagoes, while the leader becomes an unambivalently loved, idealized savior or Messiah—or the illusionary lost mother or all-powerful father—that heroically signifies divinity, immortality, and timelessness (Bion, 1961; Green, 2001; see also Freud, 1921). A *destructive-populist* fit is formed that permits both the leader and his followers to "indulge their hatred of thinking" (Kravis, 2021, p. 550).

Lies, misunderstandings, and conspiratorial delusions override truth and comprehension as this aberrant, reversed reality aims to restore order, meaning, and security by means of oppression, fear, and a virulent "move away from shared standards of truth" (S. Rosenfeld, 2019, p. 5). Rather than detoxifying and containing the mad, psychotic elements within the group, destructive processes are fueled and a love of destroying is idealized, as in the mob violence evident in the January 6 insurrection. Unfortunately, violence and war are the likely end products of this timeless "psychotic process" (Money-Kyrle, 1937, p. 153).

In my closing section, I will briefly share a few concluding thoughts to help us think about how we might employ psychoanalytic understandings to help deal with fascism's allure and destructive potency, especially in view of an increasing number of autocratic and fascistic movements worldwide.

Closing Thoughts on Dealing with the Allure of Fascism

In facing today's world and its attempted colonization by rising autocratic leadership and fascistic group movements, we might ask whether or not psychoanalytic understanding can help us mitigate the dangers of fascism, especially since a nation flooded by psychotic dynamics often finds it "very difficult to understand and acknowledge this as madness" (Rosenfeld, 1984b, p. 161).

Once socially destructive forces are unleashed, considerable time and effort are needed to contain such powers (Freud, 1933).[23]

We might ask ourselves whether we possess viable safeguards to recognize and tame the alluring seductiveness of fascistic states, especially within large group movements. As I've indicated, in addressing the political crises of our times, conscious reasoning alone is inadequate to rein in the destructive forces that have been unleashed. Taming these forces cannot occur if we refuse to understand what makes them enticing as well as formidable. For instance, as Hinshelwood (2024) so aptly reminds us, thinking about Trumpism, nationalism, and fascism requires that we go beyond conscious reasoning and the rational mind to recognize the unconscious dynamics at play; clearly, these dynamics are providing relief from intolerable, unconscious states of mind that are driving the identifications with and enduring emotional bonds with authoritarian and fascist leadership. By realizing what makes these bonds so formidable and renders them less amenable to verifiable information and rational dialogue, we can better position ourselves to reckon with the rising waves of fascism.

My aim here has been to help us in this recognition, in part through more honestly recognizing within ourselves and our own groups the fascistic allure, rather than more arrogantly believing that we—or our progressive-thinking groups, including psychoanalytic organizations—can somehow operate beyond, and/or are not subject to, such violently absolutist states. As this article makes implicit, we are left with several important questions to ponder that pertain to both individual and group psyches.

For instance, we might ask what checks and balances within both an individual and a group mind can help us recognize, stand up to, and better regulate the Mafia-mind within each of us. Can we bear witness to and yet keep the grandiose inner Fuhrer from bullying, securing, and taking over the healthier, democratic parts of the individual and group ego, in order to reinstate the reality principle and manage the death drive itself? Are we able to collectively mourn our lost omnipotence, accept our limitations and dependencies, and—in gender-based terminology—can we relinquish our individual and group-based, unconsciously sexualized and hypermasculine phallic identifications to value our so-called *feminine receptivity* (Steiner, 2022) and empathic capabilities?[24]

Are we capable of facing and sufficiently detonating our unconscious conflicts, identifications, and destructive narcissism that might otherwise prevent us from making necessary reparations and restitutions? And finally, can we, along with enough of the polity, truly become *anti-fascists*, so that we might live and engage with emotionally charged differences in a respectful, more empathic manner?[25]

Needless to say, healthy leadership is essential in appealing to libidinal instincts that promote the containment of primitive anxieties and fantasies rather than invoking images of fear, hatred, and distrust; thereby, reflecting our "better angels" (Lincoln, 1861) that can help us live up to America's *creed* (King, 1963).[26] Indeed, I find it helpful to echo Hannah Arendt's (1951) insistence that fascistic totalitarianism can only be combatted through our capacity to *think*, to *bear guilt and tensions*, and to retain *moral engagement*. This entails taming the anti-life facets of the death drive in order to ensure that love, or Eros, remains sufficiently integrated with the unbinding hate-fueled destructiveness of Thanatos. In particular, activism is required to prevent the domination of idealizing identifications in which leadership embodies a shameless, harsh, and cruel superego aimed at destroying the collective ego that democracy requires.

In conclusion, to foster cautious yet realistic hope that fascism can be held in check, steadfast efforts are required to understand fascism's unconscious dynamics, particularly as they inform the impenetrable emotional bond between the group and its leader. The challenge is to engage in persistent questioning of ourselves and the world around us, prioritizing truth-seeking, activism against injustice, and the de-objectification of others instead of malignant *othering*. Finally, in reckoning with American democracy's unconscious tensions, guilt, and insufficiently mourned losses, we must especially call to account and reject fascistic leadership within ourselves and the body politic.

Disclosure Statement

The author does not have any relevant financial or non-financial competing interest.

Notes

1 Durkheim's (1893) notion of *anomie* is useful in understanding the conditions currently in place throughout much of the world in which a breakdown of standards, norms, and values leads to a state of *normlessness* that favors the rise of autocracies and fascistic movements.
2 Stenner and her colleagues (Stenner, 2005; Stenner and Haidt, 2018) found that approximately one-third of those studied in Western democracies showed a predilection for authoritarianism in their limited ability to tolerate ambiguity, complexity, and sociocultural diversity. Interestingly, an equal percentage of the US polity seems to represent the hardcore, MAGA base. This isn't surprising given the clashing, complex cacophony of views that render the U.S. in the 21st century particularly ripe for the rise of authoritarian movements that profess to hold together societal unity by offering a single, more utopian vision, including an ultimate solution to complex problems (Diamond, 2022; see also Applebaum, 2020).
3 The following two page citations are also from Prince (2023).
4 Fascism's violent omnipotence and destructive narcissism contrast with a more authoritarian state of mind that seems somewhat more neurotically organized and closer to the depressive position (Money-Kyrle, 1937).
5 However, given the results of the 2024 election in which both houses of Congress as well as the Presidency itself are in the hands of Trump and his Republican enablers, and considering the complete loyalty of nominated cabinet members to Trump

himself rather than to the Constitution or to democracy's norms and guardrails, it is quite conceivable that dictatorial powers could be acquired after Trump takes office in 2025.

6 Figlio (2006) described this as the *absolute state of mind*. Its absolutism results from "a state of idealization of self, merged with an idealized object as an ego-ideal, withdrawn from external reality and from its constraints, such as time, space, difference, frustration, work, [and] the otherness of objects" (2006, p. 120). Moreover, as I will point out, omnipotent phantasies prevail in the absolutist, fascistic state of mind in which the individual subject is protected from experiencing either shame or guilt (Steiner, 2022).

7 Though deeply unconscious, this seemingly plays a formative role in stranger anxiety, oedipal fears, racism, and bigotry, as well as subsequent proto-fascistic group movements across a wide spectrum. Beginning with the experience of initially encountering the stranger, the dangers of separation anxiety and object loss are accompanied by compensatory unconscious fantasies that can subsequently emerge in nationalistic and fundamental ideologies (Bohleber, 2024).

8 Bohleber (2024) suggests that ubiquitous unconscious fantasies underlie such longings and pertain to caretaking and sibling rivalry, homogeneity vis-a-vis the other, and wishes for an illusionary substitute for the lost mother of infancy.

9 Unfortunately, since the attack on Israel by Hamas on October 7, 2023, we have seen such passionate, demonizing forms of splitting and fascistic-friendly leanings among extremists in both the pro-Israeli and pro-Palestinian enclaves. In this context, existential threats contribute to foreclosing both nuanced, critical thinking (with its historical awareness) and empathic humanizing of the out-group or *enemy*.

10 This is evident in a close reading of fifty-eight religious, primarily evangelical prayers offered at Trump's campaign events between November 2022 and June 2024. Extolling Trump's righteousness as a *spiritual warrior* fighting against a demonic force, these prayers mentioned Trump's name eighty-seven times, in contrast to Jesus Christ's at sixty-one. A common narrative was: "Lord, you have an instrument in Donald J. Trump. … Help us overcome any obstacles … so that we may deliver victory to your warrior" (Coppins, 2024, p. 10).

11 Such leadership is aptly described by activist and Harvard Law School professor Sherrilyn Ifill (2023) in addressing the monumental changes in the US over the last decade, in which millions of Americans have embraced and reelected Donald Trump despite his being "of such degraded moral character … so void of a spirit of public service … so fundamentally inclined toward theft, mendacity, cruelty, and criminality that we can scarcely absorb the breadth of his transgressions" (2023, p. 58). Flying in the face of rationality is the recent phenomenon that millions more Americans threw their weight behind Trump *after* he was convicted of thirty-four felony counts in May 2024.

12 It is noteworthy that states of mind seen as evidence of severe disturbance in an individual—for instance, paranoia, omnipotence, manic elation, excessive idealization, and unquestioned loyalty to a leader—are easily normalized in regressed groups that actually promote such disturbed psychic states.

13 Besides eradicating critical thinking, both the capacity for concern and the ability to empathize with the other or out-group are destroyed, especially under conditions of excessive fear (Diamond, 2022; Nussbaum, 2018). Compassion is not valued but instead is derided as weak, feminine, and a slippery slope paving the way to a welfare state.

14 *Thanatos*, a metaphysical concept, is the Greek word for *death*, as well as the name of an ancient god who was the twin of Hypnos, the god of sleep. The close

relationship between death and sleep is well known, and in fact death is sometimes described colloquially as the *Big Sleep*.

15 This brings to mind Freud's 1932 correspondence with Albert Einstein in pursuit of understanding the hatred and destructiveness manifested by war. Freud's (1933) letters advised civilized societies to deal with psychotic-level, primitive group processes through a "strengthening of the intellect" (p. 214)—a function that, sadly, cannot in itself adequately regulate or contain the malignant, primitive, and archaic forces operative in regressed large groups. It is woefully apparent today that Freud was overly optimistic in this regard.

16 In formulating these ideas, I have drawn from the writings of several 21st-century analytic writers, including David Bell (2015, 2022), Andre Green (1999, 2001, 2023), Sarah Ackerman, Lynne Zeavin, Derek Hook, David Lichtenstein, and Mark Goldblatt (2023).

17 Along similar lines, prior to Klein's work Freud (1923) posited that the superego emerges from the death drive, which operates in its pure culture to drive the ego to its death in melancholia.

18 Both Green and Lacan address *negation* in either healthy or unhealthy forms, in its mixing of libido and suffering, which can creatively serve as a foundation for individuation, often through the "compulsive enjoyment incurred by self-damaging acts" (Ackerman et al., 2023, p. 698). However, the destructiveness of the *negative* or *death narcissism* that aims for non-existence, anesthesia, and indifference, all of which are linked to the omnipotence of immortality and timelessness, finds its pleasurable allure in the *negative* that glorifies psychic death to escape life by returning to level zero (Green, 1999).

19 Here, we might recognize the aptness of the longstanding aphorism that *there are no atheists in foxholes*, along with the extreme popularity of the World War II era's song, "Praise the Lord and Pass the Ammunition," written by Frank Loesser in response to the attack on Pearl Harbor.

20 We might note how close this is to the death drive's pull toward zero and mindlessness, in which the allure is to inhabit a pain-free and conflict-free universe. Moreover, omnipotent phantasies in the form of narcissistic idealizations harness the forces used by a mental agency to aggressively oppose the self's attraction to good objects that tend to rule passionately (Rosenfeld, 1971, 1987). For instance, in its group countenance, the MAGA world under the sway of its phallically superior leader accesses the phantasy of returning to the Garden of Eden's primordial state, where the *poisons* and *vermin* within the object relational world that complicate life by creating tension and conflict no longer exist. In this realm, there is an absence of benign othering, and the negative governs in complete autonomy.

21 Bion (1962b) describes this as a *minus container* that pastes together fragmented elements through what he terms a *beta-screen*, which is impermeable to reality because it screens out what might be transformative from outside the barrier, while holding in inadequately processed sense impressions that remain agglomerated inside the barrier. Wieland (2015) suggests that fascism in the individual and societal mind operates much like a beta-screen that evokes strong emotions by gluing together "fragments of a disintegrating personality/community/nation" (2015, p. 162), which provides an alternative form of meaning in order to avert annihilation anxiety (Wieland, 2024; see also Zienert-Eilts, 2024).

22 Britton (2024) characterizes such destructive narcissism as split off from the rest of the personality, similarly to the way that Milton (1667) in *Paradise Lost* portrayed satanic pursuit as "Evil be my good" (1667, p. 105). This fascistic form of destructiveness, which aims to abolish anything other than the self (or group's self),

is distinguished from *defensive* or *libidinal* narcissism that protects against loving relationships out of fear of being hurt or annihilated.

23 In Freud's (1933) pessimistic wording, an unpleasant picture was painted of "mills that grind so slowly that people may starve before they get their flour" (1933, p. 213). Fascist, nationalistic movements have tended to be defeated over time by anti-fascist movements, often using violence and war—for instance, in the Second World War's defeat of Nazi Germany, fascist Italy, and imperial Japan. However, the use of violence in today's nuclear, biological, and technological era is especially precarious. We may be living in a time when it is critical to consider whether a deeper, more specifically psychoanalytic understanding of the forces that make fascism so alluring is vital to our survival.

24 Both in an individual mind and in a group context—for instance, as seen in post-Nazi Germany through the collective sharing of guilt, remorse, and regret—loss of omnipotence can be mourned, and it then becomes more likely that we will adopt a less destructive view of masculinity, as well as a less pejorative view of receptive femininity (Steiner, 2022).

25 Because humans are social animals who inherently incorporate collective unconscious dynamics rooted in otherness that entails fascist and racist mental states, we must humbly recognize that we can never be *non-fascists*, much as we can only be *anti*-racist rather than believing that our psyches contain neither racist (nor fascist) impulses of any kind.

26 Lincoln (1861), in his First Inaugural Address, concluded his remarks at the moment of an impending civil war with these timeless words, calling for our "better angels":

> *We are not enemies, but friends*. We must not be enemies. Though passion may have strained, it must not break our bonds of affection. The mystic chords of memory, stretching from every battlefield and patriot grave … all over this broad land, will yet swell the chorus of the Union, when again touched, as surely they will be, *by the better angels of our nature*.
>
> (italics added)

A century later, Martin Luther King (1963) gave his "I Have A Dream" speech in which he declared,

> Even though we face the difficulties of today and tomorrow, I still have a dream … [that] one day the nation will rise up, live out the true meaning of its creed: '… that all men are created equal. … We are free at last.'

References

Ackerman, S., Zeavin, L., Hook, D., Lichtenstein, D., & Goldblatt, D. (2023) 'Thanatos: Is Freud's concept still relevant?', *The Journal of the American Psychoanalytic Association*, 71, pp. 669–702.

Adorno, T. W. (1951) 'The Freudian theory and the patterns of fascist propaganda', in A. Arato & E. Gebhardt (eds.) *The Essential Frankfurt School Reader*. New York, Continuum.

Adorno, T. W., Frenkel-Brunswik, E., Levinson, D., & Sanford, N. (1950) *The Authoritarian Personality*. New York. W. W. Norton.

Applebaum, A. (2020) *Twilight of Democracy: The Seductive Lure of Authoritarianism*. New York, Doubleday.

Arendt, H. (1951) *The Origins of Totalitarianism*. New York, Harcourt Brace Jovanovich, 1968.

Beland, H. (2024) 'Herbert Rosenfeld's transposition of the individual into the collective: cultural spurs to further thinking—interview with Hermann Beland', in K. J. Zienert-Eilts & W. Hegener (eds.) *Herbert Rosenfeld: Then and Now*. London, Karnac.

Bell, D. (2015) 'The death drive: phenomenological perspectives in Kleinian theory', *International Journal of Psychoanalysis*, 96, pp. 411–423.

Bell, D. (2022) 'Psychoanalytic reflections on the conditions of possibility of human destructiveness', *International Journal of Psychoanalysis*, 103, pp. 674–691.

Ben-Ghiat, R. (2020) *Strongmen: Mussolini to the Present*. New York, W. W. Norton.

Bion, W. (1961) *Experiences in Groups and Other Papers*. London, Tavistock.

Bion, W. (1962a) *Learning from Experience*. London, Heinemann.

Bion, W. (1962b) 'The psycho-analytic study of thinking', *International Journal of Psychoanalysis*, 43, pp. 306–310.

Bohleber, W. (2024) 'Purity and unity: Narcissism and destructiveness in nationalistic and fundamentalistic ideologies', *American Imago*, 81, pp. 1–16.

Bollas, C. (1992) 'The fascist state of mind', in C. Bollas, *Being a Character: Psychoanalysis and Self Experience*. New York, Hill & Wang.

Brennan, T. C. (2022) *The Fasces: A History of Ancient Rome's Most Dangerous Political Symbol*. Oxford, UK, Oxford University Press.

Britton, R. (2021) *Sex, Death, and the Superego: Updating Psychoanalytic Experience and Development in Neuroscience*. London, Routledge.

Britton, R. (2024) 'Herbert Rosenfeld and the distinction between "defensive" and "destructive" narcissism', in K. J. Zienert-Eilts & W. Hegener (eds.) *Herbert Rosenfeld: Then and Now*. London, Karnac.

Coppins, M. (2024) 'The Most Revealing Moment of a Trump Rally', *The Atlantic*, July 29. Available at: https://www.theatlantic.com/magazine/archive/2024/09/trump-rally-prayers/679152/

Diamond, M. J. (2022) *Ruptures in the American Psyche: Containing Destructive Populism in Perilous Times*. Oxfordshire, UK, Phoenix Publishing House.

Diamond, M. J. (2023) 'Perverted containment: Trumpism, cult creation, and the rise of destructive American populism', *Psychoanalytic Inquiry*, 43, pp. 96–109.

Diamond, M. J. (2024) 'The power of certitude, mindlessness, and destruction: Discussion of Era Loewenstein's "The Allure of Fascism and the 'Appointment in Samarra'"', *Fort Da*, 30, pp. 27–41.

Durkheim, E. (1893) *The Division of Labor in Society*. New York, Free Press.

Eco, U. (1995) 'Ur-fascism', *The New York Review of Books*, 42, pp. 12–15.

Feldman, M. (2022) 'The appeal of omnipotence', in J. Arundale (ed.) *The Omnipotent State of Mind: Psychoanalytic Perspectives*. London, Routledge.

Figlio, K. (2006) 'The absolute state of mind in society and the individual', *Psychoanalysis, Culture & Society*, 11, pp. 119–143.

Finchelstein, F. (2024) *The Wannabe Fascists: A Guide to Understanding the Greatest Threat to Democracy*. Oakland, CA, University of California Press.

Freud, S. (1914) 'On Narcissism: An Introduction', in J. Strachey, A. Freud, A. Strachey, & A. Tyson (eds.) *The Standard Edition of the Complete Psychological Works of Sigmund Freud, Volume XIV (1914–1916): On the History of the Psycho-Analytic Movement, Papers on Metapsychology and Other Works*. London, Hogarth Press, pp. 67–102.

Freud, S. (1920) 'Beyond the Pleasure Principle', in J. Strachey, A. Freud, A. Strachey, & A. Tyson (eds.) *The Standard Edition of the Complete Psychological Works of Sigmund Freud, Volume XVIII (1920–1922): Beyond the Pleasure Principle, Group Psychology and Other Works*. London, Hogarth Press, pp. 1–64.

Freud, S. (1921) 'Group Psychology and the Analysis of the Ego', in J. Strachey, A. Freud, A. Strachey, & A. Tyson (eds.) *The Standard Edition of the Complete Psychological Works of Sigmund Freud, Volume XVIII (1920–1922): Beyond the Pleasure Principle, Group Psychology and Other Works*. London, Hogarth Press, pp. 65–144.

Freud, S. (1923) 'The ego and the id', in J. Strachey, A. Freud, A. Strachey, & A. Tyson (eds.) *The Standard Edition of the Complete Psychological Works of Sigmund Freud, Volume XIX (1923–1925): The Ego and the Id and Other Works*. London, Hogarth Press, pp. 3–68.

Freud, S. (1930) 'Civilization and its Discontents', in J. Strachey, A. Freud, A. Strachey, & A. Tyson (eds.) *The Standard Edition of the Complete Psychological Works of Sigmund Freud, Volume XXI (1927–1931): The Future of an Illusion, Civilization and its Discontents and Other Works*. London, Hogarth Press, pp. 59–148.

Freud, S. (1933) 'Why war?', in J. Strachey, A. Freud, A. Strachey, A. Tyson, & A. Richards (eds.) *The Standard Edition of the Complete Psychological Works of Sigmund Freud, Volume XXII (1932–1936): New Introductory Works on Psycho-Analysis and Other Works*. London, Hogarth Press, pp. 197–218.

Fromm, E. (1941) *Escape from Freedom*. New York, Farrar & Rinehart.

Gandesha, S. (2019) 'The "authoritarian personality" reconsidered: The phantom of "left fascism"', *The American Journal of Psychoanalysis*, 79, pp. 601–624.

Gopnik, A. (2024) 'The enablers: Hitler didn't grab power; he was given it', *The New Yorker*, March 25, pp. 72–76.

Green, A. (1999) 'The death drive, negative narcissism, and the disobjectalising function', in A. Green, *The Work of the Negative*. London, Free Association Books.

Green, A. (2001) *Life Narcissism, Death Narcissism*. London, Free Association Books.

Green, A. (2023) *On the Destruction and the Death Drives*. Oxfordshire, UK, Phoenix Publishing House.

Haas, C. A. & Topfer, N. F. (2024). A tale of scorpions and frogs: Clinical considerations and the social dynamics of destructive narcissism. In K. J. Zienert-Eilts & W. Hegener (eds.) *Herbert Rosenfeld: Then and Now*. London, Karnac.

Havel, V. (1979) 'The power of the powerless', in J. Keane (ed.) *The Power of the Powerless: Citizens Against the State in Central-Eastern Europe*. London, Routledge.

Hinshelwood, R. D. (2023) 'Populism: The politics of emotions', *Psychoanalytic Inquiry*, 43, pp. 110–118.

Hinshelwood, R. D. (2024) The allure of populism and fascism. *Paper presented at the 113th Annual Conference of the American Psychoanalytic Association*, June.

Hinshelwood, R. D. (2025) *Unconscious Politics: Alienation, Social Science and Psychoanalysis*. London, Karnac.

Hoffer, E. (1951) *The True Believer: Thoughts on the Nature of Mass Movements*. Harper, New York.

Hofstadter, R. (1965) *The Paranoid Style in American Politics and Other Essays*. New York, Knopf.

Ifill, S. (2023) 'How America ends and begins again', *New York Review of Books*, 70(December 2), pp. 58–60.

Kernberg, O. F. (2020) 'Malignant narcissism and large group regression', *Psychoanalytic Quarterly*, 89, pp. 1–24.

King, M. L. (1963) *I have a dream*. Available at: https://www.npr.org/2010/01/18/122701268/i-have-a-dream-speech-in-its-entirety (open in a new window).

Klein, M. (1933) 'The early development of conscience in the child', in M. Klein, *Love, Guilt and Reparation and Other Works, 1921–1945*. New York, Free Press.

Klein, M. (1946) 'Notes on some schizoid mechanisms', *International Journal of Psychoanalysis*, 27, pp. 99–110.

Klein, M. (1958) 'On the development of mental functioning', in M. Klein, *Envy, Gratitude and Other Works, 1946–1963*. New York, Free Press.

Kravis, N. (2021) 'Charisma', *Psychoanalytic Quarterly*, 90, pp. 523–554.

Kristofferson, K. & Foster, F. L. (1969) *Me and Bobby McGee*. Nashville, TN, Combine Music Corporation.

Lacan, J. (1966) *Écrits: The First Complete Edition in English*. New York, Norton.

Lincoln, A. (1861) *First Inaugural Address*. Available at: https://avalon.law.yale.edu/19th_century/lincoln1.asp (open in a new window).
Loewenstein, E. A. (2023) 'In dark times: Psychoanalytic praxis as a form of resistance to fascist propaganda', *Psychoanalytic Inquiry*, 43, pp. 130–144.
Loewenstein, E. A. (2024a) 'The allure of fascism and "The appointment in Samarra"', *fort da*, 30, pp. 8–26.
Loewenstein, E. A. (2024b) The leader and his followers: The allure of fascistic states of mind. *Paper presented at the 113th Annual Conference of the American Psychoanalytic Association*, June.
Löwenthal, L. & Guterman, N. (1949) *Prophets of Deceit: A Study of the Techniques of the American Agitator*. London, Verso.
Milton, J. (1667) *Paradise Lost*. New York, Dutton.
Money-Kyrle, R. (1934) 'A psychological analysis of the causes of war', in D. Meltzer (ed.) *The Collected Papers of Roger Money-Kyrle*. London, Karnac.
Money-Kyrle, R. (1937) 'The development of war', in D. Meltzer (ed.) *The Collected Papers of Roger Money-Kyrle*. London, Karnac.
Money-Kyrle, R. (1941) 'The psychology of propaganda', in D. Meltzer (ed.) *The Collected Papers of Roger Money-Kyrle*. London, Karnac.
Money-Kyrle, R. (1968) 'Cognitive development', *The International Journal of Psychoanalysis*, 49, pp. 691–698.
Musil, R. (1976) *Diaries, 1899–1942*. New York, Basic Books.
Nussbaum, M. C. (2018) *The Monarchy of Fear: A Philosopher Looks at our Political Crisis*. New York, Simon & Schuster.
Paxton, R. (2004) *The Anatomy of Fascism*. London, Penguin Books.
Prince, R. M. (2023) Locating the fascist mind. *Psychoanalytic Inquiry*, 43, pp. 70–83.
Reich, W. (1933) *The Mass Psychology of Fascism*. New York, Farrar, Strauss & Giroux.
Rosenfeld, H. (1971) 'A clinical approach to the psychoanalytic theory of the life and death instincts: An investigation into the aggressive aspects of narcissism', *International Journal of Psychoanalysis*, 52, pp. 169–178.
Rosenfeld, H. (1984a) 'Narcissism and aggression: Clinical and theoretical considerations', in H. S. Hart (ed.) *Narcissism and Aggression: Working Conference of the DPV 1984 in Wiesbaden*. DPV Conference Publication. [Originally published in German as: 'Narzißmus und aggression', in P. Kutter, R. Páramo-Ortega & P. Zagermann (eds.) *Die psychoanalytische haltung: Auf der suche nach dem selbstbild der psychoanalyse* (*The psychoanalytic attitude: In search of the self-image of psychoanalysis*). Munich, Verlag Internationale Psychoanalyse.]
Rosenfeld, H. (1984b) 'Applying my theory of psychosis to the Nazi phenomenon', in K. J. Zienert-Eilts & W. Hegener (eds.) *Herbert Rosenfeld: Then and Now*. London, Karnac.
Rosenfeld, H. (1987) *Impasse and Interpretation: Therapeutic and Anti-Therapeutic Factors in the Psychoanalytical Treatment of Psychotic, Borderline, and Neurotic Patients*. London, Routledge.
Rosenfeld, S. (2019) *Democracy and Truth: A Short History*. Philadelphia, PA, University of Pennsylvania Press.
Segal, H. (1987) 'Silence is the real crime', *The International Review of Psychoanalysis*, 14, pp. 3–12.
Segal, H. (2006) 'September 11', *Psychoanalytic Psychotherapy*, 20, pp. 115–121.
Steiner, J. (2022) 'Overcoming obstacles in analysis: Is it possible to relinquish omnipotence and accept receptive femininity?', in J. Arundale (ed.) *The Omnipotent State of Mind: Psychoanalytic Perspectives*. London, Routledge.
Stenner, K. (2005) *The Authoritarian Dynamic*. Cambridge, UK, Cambridge University Press.

Stenner, K. & Haidt, J. (2018) 'Authoritarianism is not a momentary madness, but an eternal dynamic within liberal democracies', in C. R. Sunstein (ed.) *Can It Happen Here? Authoritarianism in America*. New York, Harper Collins.
Volkan, V. D. (2020) *Large Group Psychology: Racism, Societal Divisions, Narcissistic Leaders, and Who We Are Now*. Oxfordshire, UK, Phoenix Publishing House.
Wieland, C. (2015) *The Fascist State of Mind and the Manufacturing of Masculinity: A Psychoanalytic Approach*. London, Routledge.
Wieland, C. (2024) Fascism as religion—The great allure. *Paper presented at the 113th Annual Conference of the American Psychoanalytic Association*, June.
Winnicott, D. W. (1962) 'Ego integration in child development', in D. W. Winnicott, *The Maturational Processes and the Facilitating Environment*. New York, International University Press.
Zienert-Eilts, K. J. (2020) 'Destructive populism as "perverted containing": A psychoanalytical look at the attraction of Donald Trump', *International Journal of Psychoanalysis*, 101, pp. 971–991.
Zienert-Eilts, K. J. (2024) 'Destructive narcissism and the susceptibility to "perverted containing" using the example of destructive populism: Further psychoanalytical considerations', in K. J. Zienert-Eilts & W. Hegener (eds.) *Herbert Rosenfeld: Then and Now*. London, Karnac, pp. 195–209.

Chapter 3

Trump and the Paranoid-Schizoid Politics of Ideality

Noëlle C. McAfee

Reasons for Inclusion

Noëlle McAfee is one of the foremost theorists of psychoanalysis and authoritarian political movements working today, authoring a variety of excellent books, chapters, and articles on the topic (see "Directions for Future Research and Further Readings"). One of McAfee's major contributions is to link authoritarian politics to Winnicott's "fear of breakdown", theorizing the link between mass social crises, individual psychic defences, and political beliefs and movements. Written soon after Donald Trump first took the Oval Office, this brief paper serves as an introduction to McAfee's thinking. The paper critically considers Trumpism, identifying the Kleinian paranoid-schizoid mechanisms and the Kristevan syndrome of "ideality" at play in the movement's rhetoric and policies. McAfee concludes by contrasting Trumpism with a psychoanalytically-informed politics of "working through" that leads "toward a position that can tolerate loss, ambiguity, and uncertainty, that is, the human condition" (this reader, p. 68). Like Salberg's contribution below (see Chapter 12), McAfee's work is essential for those who hope to theorize contemporary fascism, and to those who aim to develop a psychoanalytically-informed mode of resistance.

***

The phenomenon of Donald Trump's ascendancy to become the forty-fifth President of the United States is surely overdetermined, meaning that there are likely many different causes for this. The one I entertain here is I believe significant, though I do not argue that it is the main or only cause. But it is one we should consider and address. In short, I argue that the rise of Trump is in part due to a paranoid-schizoid politics found both in the personality of Trump himself and in a large-scale regression of many in the populace to a more primitive state of denial, splitting, and demonization, coupled with a syndrome of ideality. In other words, both Trump and his supporters split the world into good and bad (or "SAD!!!!" as Trump likes to tweet). In his inaugural speech, he repeatedly demonized foreign powers and idealized America. His *America First* policy is textbook paranoid-schizoid: "We must protect our borders from

DOI: 10.4324/9781003742876-5

the ravages of other countries making our products, stealing our companies and destroying our jobs."

The Trump phenomenon shares much with many other nationalist politics on the rise around the world, but mostly an inability to tolerate difference and loss, including loss of a romanticized past or an idealized future. Hence our politics today needs something that psychoanalytic theory has tried to offer: an understanding of how to work through trauma, loss, and persecutory fantasies. A politics of working through difficult choices and misrepresentations of others in our midst could help allay the paranoid politics that dominates politics today.

After giving an account of the concept of *working through* in Freud, Klein, and Kristeva, I turn to the Trump phenomenon and then close with a brief account of *a politics of working through*.

I

Globally, our politics needs something that only psychoanalysis has been able to promise: the capacity to work through trauma, loss, and persecutory fantasies. A politics of working through difficult choices and misrepresentations of others in our midst could help allay the paranoid politics that dominates politics today. How might psychoanalytic insights help bodies politic? To explore this question, this paper is loosely structured around Freud's essay, "Remembering, Repeating, and Working Through." Part I of this paper takes up Freud's model that aimed to free up resistances to remembering past trauma; part II moves beyond Freud to Klein's and Kristeva's insights about the pathologies that have little to do with external traumas and more to do with early primitive defense mechanisms; and the final part focuses on how—whether our troubles originate from trauma, loss, or primitive defenses—our deliberative practices can better cultivate modes of mourning and working through, beyond lost ideals and fantasies, towards dealing with life's ambiguities.

Freud grappled with the process of working through in his 1914 essay, "Remembering, Repeating, and Working Through," and later in his 1926 essay, "Inhibitions, Symptoms, and Anxiety." In the former he gives the first direct account of the process of working through trauma, loss, and remember-less repetition. He found that catharsis and knowledge were insufficient in overcoming neuroses, especially in the case of repeating, the phenomenon where the "patient does not *remember* anything of what he has forgotten and repressed, but *acts* it out. He reproduces it not as a memory but as an action; he *repeats* it, without, of course, knowing that he is repeating it" (Freud, 1914, p. 150). In repeating, there is a powerful resistance at work that the analysand must work through.

Even if the ego decides to give up resistance, he notes, repression can remain because of unconscious sources of resistance, and so the analysand enters a period of "strenuous effort … the phase of 'working through'" because "the compulsion to repeat—the attraction exerted by the unconscious prototypes upon the repressed instinctual process—has still to be overcome" (Freud, 1926, p. 159).

In the 1926 essay, he returns to the matter of resistance, especially the resistance that emanates from the id, the most primitive part of oneself. And also, here he is considering anxiety more than repression. In fact, he has reversed the formula: rather than repression leading to anxiety, now anxiety leads to repression. Anxiety arises after a trauma in which one has been rendered helpless and bereft. All subsequent anxiety is a "repetition of the situation of danger" (Freud, 1926, p. 137). But why repeat this and not simply forget it? In order, perhaps, to master it, undo it. Maybe this time it will turn out differently. Undoing, Freud also notes in this essay, is the obsessional neurotic's attempt to "blow away" the original event. Akin to a magical act, repeating offers the possibility of trying again in order to undo what was done, to undo the terror of the loss of the primary object, mother (1926, pp. 137–138).

So each fresh bout of anxiety, that is, repetition, offers an opportunity to undo the damage done. What is different going forward is the formation of neurotic symptoms, which, according to a view that Freud seems to favor, are "formed in order to avoid anxiety: they bind the psychical energy which would otherwise be discharged as anxiety. Thus, anxiety would be the fundamental phenomenon and main problem of neurosis" (Freud, 1926, p. 144). Or in other words, "symptoms are created in order to remove the ego from a situation of danger" (1926, p. 144).

Most people grow out of their childhood terrors—of the dark, of being alone—but many do not, and they hang on to their neurotic mechanisms of defense against anxiety. The former have worked through the loss of light and of the mother's constant presence; they have somehow internalized the good objects that can see them through. But in various situations any one of us, or all of us, can be thrown back into terror and once again we need to work through loss. As I will now begin to tie together, working through resistance and working through loss operate hand in glove with effects that are both personal and political. Without these processes, we are stuck with infantile phobias and delusions. A politics that defers the work of mourning and trades in idealities is a politics on a treacherous periphery of fanaticism.

Coming on the scene a generation after Freud's first initial discoveries, Melanie Klein identified the need for mourning at a very early point in the infant's development, when the infant begins to experience awareness that its "objects" are complex and whole and that the child's earlier sadistic rages against the absent "bad breast" could lead to loss of any love and its own death. In the earlier "paranoid-schizoid position," the young infant experiences the world at one moment as nourishing and fulfilling and another moment as terrifying and death-dealing. It imagines revenge through annihilating the persecuting bad breast, devouring the good breast, depositing its bad parts in the other, or any number of infantile splitting and projection towards these good and bad others. As the child begins to fathom that the good breast and bad breast belonged to one complex person, sometimes present and sometimes not, it begins to see this other person as a whole object, begins to introject this whole other, and then feels anguish and guilt about its sadistic impulses. Now the child pines for the internalized whole object, wants to make reparations, and feels intense grief. This Klein calls the depressive position. In this second position, if all goes well, the infant's internal world becomes populated with good introjected objects, first mother, then father, then others, and the infant also begins testing these internal realities against external ones.

But this is not an easy path. In the process of coming to terms with its earlier and perhaps continuing destructive fantasies the infant becomes a bit manic. "When the depressive position arises, the ego is forced (in addition to earlier defences) to develop methods of defence which are essentially directed against the 'pining' for the loved object. These are fundamental to the whole ego organization" (Klein, 1986, p. 151). Klein calls these the manic defenses. Worried that its loved object or even itself will be destroyed by its own sadistic tendencies, the ego builds up "omnipotent and violent fantasies, partly for the purpose of controlling and mastering the 'bad', dangerous objects, partly in order to save and restore the loved ones" (Klein, 1986, p. 151).

While the journey is perilous, it can and often does go well. By populating its internal world with good objects, the infant can come to have a more integrated sense of self. Our internal good objects become a ballast through life. Internal good objects validate oneself, keep one from feeling entirely alone and unmoored (and, as Winnicott observed, allow the baby to play happily alone in the next room), provide validation of one's own worth and experiences. But then the journey might not go well. "Who or what accompanies or deserts one on this journey through life," writes Eric Brenman, "makes all the difference" (Brenman, 2006, 1st p. ch. 8). If there is a failure early in life, due, for example to a parent's illness and long absence, the infant may not be able to introject the good object of a loving parent. The child may grow up and become manic, melancholic, or obsessive (Klein, 1986, p. 173).

Like Klein, Julia Kristeva argues that the paranoid-schizoid position is a constant temptation throughout life, but also that it appears in adolescence where a similar but exponentially stronger form of splitting occurs between good and bad objects. Where the small child is a researcher and questioner ("Who am I?", "Where do I come from?", "What do I want?"), on the path toward object relations, the adolescent is a believer: "Faith implies a passion for the object relation: Faith is potentially fundamentalist, as is the adolescent" (Kristeva, 2007, p. 717). But because of the sadomasochistic nature of the drives, the adolescent's belief in the ideal object is constantly threatened. Accordingly, Kristeva argues, "the adolescent is a believer of the object relation and/or of its impossibility" (pp. 717–718). This gives rise to the ideality syndrome, the belief that there is a Great Other that exists and can provide absolute satisfaction. This is not just a syndrome that plagues teenagers: "We are all adolescents when we are enthralled by the absolute" (Kristeva, 2007,

p. 717). Just as anyone can regress back to a paranoid-schizoid position, the temptation of ideality or its flip side of nihilism can tempt any adult as well as political bodies.

II

Trump and many of his followers are prime examples of both the syndrome of ideality and the repetition compulsion, caught up in playing out over and over an attempt to undo what they imagine they have lost, whether a good mother or a perfect country. The cry Trump repeats at every opportunity—"Let's Make America Great Again"—taps into a dual wager: (1) that those who imagine themselves as the dominant and quintessential "American" people need not mourn the loss of their presumed dominance at home and abroad and (2) that those who are undermining the old status quo can be undone, thrown out, excised from the body politic, making possible an ideal and perfect state. Those who will not mourn their losses nor tarry with indeterminacy, uncertainty, and democracy demand a politics of black and white and good and evil; and they presume that those who oppose them are the enemies of all things perfect and true.

Let me offer a psychoanalytic, though hypothetical account of the genesis of Trump's character: Just after his second birthday, his mother gave birth to a baby brother and then she almost died. After childbirth she got an infection, had to have a hysterectomy then several other surgeries. What trauma. First there was this brute fact that his mother was going to give birth to a rival, then there's possibly some murderous rage for her doing this, then after that murderous rage she does in fact almost die, and then she's gone—for how long?—in the hospital, almost dead, almost gone. The boy's one true love has first defied him, then in fantasy been killed by him, then almost dies and is gone, perhaps he felt terrible guilt that he could not repair and so he could not internalize a good mother.

He grows up to be a bully. At his private school where his wealthy father is a benefactor, he becomes a troublemaker and tyrant, and eventually his teachers persuade the father to send him elsewhere. At military school, the boy learns the lessons that he is special and great and in the course of this, he almost kills his roommate for not folding the linens correctly. He becomes fastidiously neat and develops a fear of germs, of anything that might invade his body. He goes on in life to purge any imagined invaders, including in his fantasies Muslims, Mexicans, and those who've deigned to ruin his imagined perfect kingdom.

And he imagines that he is the king! He takes up the great defense of undoing. This is the defense against felt harm that involves trying to do something all over again in a way that turns out better. How to undo mother's death from his life when he was just beginning to become a little self? Maybe he could be a big self, maybe he could be so perfect and important and big and great that she would finally notice and love him. Maybe he could be so important and smart and wealthy that she would love him more than anyone else in the world.

Maybe also he could avenge his father's loss, his father who had to grow up and take over the family business as a young adolescent when his own father died, the grandfather who made his wealth as a poor immigrant by setting up brothels where fools went looking for gold. And in the process maybe he could avenge his mother's shame, a poor immigrant "domestic" from Scotland, leaving home at 17, arriving at 18, with only $50 in her pocket.

So the child who suffers these losses sets out to avenge and to undo the harm. He cannot help himself; he isn't even conscious of what he is doing. His loss turns into narcissism and grandiosity. At his rallies, he throws out protesters and crying babies. He doesn't see his effects on other people, though most everyone around him is painfully aware of this great malformation. There's an immense disjunct between how he acts and how he thinks of himself. Something is terribly wrong. In public, he makes great proclamations about his greatness, intelligence, and bigness, and has no sense of how bizarre all this sounds. He insults other people for their "smallness," and seems totally oblivious that he is exhibiting his own obliviousness. In this respect, he is delusional.

He has no tolerance for criticism, no ability to appreciate other points of view, no capacity for self-reflection. He is like a person play-acting being a person, a person who is big and great and wonderful, whose enemies ought to be purged or imprisoned.

Or as Freud described his type of character:

> In obsessional neurosis and paranoia the forms which the symptoms assume become very valuable to the ego because they obtain for it, not certain advantages, but a narcissistic satisfaction which it would otherwise be without. The systems which the obsessional neurotic constructs flatter his self-love by making him feel that he is better than other people because he is specially cleanly or specially conscientious. The delusional constructions of the paranoic offer to his acute perceptive and imaginative powers a field of activity which he could not easily find elsewhere.
>
> (Freud, 1926, p. 99)

In all his attempts to purge his imagined perfect world of invaders, he purges his own internal shames and demons: the mother who entered the country as a poor domestic servant, the grandfather who made millions by prostituting land and women, all those immigrant foreigners who are trying to infect us. He purges anyone who interrupts him.

He befriends those like him, other authoritarian figures. He belittles anyone who doesn't try to be as strong as him. And because of his appeal to all those in his country who harbor similar wounds, who feel cheated, infiltrated, abandoned, and wronged, the people project their own anxieties into his anxieties and identify with his ways of acting out. He does for them what they cannot do for themselves. Where they are trapped in powerlessness, he can be their power player, their avenger, their hero. And so they elect him to be the president of their country.

The Trump phenomenon taps into a global political problem: a lack of public and shared means for working through ambiguity and loss, for coming to understand the strangers in our midst, that is, for moving from a paranoid-schizoid politics to and through a Kleinian depressive kind of politics.

III

In her work on revolt and the adolescent syndrome of ideality, Julia Kristeva calls for a process of such work. The iconic scene is the analytic space: patient on the couch, analyst behind, and the analytic third to their dyad where Manichaean divides can transform into shades of grey; where projected demons can be taken back and metabolized; where the adolescent selves we all are at one time or another might grow up and realize the world is not made of saints and sinners but of complex and imperfect people; and most importantly that there are no perfect solutions that will solve all our troubles. The task is how to take this micro-politics to a macro level, how to move to a politics of mourning and working though.

To deal with the adolescent syndrome of ideality, Kristeva argues that, first, the analyst must recognize and not dismiss the need to believe, for this idealization is in fact a source of extreme pleasure. This allows for a positive transference that the analyst can use to model another way of thinking that is also pleasurable. As Kristeva writes,

> only the analyst's capacity to see through the idealizing course of adolescent drives will allow him to provide a credible and effective transference—and thus be capable of metabolizing the need to believe not through acting out but through the pleasure that comes with thinking, questioning and analyzing.
>
> (Kristeva, 2007, pp. 724–725)

In other words, to overcome the syndrome of ideality, we need to transform the need to believe into an urge to question and think, that is, to move from seeing the world in black and white to seeing its variegated and complex hues. In a dyad of analyst and analysand, this can occur through the transference.

What might be the analog for the political body, when the adolescent syndrome sweeps up broad swaths of people? As I discuss elsewhere, public discourse of a certain frame can provide something close to, however imperfect, a "talking cure" that involves mourning the loss of ideality through the kind of deliberation that elucidates what is gained and what is lost in any course of action we might take. In all our deliberations, private and public, we have to weigh, as on a scale, what will be gained and what will be lost. In making a choice to go in one direction rather than another, we also need to metabolize the loss in advance thereby giving ourselves the will to move this way rather than that. Otherwise we will be glued in place, unable to take either fork in the road. Despite what a lot of political philosophers say, political deliberation is fundamentally an affective process that helps people work through fantasies of denial, splitting, and revenge and toward a position that can tolerate loss, ambiguity, and uncertainty, that is, the human condition.

References

Brenman, E. (2006). *Recovery of the Lost Good Object*. Ed. Dana Birksted-Breen. London and New York: Routledge.

Freud, S. (1914). Remembering, Repeating and Working-Through (Further Recommendations on the Technique of Psycho-Analysis II). *The Standard Edition of the Complete Psychological Works of Sigmund Freud. Volume XII (1911–1913): The Case of Schreber, Papers on Technique and Other Works*. Trans. Joan Riviere. Ed. James Strachey. London: The Hogarth Press and the Institute of Psychoanalysis. 145–156.

Freud, S. (1926). Inhibitions, Symptoms and Anxiety. *The Standard Edition of the Complete Psychological Works of Sigmund Freud. Volume XX (1925–1926): An Autobiographical Study, Inhibitions, Symptoms and Anxiety, The Question of Lay Analysis and Other Works*. Ed. James Strachey. London: The Hogarth Press and the Institute of Psychoanalysis, 75–176.

Klein, M. (1986). *The Selected Melanie Klein*. Ed. Juliet Mitchell. New York: The Free Press.

Kristeva, J. (2007). Adolescence, a Syndrome of Ideality. *Psychoanalytic Review* 94: 715–725.

Part II

Mass Psychology

Chapter 4

Freudian Theory and the Pattern of Fascist Propaganda*

Theodor W. Adorno

Reasons for Inclusion

This is a seminal text in the history of psychoanalytic writing about fascism, which powerfully synthesises Freud's work on mass psychology with early critical theory. Adorno presents a remarkably lucid account of Freud's almost clairvoyant anticipation of fascism in European societies in the wake of the First World War, arguing that Freud "clearly foresaw the rise and nature of fascist mass movements". While readers should engage separately with Freud's essay (not included in this reader), Adorno's essay more clearly relates the psychological formation of the mass to the "pattern of fascist propaganda", with sustained historical reference to Nazi Germany. Adorno originally published this essay in English in 1951, in a US journal founded by émigré Hungarian-Jewish psychoanalyst Géza Róheim in order to bridge the gap between psychoanalysis and the social sciences. Adorno begins his essay with a reference to "American fascist agitators", and ends with a warning to "those who keep their eyes shut though they are no longer asleep." We are grateful to Suhrkamp Verlag for permission to include this essay in the reader.

***

During the past decade, the nature and content of the speeches and pamphlets of American fascist agitators have been subjected to intensive research by social scientists. Some of these studies, undertaken along the lines of content analysis, have finally led to a comprehensive presentation in the book, *Prophets of Deceit*, by L. Lowenthal and N. Guterman (1949).[1] The overall picture obtained is characterized by two main features. First, with the exception of some bizarre and completely negative recommendations: to put aliens into concentration camps or to expatriate Zionists, fascist propaganda material in this country is little concerned with concrete and tangible political issues. The overwhelming majority of all agitators' statements are directed *ad hominen*. They are obviously based on psychological calculations rather than on the

* This chapter forms part of the author's continuing collaboration with Max Horkheimer.

DOI: 10.4324/9781003742876-7

intention to gain followers through the rational statement of rational aims. The term 'rabble-rouser', though objectionable because of its inherent contempt of the masses as such, is adequate in so far as it expresses the atmosphere of irrational emotional aggressiveness purposely promoted by our would-be Hitlers. If it is an impudence to call people 'rabble', it is precisely the aim of the agitator to transform the very same people into 'rabble', that is, crowds bent on violent action without any sensible political aim, and to create the atmosphere of the pogrom. The universal purpose of these agitators is to instigate methodically what, since Gustave Le Bon's famous book, *Psychologie des Foules* (1895), is commonly known as 'the psychology of the masses'.

Second, the agitators' approach is truly systematical and follows a rigidly set pattern of clear-cut 'devices'. This does not merely pertain to the ultimate unity of the political purpose: the abolition of democracy through mass support against the democratic principle, but even more so to the intrinsic nature of the content and presentation of propaganda itself. The similarity of the utterances of various agitators, from much publicized figures such as Coughlin and Gerald Smith to provincial small-time hate-mongers, is so great that it suffices in principle to analyse the statements of one of them in order to know them all.[2] Moreover, the speeches themselves are so monotonous that one meets with endless repetitions as soon as one is acquainted with the very limited number of stock devices. As a matter of fact, constant reiteration and scarcity of ideas are indispensable ingredients of the entire technique.

While the mechanical rigidity of the pattern is obvious and itself the expression of certain psychological aspects of fascist mentality, one cannot help feeling that propaganda material of the fascist brand forms a structural unit with a total common conception, be it conscious or unconscious, which determines every word that is said. This structural unit seems to refer to the implicit political conception as well as to the psychological essence. So far, only the detached and in a way isolated nature of each device has been given scientific attention; the psychoanalytic connotations of the devices have been stressed and elaborated. Now that the elements have been cleared up sufficiently, the time has come to focus attention on the psychological system as such—and it may not be entirely accidental that the term summons the association of paranoia—which comprises and begets these elements. This seems to be the more appropriate since otherwise the psychoanalytical interpretation of the individual devices will remain somewhat haphazard and arbitrary. A kind of theoretical frame of reference will have to be evolved. Inasmuch as the individual devices call almost irresistibly for psychoanalytic interpretation, it is but logical to postulate that this frame of reference should consist of the application of a more comprehensive, basic psychoanalytic theory to the agitators' overall approach.

Such a frame of reference has been provided by Freud himself in his book *Group Psychology and the Analysis of the Ego*, published in English as early as 1922, and long before the danger of German fascism appeared to be acute.[3] It is not an overstatement if we say that Freud, though he was hardly interested in the political phase of the problem, clearly foresaw the rise and nature of fascist mass movements in purely psychological categories. If it is true that the analyst's unconscious perceives the unconscious of the patient, one may also presume that his theoretical intuitions are capable of anticipating tendencies still latent on a rational level but manifesting themselves on a deeper one. It may not have been perchance that after the First World War Freud turned his attention to narcissism and ego problems in the specific sense. The mechanisms and instinctual conflicts involved evidently play an increasingly important role in the present epoch, whereas, according to the testimony of practising analysts, the 'classical' neuroses such as conversion hysteria, which served as models for the method, now occur less frequently than at the time of Freud's own development when Charcot dealt with hysteria clinically and Ibsen made it the subject matter of some of his plays. According to Freud, the problem of mass psychology is closely related to the new type of psychological affliction so characteristic of the era which for socio-economic reasons witnesses the decline of the individual and his subsequent weakness. While Freud did not concern himself with the social changes, it may be said that he developed within the monadological confines of the individual the traces of its profound crisis and willingness to yield unquestioningly to powerful outside, collective agencies. Without ever devoting himself to the study of contemporary social developments, Freud has pointed to historical trends through the development of his own work, the choice of his subject matters, and the evolution of guiding concepts.

The method of Freud's book constitutes a dynamic interpretation of Le Bon's description of the mass mind and a critique of a few dogmatic concepts—magic words, as it were—which are employed by Le Bon and other pre-analytic psychologists as though they were keys for some startling phenomena. Foremost among these concepts is that of suggestion which, incidentally, still plays a large role as a stop-gap in popular thinking about the spell exercised by Hitler and his like over the masses. Freud does not challenge the accuracy of Le Bon's well-known characterizations of masses as being largely de-individualized, irrational, easily influenced, prone to violent action and altogether of a regressive nature. What distinguishes him from Le Bon is rather the absence of the traditional contempt for the masses which is the *thema probandum* of most of the older psychologists. Instead of inferring from the usual descriptive findings that the masses are inferior per se and likely to remain so, he asks in the spirit of true enlightenment: what makes the masses into masses? He rejects the easy hypothesis of a social or herd instinct, which for him denotes the problem and not its solution. In addition to the purely psychological reasons he gives for this rejection, one might say that he is on safe ground also from the sociological point of view. The straightforward comparison of modern mass formations with biological phenomena can hardly be regarded as valid since the members of contemporary masses are at least *prima facie* individuals, the children of a liberal, competitive and individualistic society, and conditioned to maintain themselves as independent, self-sustaining units; they are continuously admonished to be 'rugged' and warned against surrender. Even if one were to assume that archaic, pre-individual instincts survive, one could not simply point to this inheritance but would have to explain why modern men revert to patterns of behaviour which flagrantly contradict their own rational level and the present stage of enlightened technological civilization. This is precisely what Freud wants to do. He tries to find out which psychological forces result in the transformation of individuals into a mass. 'If the individuals in the group are combined into a unity, there must surely be something to unite them, and this bond might be precisely the thing that is characteristic of a group' (Freud, 1922, p. 7). This quest, however, is tantamount to an exposition of the fundamental issue of fascist manipulation. For the fascist demagogue, who has to win the support of millions of people for aims largely incompatible with their own rational self-interest, can do so only by artificially creating the *bond* Freud is looking for. If the demagogues' approach is at all realistic—and their popular success leaves no doubt that it is—it might be hypothesized that the bond in question is the very same the demagogue tries to produce synthetically; in fact, that it is the unifying principle behind his various devices.

In accordance with general psychoanalytic theory, Freud believes that the bond which integrates individuals into a mass, is of a *libidinal* nature. Earlier psychologists have occasionally hit upon this aspect of mass psychology.

> In McDougall's opinion, men's emotions are stirred in a group to a pitch that they seldom or never attain under other conditions; and it is a pleasurable experience for those who are concerned to surrender themselves so unreservedly to their passions and thus to become merged in the group and to lose the sense of the limits of their individuality.
>
> (Freud, 1922, p. 27)

Freud goes beyond such observations by explaining the coherence of masses altogether in terms of the pleasure principle, that is to say, the actual or vicarious gratifications individuals obtain from surrendering to a mass. Hitler, by the way, was well aware of the libidinal source of mass formation through surrender when he attributed specifically female, passive features to the participants of his meetings, and thus also hinted at the role of unconscious homosexuality in mass psychology.[4] The most important consequence of Freud's introduction of libido into group psychology is that the traits generally ascribed to masses lose the deceptively primordial and irreducible character reflected by the arbitrary construct of specific mass or herd instincts. The latter are effects rather than causes. What is peculiar to the masses is, according to Freud, not so much a new quality as the manifestation of old ones usually hidden.

> From our point of view we need not attribute so much importance to the appearance of new characteristics. For us it would be enough to say that in

a group the individual is brought under conditions which allow him to throw off the repressions of his unconscious instincts.

(Freud, 1922, pp. 9–10)

This does not only dispense with auxiliary hypotheses *ad hoc* but also does justice to the simple fact that those who become submerged in masses are not primitive men but display primitive attitudes contradictory to their *normal* rational behaviour. Yet, even the most trivial descriptions leave no doubt about the affinity of certain peculiarities of masses to archaic traits. Particular mention should be made here of the potential short-cut from violent emotions to violent actions stressed by all authors on mass psychology, a phenomenon which in Freud's writings on primitive cultures leads to the assumption that the murder of the father of the primary horde is not imaginary but corresponds to prehistoric reality. In terms of dynamic theory, the revival of such traits has to be understood as the result of a *conflict*. It may also help to explain some of the manifestations of fascist mentality which could hardly be grasped without the assumption of an antagonism between varied psychological forces. One has to think here above all of the psychological category of destructiveness with which Freud dealt in his *Civilization and its Discontents*. As a rebellion against civilization, fascism is not simply the reoccurrence of the archaic but its reproduction in and by civilization itself. It is hardly adequate to define the forces of fascist rebellion simply as powerful id energies which throw off the pressure of the existing social order. Rather, this rebellion borrows its energies partly from other psychological agencies which are pressed into the service of the unconscious.

Since the libidinal bond between members of masses is obviously not of an uninhibited sexual nature, the problem arises as to which psychological mechanisms transform primary sexual energy into feelings which hold masses together. Freud copes with the problem by analysing the phenomena covered by the terms suggestion and suggestibility. He recognises suggestion as the 'shelter' or 'screen' concealing 'love relationships'. It is essential that the 'love relationship' behind suggestion remains unconscious.[5] Freud dwells on the fact that in organized groups such as the Army or the Church there is either no mention of love whatsoever between the members, or it is expressed only in a sublimated and indirect way, through the mediation of some religious image in the love of whom the members unite and whose all-embracing love they are supposed to imitate in their attitude towards each other. It seems significant that in today's society with its artificially integrated fascist masses, reference to love is almost completely excluded.[6] Hitler shunned the traditional role of the loving father and replaced it entirely by the negative one of threatening authority. The concept of love was relegated to the abstract notion of *Germany* and seldom mentioned without the epithet of 'fanatical' through which even this love obtained a ring of hostility and aggressiveness against those not encompassed by it. It is one of the basic tenets of fascist leadership to keep primary libidinal energy on an unconscious level so as to divert its manifestations in a way suitable to political ends. The less an objective idea such as religious salvation plays a role in mass formation, and the more mass manipulation becomes the sole aim, the more thoroughly uninhibited love has to be repressed and moulded into obedience. There is too little in the content of fascist ideology that *could* be loved.

The libidinal pattern of fascism and the entire technique of fascist demagogues are authoritarian. This is where the techniques of the demagogue and the hypnotist coincide with the psychological mechanism by which individuals are made to undergo the regressions which reduce them to mere members of a group.

> By the measures that he takes, the hypnotist awakens in the subject a portion of his archaic inheritance which had also made him compliant towards his parents and which had experienced an individual reanimation in his relation to his father: what is thus awakened is the idea of a paramount and dangerous personality, towards whom only a passive-masochistic attitude is possible, to whom one's will has to be surrendered, while to be alone with him, 'to look him in the face', appears a hazardous enterprise. It is only in some such way as this that we can picture the relation of the individual member of the primal horde to the primal father ... The uncanny and coercive characteristics of group formations, which are shown in their suggestion phenomena, may therefore with justice be traced back to the fact of their origin from the primal horde. The leader of the group is still the dreaded primal father; the group still wishes to be governed by unrestricted force; it has an extreme passion for authority; in Le Bon's phrase, it has a thirst for obedience. The primal father is the group ideal, which governs the ego in the place of the ego ideal. Hypnosis has a good claim to being described as a group of two; there remains as a definition for suggestion—a conviction which is not based upon perception and reasoning but upon an erotic tie.[7]
>
> (Freud, 1922, pp. 99–100)

This actually defines the nature and content of fascist propaganda. It is psychological because of its irrational authoritarian aims which cannot be attained by means of rational convictions but only through the skilful awakening of 'a portion of the subject's archaic inheritance'. Fascist agitation is centred in the idea of the leader, no matter whether he actually leads or is only the mandatory of group interests, because only the psychological image of the leader is apt to reanimate the idea of the all-powerful and threatening primal father. This is the ultimate root of the otherwise enigmatic *personalization* of fascist propaganda, its incessant plugging of names and supposedly great men, instead of discussing objective causes. The formation of the imagery of an omnipotent and unbridled father figure, by far transcending the individual father and therewith apt to be enlarged into a 'group ego', is the only way to promulgate the 'passive-masochistic attitude ... to whom one's will has to be surrendered', an attitude required of the fascist follower the more his political behaviour becomes irreconcilable with his own rational interests as a private person as well as those of the group or class to which he actually belongs.[8] The follower's reawakened irrationality is, therefore, quite rational from the leader's viewpoint: it necessarily has to be 'a conviction which is not based upon perception and reasoning but upon an erotic tie'.

The mechanism which transforms libido into the bond between leader and followers, and between the followers themselves, is that of *identification*. A great part of Freud's book is devoted to its analysis (Freud, 1922, pp. 58). It is impossible to discuss here the very subtle theoretical differentiation, particularly the one between identification and introjection. It should be noted, however, that the late Ernst Simmel, to whom we owe valuable contributions to the psychology of fascism, took up Freud's concept of the ambivalent nature of identification as a derivative of the oral phase of the organization of the libido (Freud, 1922, p. 61), and expanded it into an analytic theory of anti-Semitism.

We content ourselves with a few observations on the relevancy of the doctrine of identification to fascist propaganda and fascist mentality. It has been observed by several authors and by Erik Homburger Erikson in particular, that the specifically fascist leader type does not seem to be a father figure such as for instance the king of former times. The inconsistency of this observation with Freud's theory of the leader as the primal father, however, is only superficial. His discussion of identification may well help us to understand, in terms of subjective dynamics, certain changes which are actually due to objective historical conditions. Identification is 'the *earliest* expression of an emotional tie with another person, "playing" a part in the early history of the Oedipus complex' (Freud, 1922, p. 60). It may well be that this pre-oedipal component of identification helps to bring about the separation of the leader image as that of an all-powerful primal father, from the actual father image. Since the child's identification with his father as an answer to the Oedipus complex is only a secondary phenomenon, infantile regression may go beyond this father image and through an 'anaclitic' process reach a more archaic one. Moreover, the primitively narcissistic aspect of identification as an act of *devouring*, of making the beloved object part of oneself, may provide us with a clue to the fact that the modern leader image sometimes seems to be the enlargement of the subject's own personality, a collective projection of himself, rather than the image of the father whose role during the later phases of the subject's infancy may well have decreased in present day society (cf. Horkheimer, 1949). All these facets call for further clarification.

The essential role of narcissism in regard to the identifications which are at play in the formation of fascist groups, is recognised in Freud's theory of *idealization*.

> We see that the object is being treated in the same way as our own ego, so that when we are in love a considerable amount of narcissistic libido overflows on the object. It is even obvious, in many forms of love choice, that the object serves as a substitute for some unattained ego ideal of our own. We love it on account of the perfections which we have striven to reach for our own ego, and which we should now like to procure in this roundabout way as a means of satisfying our narcissism.
>
> (Freud, 1922, p. 74)

It is precisely this idealization of himself which the fascist leader tries to promote in his followers, and which is helped by the *Führer* ideology. The people he has to reckon with generally undergo the characteristic modern conflict between a strongly developed rational, self-preserving ego agency[9] and the continuous failure to satisfy their own ego demands. This conflict results in strong narcissistic impulses which can be absorbed and satisfied only through idealization as the partial transfer of the narcissistic libido to the object. This, again, falls in line with the semblance of the leader image to an enlargement of the subject: by making the leader his ideal he loves himself, as it were, but gets rid of the stains of frustration and discontent which mar his picture of his own empirical self. This pattern of identification through idealization, the caricature of true conscious solidarity, is, however, a collective one. It is effective in vast numbers of people with similar characterological dispositions and libidinal leanings. The fascist *community of the people* corresponds exactly to Freud's definition of a group as being 'a number of individuals who have substituted one and the same object for their ego ideal and have consequently identified themselves with one another in their ego' (Freud, 1922, p. 80). The leader image, in turn, borrows as it were its primal father-like omnipotence from collective strength.

Freud's psychological construction of the leader imagery is corroborated by its striking coincidence with the fascist leader type, at least as far as its public build-up is concerned. His descriptions fit the picture of Hitler no less than idealizations into which the American demagogues try to style themselves. In order to allow narcissistic identification, the leader has to appear himself as absolutely narcissistic, and it is from this insight that Freud derives the portrait of the 'primal father of the horde' which might as well be Hitler's.

> He, at the very beginning of the history of mankind, was the *Superman*[10] whom Nietzsche only expected from the future. Even today, the members of a group stand in need of the illusion that they are equally and justly loved by their leader; but the leader himself need love no one else, he may be of a masterly nature, absolutely narcissistic, but self-confident and independent. We know that love puts a check upon narcissism, and it would be possible to show how, by operating in this way, it became a factor of civilization.
>
> (Freud, 1922, p. 93)

One of the most conspicuous features of the agitator's speeches, namely the absence of a positive programme and of anything they might 'give', as well as the paradoxical prevalence of threat and denial, is thus being accounted for; the leader can be loved only if he himself does not love. Yet Freud is aware of another aspect of the leader image which apparently contradicts the first one. While appearing as a superman, the leader must at the same time work the miracle of appearing as an average person, just as Hitler posed as a composite of King Kong and the suburban barber. This too, Freud explains through his theory of narcissism. According to him,

> the individual gives up his ego ideal and substitutes for it the group ideal as embodied in the leader. [However,] in many individuals the separation between the ego and the ego ideal is not very far advanced; the two still coincide readily; the ego has often preserved its earlier self-complacency. The selection of the leader is very much facilitated by this circumstance. He need only possess the typical qualities of the individuals concerned in a particularly clearly marked and pure form, and need only give an impression of greater force and of more freedom of libido; and in that case the need for a strong chief will often meet him half-way and invest him with a predominance to which he would otherwise perhaps have had no claim. The other members of the group, whose ego ideal would not, apart from this, have become embodied in his person without some correction, are then carried away with the rest by 'suggestion', that is to say, by means of identification.
>
> (Freud, 1922, p. 102)

Even the fascist leader's startling symptoms of inferiority, his resemblance to ham actors and asocial psychopaths, is thus anticipated in Freud's theory. For the sake of those parts of the follower's narcissistic libido which have not been thrown into the leader image but remain attached to the follower's own ego, the superman must still resemble the follower and appear as his 'enlargement'. Accordingly, one of the basic devices of personalized fascist propaganda is the concept of the 'great little man', a person who suggests both omnipotence and the idea that he is just one of the folks, a plain, red-blooded American, untainted by material or spiritual wealth. Psychological ambivalence helps to work a social miracle. The leader image gratifies the follower's twofold wish to submit to authority and to be the authority himself. This fits into a world in which irrational control is exercised though it has lost its inner conviction through universal enlightenment. The people who obey the dictators also sense the latter are superfluous. They reconcile this contradiction through the assumption that they are themselves the ruthless oppressor.

All the agitators' standard devices are designed along the line of Freud's expose of what became later the basic structure of fascist demagoguery, the technique of personalization,[11] and the idea of the great little man. We limit ourselves to a few examples picked at random.

Freud gives an exhaustive account of the hierarchical element in irrational groups. 'It is obvious that a soldier takes his superior, that is, really, the leader of the army, as his ideal, while he identifies himself with his equals, and derives from this community of their egos the obligations for giving mutual help and for sharing possessions which comradeship implies. But he becomes ridiculous if he tries to identify himself with the general' (Freud, 1922, p. 110), to wit, consciously and directly. The fascists, down to the last small-time demagogue, continuously emphasize ritualistic ceremonies and hierarchical differentiations. The less hierarchy within the set-up of a highly rationalized and quantified industrial society is warranted, the more artificial hierarchies with no objective *raison d'être* are built up and rigidly imposed by fascists for purely psycho-technical reasons. It may be added, however, that this is not the only libidinous source involved. Thus, hierarchical structures are in complete keeping with the wishes of the sado-masochistic character. Hitler's famous formula, *Verantwortung nach oben, Autorität nach unten* (responsibility towards above, authority towards below), nicely rationalizes this character's ambivalence.[12]

The tendency to tread on those below, which manifests itself so disastrously in the persecution of weak and helpless minorities, is as outspoken as the hatred against those outside. In practice, both tendencies quite frequently fall together. Freud's theory sheds light on the all-pervasive, rigid distinction between the beloved in-group and the rejected out-group. Throughout our culture, this way of thinking and behaving has come to be regarded as self-evident to such a degree that the question of why people love what is like themselves and hate what is different is rarely asked seriously enough. Here as in many other instances, the productivity of Freud's approach lies in his questioning that which is generally accepted. Le Bon had noticed that the irrational crowd 'goes directly to extremes' (Freud, 1922, p. 16). Freud expands this observation and points out that the dichotomy between in- and out-groups is of so deep-rooted a nature that it affects even those groups whose 'ideas' apparently exclude such reactions. By 1921, he was therefore able to dispense with the liberalistic illusion that the progress of civilization would automatically bring about an increase of tolerance and a lessening of violence against out-groups.

> Even during the kingdom of Christ, those people who do not belong to the community of believers, who do not love him, and whom he does not love, stand outside this tie. Therefore, so religion, even if it calls itself the religion of love, must be hard and unloving to those who do not belong to it. Fundamentally, indeed, every religion is in this same way a religion of love for all those whom it embraces; while cruelty and intolerance towards those who do not belong to it are natural to every religion. However difficult we may find

> it personally, we ought not to reproach believers too severely on this account: people who are unbelieving or indifferent are so much better off psychologically in this respect. If today that intolerance no longer shows itself so violent and cruel as in former centuries, we can scarcely conclude that there has been a softening in human manners. The cause is rather to be found in the undeniable weakening of religious feelings and the libidinal ties which depend upon them. If another group tie takes the place of the religious one—and the socialistic tie seems to be succeeding in doing so—then there will be the same intolerance towards outsiders as in the age of the Wars of Religion.
>
> (Freud, 1922, pp. 50–1)

Freud's error in political prognosis, his blaming the 'socialists' for what their German arch-enemies did, is as striking as his prophecy of fascist destructiveness, the drive to eliminate the out-group.[13] As a matter of fact, neutralization of religion seems to have led to just the opposite of what the enlightener Freud anticipated: the division between the believers and the non-believers has been maintained and reified. However, it has become a structure in itself, independent of any ideational content, and is even more stubbornly defended since it lost its inner conviction. At the same time, the mitigating impact of the religious doctrine of love vanished. This is the essence of the 'sheep and goat' device employed by all fascist demagogues. Since they do not recognize any spiritual criterion in regard to who is chosen and who is rejected, they substitute a pseudo-natural criterion such as the race,[14] which seems to be inescapable and can therefore be applied even more mercilessly than was the concept of heresy during the Middle Ages. Freud has succeeded in identifying the libidinal function of this device. It acts as a negatively integrating force. Since the positive libido is completely invested in the image of the primal father, the leader, and since few positive contents are available, a negative one has to be found.

> The leader or the leading idea might also, so to speak, be negative; hatred against a particular person or institution might operate in just the same unifying way, and might call up the same kind of emotional ties as positive attachment.
>
> (Freud, 1922, p. 53)

It goes without saying that this negative integration feeds on the instinct of destructiveness to which Freud does not explicitly refer in his *Group Psychology*, the decisive role of which he has, however, recognized in his *Civilization and Its Discontents*. In the present context, Freud explains the hostility against the out-group with narcissism:

> In the undisguised antipathies and aversions which people feel towards strangers with whom they have to do, we may recognize the expression of

> self-love—of narcissism. This self-love works for the self-assertion of the individual, and behaves as though the occurrence of any divergence from his own particular lines of development involved a criticism of them and a demand for their alteration.
>
> (Freud, 1922, pp. 55–6)

The narcissistic *gain* provided by fascist propaganda is obvious. It suggests continuously and sometimes in rather devious ways, that the follower, simply through belonging to the in-group, is better, higher and purer than those who are excluded. At the same time, any kind of critique or self-awareness is resented as a narcissistic loss and elicits rage. It accounts for the violent reaction of all fascists against what they deem *zersetzend*, that which debunks their own stubbornly maintained values, and it also explains the hostility of prejudiced persons against any kind of introspection. Concomitantly, the concentration of hostility upon the out-group does away with intolerance in one's own group to which one's relation would otherwise be highly ambivalent.

> But the whole of this intolerance vanishes, temporarily or permanently, as the result of the formation of a group, and in a group. So long as a group formation persists or so far as it extends, individuals behave as though they were uniform, tolerate other people's peculiarities, put themselves on an equal level with them, and have no feeling of aversion towards them. Such a limitation of narcissism can, according to our theoretical views, only be produced by one factor, a libidinal tie with other people.
>
> (Freud, 1922, p. 56)

This is the line pursued by the agitators' standard 'unity trick'. They emphasize their being different from the outsider but play down such differences within their own group and tend to level out distinctive qualities among themselves with the exception of the hierarchical one. 'We are all in the same boat'; nobody should be better off—the snob, the intellectual, the pleasure seeker are always attacked. The undercurrent of malicious egalitarianism, of the brotherhood of all-compromising humiliation, is a component of fascist propaganda and fascism itself. It found its symbol in Hitler's notorious command of the *Eintopfgericht*. The less they want the inherent social structure changed, the more they prate about social justice, meaning that no member of the 'community of the people' should indulge in individual pleasures. Repressive egalitarianism instead of realization of true equality through the abolition of repression is part and parcel of the fascist mentality and reflected in the agitators' 'if-you-only-knew' device which promises the vindictive revelation of all sorts of forbidden pleasures enjoyed by others. Freud interprets this phenomenon in terms of the transformation of individuals into members of a psychological 'brother horde'. Their coherence is a reaction formation against their primary jealousy of each other, pressed into the service of group coherence.

> What appears later on in society in the shape of *Gemeingeist, esprit de corps*, 'group spirit', etc. does not belie its derivation from what was originally envy. No one must want to put himself forward, every one must be the same and have the same. Social justice means that we deny ourselves many things so that others may have to do without them as well, or, what is the same thing, may not be able to ask for them.
>
> (Freud, 1922, pp. 87–8)

It may be added that the ambivalence towards the brother has found a rather striking, ever-recurring expression in the agitators' technique. Freud and Rank have pointed out that in fairy tales, small animals such as bees and ants 'would be the brothers in the primal horde, just as in the same way in dream symbolism insects or vermin signify brothers and sisters (contemptuously, considered as babies)' (Freud, 1922, p. 114). Since the members of the in-group have supposedly 'succeeded in identifying themselves with one another by means of similar love for the same object' (Freud, 1922, p. 87), they cannot admit this contempt for each other. Thus, it is expressed by completely negative cathexis of these low animals, fused with hatred against the out-group, and projected upon the latter. Actually it is one of the favourite devices of fascist agitators—examined in great detail by Leo Lowenthal (cf. also: Lowenthal and Guterman, 1948)—to compare out-groups, all foreigners and particularly refugees and Jews, with low animals and vermin.

If we are entitled to assume a correspondence of fascist propagandist stimuli to the mechanisms elaborated in Freud's *Group Psychology*, we have to ask ourselves the almost inevitable question how did the fascist agitators, crude and semi-educated as they were, obtain knowledge of these mechanisms? Reference to the influence exercised by Hitler's *Mein Kampf* upon the American demagogues would not lead very far, since it seems impossible that Hitler's theoretical knowledge of group psychology went beyond the most trivial observations derived from a popularized Le Bon. Neither can it be maintained that Goebbels was a mastermind of propaganda and fully aware of the most advanced findings of modern depth-psychology. Perusal of his speeches and selections from his recently published diaries give the impression of a person shrewd enough to play the game of power politics but utterly naive and superficial in regard to all social or psychological issues below the surface of his own catchwords and newspaper editorials. The idea of the sophisticated and 'radical' intellectual Goebbels is part of the devil's legend associated with his name and fostered by eager journalism; a legend, incidentally, which itself calls for psychoanalytic explanation. Goebbels himself thought in stereotypes and was completely under the spell of personalization. Thus, we have to seek for sources other than erudition for the much advertised fascist command of psychological techniques of mass manipulation. The foremost source seems to be the already mentioned basic identity of leader and follower which circumscribes one of the aspects of identification. The leader can guess the psychological wants and needs of those susceptible to his propaganda because he resembles them psychologically, and is distinguished from them by a capacity to express without inhibitions what is latent in them, rather than by any intrinsic superiority. The leaders are generally oral character types, with a compulsion to speak incessantly and to befool the others. The famous spell they exercise over their followers seems largely to depend on their orality: language itself, devoid of its rational significance, functions in a magical way and furthers those archaic regressions which reduce individuals to members of crowds. Since this very quality of uninhibited but largely associative speech presupposes at least a temporary lack of ego control, it may well indicate weakness rather than strength. The fascist agitators' boasting of strength is indeed frequently accompanied by hints at such weakness, particularly when begging for monetary contributions—hints which, to be sure, are skilfully merged with the idea of strength itself. In order successfully to meet the unconscious dispositions of his audience, the agitator so to speak simply turns his own unconscious outward. His particular character syndrome makes it possible for him to do exactly this, and experience has taught him consciously to exploit this faculty, to make rational use of his irrationality, similarly to the actor, or a certain type of journalist who knows how to sell their innervations and sensitivity. Without knowing it, he is thus able to speak and act in accord with the psychological theory for the simple reason that the psychological theory is true. All he has to do in order to make the psychology of his audience click, is shrewdly to exploit his own psychology.

The adequacy of the agitators' devices to the psychological basis of their aim is further enhanced by another factor. As we know, fascist agitation has by now come to be a profession, as it were, a livelihood. It had plenty of time to test the effectiveness of its various appeals and, through what might be called natural selection, only the most catchy ones have survived. Their effectiveness is itself a function of the psychology of the consumers. Through a process of 'freezing', which can be observed throughout the techniques employed in modern mass culture, the surviving appeals have been standardized, similarly to the advertising slogans which proved to be most valuable in the promotion of business. This standardization, in turn, falls in line with the stereotypical thinking, that is to say, with the 'stereopathy' of those susceptible to this propaganda and their infantile wish for endless, unaltered repetition. It is hard to predict whether the latter psychological disposition will prevent the agitators' standard devices from becoming blunt through excessive application. In National Socialist Germany, everybody used to make fun of certain propagandistic phrases such as 'blood and soil' (*Blut und Boden*), jokingly called *Blubo*, or the concept of the nordic race from which the verb *aufnorden* (to 'northernize') was derived. Nevertheless, these appeals do not seem to have lost their attractiveness. Rather, their very 'phoniness' may have been relished cynically and sadistically as an index for the fact that power alone decided one's fate in the Third Reich, that is, power unhampered by rational objectivity.

Furthermore, one may ask: why is the applied group psychology discussed here peculiar to fascism rather than to most other movements that seek mass support? Even the most casual comparison of fascist propaganda with that of liberal, progressive parties will show this to be so. Yet, neither Freud nor Le Bon envisaged such a distinction. They spoke of crowds 'as such', similar to the conceptualizations used by formal sociology, without differentiating between the political aims of the groups involved. As a matter of fact, both thought of traditional socialistic movements rather than of their opposite, though it should be noted that the Church and the Army—the examples chosen by Freud for the demonstration of this theory—are essentially conservative and hierarchical. Le Bon, on the other hand, is mainly concerned with nonorganized, spontaneous, ephemeral crowds. Only an explicit theory of society, by far transcending the range of psychology, can fully answer the question raised here. We content ourselves with a few suggestions. First, the objective aims of fascism are largely irrational in so far as they contradict the material interest of great numbers of those whom they try to embrace, notwithstanding the pre-war boom of the first years of the Hitler regime. The continuous danger of war inherent in fascism spells destruction and the masses are at least preconsciously aware of it. Thus, fascism does not altogether speak the untruth when it refers to its own irrational powers, however faked the mythology which ideologically rationalizes the irrational may be. Since it would be impossible for fascism to win the masses through rational arguments, its propaganda must necessarily be deflected from discursive thinking; it must be oriented psychologically, and has to mobilize irrational, unconscious, regressive processes. This task is facilitated by the frame of mind of all those strata of the population who suffer from senseless frustrations and therefore develop a stunted, irrational mentality. It may well be the secret of fascist propaganda that it simply takes men for what they are: the true children of today's standardized mass culture, largely robbed of autonomy and spontaneity, instead of setting goals the realization of which would transcend the psychological *status quo* no less than the social one. Fascist propaganda has only to *reproduce* the existent mentality for its own purposes; it need not induce a change—and the compulsive repetition which is one of its foremost characteristics will be at one with the necessity for this continuous reproduction. It relies absolutely on the total structure as well as on each particular trait of the authoritarian character which is itself the product of an internalization of the irrational aspects of modern society. Under the prevailing conditions, the irrationality of fascist propaganda becomes rational in the sense of instinctual economy. For if the status quo is taken for granted and petrified, a much greater effort is needed to see through it than to adjust to it and to obtain at least some gratification through identification with the existent—the focal point of fascist propaganda. This may explain why ultra-reactionary mass movements use the 'psychology of the masses' to a much greater extent than do movements which show more faith in the masses. However, there is no doubt that even the most progressive political movement can deteriorate to the level of the 'psychology of the crowd' and its manipulation, if its own rational content is shattered through the reversion to blind power.

The so-called psychology of fascism is largely engendered by manipulation. Rationally calculated techniques bring about what is naively regarded as the 'natural' irrationality of masses. This insight may help us to solve the problem of whether fascism as a mass phenomenon can be explained at all in psychological terms. While there certainly exists potential susceptibility for fascism among the masses, it is equally certain that the manipulation of the unconscious, the kind of suggestion explained by Freud in genetic terms, is indispensable for actualization of this potential. This, however, corroborates the assumption that fascism as such is *not* a psychological issue and that any attempt to understand its roots and its historical role in psychological terms still remains on the level of ideologies such as the one of 'irrational forces' promoted by fascism itself. Although the fascist agitator doubtlessly takes up certain tendencies within those he addresses, he does so as the mandatory of powerful economic and political interests. Psychological dispositions do not actually cause fascism; rather, fascism defines a psychological area which can be successfully exploited by the forces which promote it for entirely non-psychological reasons of self-interest. What happens when masses are caught by fascist propaganda is not a spontaneous primary expression of instincts and urges but a quasi-scientific revitalization of their psychology—the artificial regression described by Freud in his discussion of organized groups. The psychology of the masses has been taken over by their leaders and transformed into a means for their domination. It does not express itself directly through mass movements. This phenomenon is not entirely new but was foreshadowed throughout the counter-revolutionary movements of history. Far from being the source of fascism, psychology has become one element among others in a superimposed system the very totality of which is necessitated by the potential mass of resistance—the masses' own rationality. The content of Freud's theory, the replacement of individual narcissism by identification with leader images, points in the direction of what might be called the appropriation of mass psychology by the oppressors. To be sure, this process has a psychological dimension, but it also indicates a growing tendency towards the abolition of psychological motivation in the old, liberalistic sense. Such motivation is systematically controlled and absorbed by social mechanisms which are directed from above. When the leaders become conscious of mass psychology and take it into their own hands, it ceases to exist in a certain sense. This potentiality is contained in the basic construct of psychoanalysis inasmuch as for Freud the concept of psychology is essentially a negative one. He defines the realm of psychology by the supremacy of the unconscious and postulates that what is id should become ego. The emancipation of man from the heteronomous rule of his unconscious would be tantamount to the abolition of his 'psychology'. Fascism furthers this abolition in the opposite sense through the perpetuation of dependence instead of the realization of potential freedom, through expropriation of the unconscious by social control instead of making the subjects conscious of their unconscious. For, while psychology always denotes some bondage of the individual, it also presupposes freedom in the sense of a certain self-sufficiency and autonomy of the individual. It is not accidental that the nineteenth century was the great era of psychological thought. In a thoroughly reified society, in which there are virtually no direct relationships between men, and in which each person has been reduced to a social atom, to a mere function of collectivity, the psychological processes, though they still persist in each individual, have ceased to appear as the determining forces of the social process. Thus, the psychology of the individual has lost what Hegel would have called substance. It is perhaps the greatest merit of Freud's book that though he restricted himself to the field of individual psychology and wisely abstained from introducing sociological factors from outside, he nevertheless reached the turning point where psychology abdicates. The psychological 'impoverishment' of the subject that 'surrendered itself to the object' which 'it has substituted for its most important constituent' (Freud, 1922, p. 76); that is, the super-ego, anticipates almost with clairvoyance the post-psychological de-individualized social atoms which form the fascist collectivities. In these social atoms the psychological dynamic of group formation have overreached themselves and are no longer a reality. The category of 'phoniness' applies to the leaders as well as to the act of identification on the part of the masses and their supposed frenzy and hysteria. Just as little as people believe in the depth of their hearts that the Jews are the devil, do they completely believe in their leader. They do not really identify themselves with him but act this identification, perform their own enthusiasm, and thus participate in their leader's performance. It is through this performance that they strike a balance between their continuously mobilized instinctual urges and the historical stage of enlightenment they have reached, and which cannot be revoked arbitrarily. It is probably the suspicion of this fictitiousness of their own 'group psychology' which makes fascist crowds so merciless and unapproachable. If they would stop to reason for a second, the whole performance would go to pieces, and they would be left to panic. Freud came upon this element of 'phoniness' within an unexpected context, namely, when he discussed hypnosis as a retrogression of individuals to the relation between primal horde and primal father.

> As we know from other reactions, individuals have preserved a variable degree of personal aptitude for reviving old situations of this kind. Some knowledge that in spite of everything hypnosis is only a game, a deceptive renewal of these old impressions, may however remain behind and take care that there is a resistance against any too serious consequences of the suspension of the will in hypnosis.
>
> (Freud, 1922, p. 99)

In the meantime, this game has been socialized, and the consequences have proved to be very serious. Freud made a distinction between hypnosis and group psychology by defining the former as taking place between two people only. However, the leaders' appropriation of mass psychology, the streamlining of their technique, has enabled them to collectivize the hypnotic spell. The Nazi battle cry of 'Germany awake' hides its very opposite. The collectivization and institutionalization of the spell, on the other hand, have made the transference more and more indirect and precarious so that the aspect of performance, the 'phoniness' of enthusiastic identification and of all the traditional dynamics of group psychology, have tremendously increased. This increase may well terminate in sudden awareness of the untruth of the spell, and eventually in its collapse. Socialized hypnosis breeds within itself the forces which will do away with the spook of regression through remote control, and in the end awaken those who keep their eyes shut though they are no longer asleep.

Notes

1 Cf. also: Leo Lowenthal and Norbert Guterman (1948) 'Portrait of the American Agitator', *Public Opinion Quarterly*, (Fall), pp. 417ff.

2 This requires some qualification. There is a certain difference between those who, speculating rightly or wrongly on large-scale economic backing, try to maintain an air of respectability and deny that they are anti-Semites before coming down to the business of Jew-baiting—and overt Nazis who want to act on their own, or at least make believe that they do, and indulge in the most violent and obscene language. Moreover, one might distinguish between agitators who play the old-fashioned, homely, Christian conservative and can easily be recognized by their hostility against the 'dole', and those who, playing a more streamlined modern version, appeal mostly to youth and sometimes pretend to be revolutionary. However, such differences should not be overrated. The basic structure of their speeches as well as their supply of devices is identical in spite of carefully fostered differences in overtones. What one has to face is a division of labour rather than genuine divergencies. It may be noted that the National Socialist party shrewdly maintained differentiations of a similar kind, but that they never amounted to anything nor led to any serious clash of political ideas within the party. The belief that the victims of 30 June 1934 were revolutionaries is mythological. The blood purge was a matter of rivalries between various rackets and had no bearing on social conflicts.

3 The German title, under which the book was published in 1921, is *Massenpsychologie und Ichanalyse*. The translator, James Strachey, rightly stresses that the term group here means the equivalent of Le Bon's *foule* and the German *Masse*. It may be added that in this book the term ego does not denote the specific psychological agency as described in Freud's later writing in contrast to the id and the super-ego; it simply means the individual. It is one of the most important implications of Freud's *Group Psychology* that he does not recognize an independent, hypostastized 'mentality of the crowd,' but reduces the phenomena observed and described by writers such as Le Bon and McDougall to regressions which take place in each one of the individuals who form a crowd and fall under its spell.

4 Freud's book does not follow up this phase of the problem but a passage in the addendum indicates that he was quite aware of it. 'In the same way, love for women breaks through the group ties of race, of national separation, and of the social class

system, and it thus produces important effects as a factor in civilization. It seems certain that homosexual love is far more compatible with group ties, even when it takes the shape of uninhibited sexual tendencies' (Freud, 1922, p. 123). This was certainly borne out under German fascism where the borderline between overt and repressed homosexuality, just as that between overt and repressed sadism, was much more fluent than in liberal middleclass society.

5 "... love relationships ... also constitute the essence of the group mind. Let us remember that the authorities make no mention of any such relations" (Freud, 1922, p. 40).

6 Perhaps one of the reasons for this striking phenomenon is the fact that the masses whom the fascist agitator—prior to seizing power—has to face are primarily not organized ones but the accidental crowds of the big city. The loosely knit character of such motley crowds makes it imperative that discipline and coherence be stressed at the expense of the centrifugal uncanalized urge to love. Part of the agitator's task consists in making the crowd believe that it is organized like the Army or the Church. Hence the tendency towards over-organization. A fetish is made of organization as such; it becomes an end instead of a means and this tendency prevails throughout the agitator's speeches.

7 This key statement of Freud's theory of group psychology incidentally accounts for one of the most decisive observations about the fascist personality: the externalization of the super-ego. The term 'ego ideal' is Freud's earlier expression for what he later called the super-ego. Its replacement through a 'group ego' is exactly what happens to fascist personalities. They fail to develop an independent autonomous conscience and substitute for it an identification with collective authority which is irrational as Freud described it, heteronomous, rigidly oppressive, largely alien to the individuals' own thinking and, therefore, easily exchangeable in spite of its structural rigidity. The phenomenon is adequately expressed in the Nazi formula that what serves the German people is good. The pattern reoccurs in the speeches of American fascist demagogues who never appeal to their prospective followers' own conscience but incessantly invoke external, conventional and stereotyped values which are taken for granted and treated as authoritatively valid without ever being subject to a process of living experience or discursive examination. As pointed out in detail in the book, *The Authoritarian Personality*, by T.W. Adorno, Else Frenkel-Brunswik, Daniel L. Levinson and R. Nevitt Sanford (1950), Harper Brothers, New York, prejudiced persons generally display belief in conventional values instead of making moral decisions of their own and regard as right 'what is being done'. Through identification, they too tend to submit to a group ego at the expense of their own ego ideal which becomes virtually merged with external values.

8 The fact that the fascist follower's masochism is inevitably accompanied by sadistic impulses is in harmony with Freud's general theory of ambivalence, originally developed in connection with the Oedipus complex. Since the fascist integration of individuals into masses satisfied them only vicariously, their resentment against the frustrations of civilization survives but is canalized to become compatible with the leader's aims; it is psychologically fused with authoritarian submissiveness. Though Freud does not pose the problem of what was later called 'sado-masochism', he was nevertheless well aware of it, as evidenced by his acceptance of Le Bon's idea that 'since a group is in no doubt as to what constitutes truth or error, and is conscious, moreover, of its own great strength, it is as intolerant as it is obedient to authority. It respects force and can only be slightly influenced by kindness, which it regards merely as a form of weakness. What it demands of its heroes is strength, or even violence. It wants to be ruled and oppressed and to fear its masters' (Freud, 1922, p. 17).

9 The translation of Freud's book renders his term '*Instantz*' by 'faculty', a word which, however, does not carry the hierarchical connotation of the German original. 'Agency' seems to be more appropriate.

10 It may not be superfluous to stress that Nietzsche's concept of the Superman has as little in common with this archaic imagery as his vision of the future with fascism. Freud's allusion is obviously valid only for the 'Superman' as he became popularized in cheap slogans.

11 For further details on personalization compare (Freud (1922) p. 44, footnote), where he discusses the relation between ideas and leader personalities, and p. 53, where he defines as 'secondary leaders' those essentially irrational ideas which hold groups together. In technological civilization, no *immediate* transference to the leader, unknown and distant as he actually is, is possible. What happens is rather a regressive repersonalization of impersonal, detached social powers. This possibility was clearly envisaged by Freud. '… A common tendency, a wish in which a number of people can have a share, may … serve as a substitute. This abstraction, again, might be more or less completely embodied in the figure of what we might call a secondary leader.'

12 German folklore has a drastic symbol for this trait. It speaks of *Radfahrernaturen*, bicyclist's characters. Above they bow, they kick below.

13 With regard to the role of 'neutralized', diluted religion in the make-up of the fascist mentality, compare *The Authoritarian Personality*. Important psychoanalytic contributions to this whole area of problems are contained in Theodor Reik's *Der eigene und der fremde Gott*, and in Paul Federn's *Die vaterlose Gesellschaft*.

14 It may be noted that the ideology of race distinctly reflects the idea of primitive brotherhood revived, according to Freud, through the specific regression involved in mass formation. The notion of race shares two properties with brotherhood: it is supposedly 'natural', a bond of 'blood', and it is desexualized. In fascism this similarity is kept unconscious. It mentions brotherhood comparatively rarely, and usually only in regard to Germans living *outside* the borders of the Reich ('Our Sudeten brothers'). This, of course, is partly due to recollections of the ideal of *fraternité* of the French Revolution, taboo to the Nazis.

References

Freud, S. (1922) *Group Psychology and the Analysis of the Ego*. London: Analytical Press.

Horkheimer, M. (1949) Authoritarianism and the Family Today. In R.N. Anshen (ed.) *The Family: Its Function and Destiny*. New York: Harper Brothers.

Le Bon, G. (1895) *Psychologie des Foules*. Paris: Félix Alcan.

Lowenthal, L. and Guterman, N. (1948) Portrait of the American Agitator. *Public Opinion Quarterly*, 12(3), pp. 417ff.

Lowenthal, L. and Guterman, N. (1949) *Prophets of Deceit*. New York: Harper Brothers.

Chapter 5

Malignant Narcissism and Large Group Regression

Otto F. Kernberg

Reasons for Inclusion

Kernberg's paper provides a contemporary psychoanalytic account of group psychology, giving special attention to mass psychic regression in times of crisis, and to the tendency of regressed groups to select narcissistic, paranoid leaders who marshal their desires and anxieties towards destructive ends. Kernberg's essay provides a helpful review of the relevant literature on group psychology, from Freud to Bion and Volkan, bridging the account of individual psychic radicalization and the phenomenon of tyrannical leadership entailed in extremist mass movements. While Kernberg's contribution points to the limits of a psychoanalytic perspective on fascism, which it deliberately blurs with totalitarianism and dictatorship, it does helpfully emphasize the social context of mass radicalization, an important facet of fascistic politics neglected by some of the other papers included in the reader. As with some of the other papers in this reader by authors based in the USA, Donald Trump is firmly in the background.

***

From a psychoanalytic perspective, we have to recognize that a psychoanalytic understanding only covers a limited area of the complex social forces triggered by the interaction of regressed large groups and the corresponding pathological leadership: the nature of historical determinants of the formation of social subgroups; the origin of cultural, social, political, religious and social bias; the cause of present traumatic circumstances, and the political system within which regressed large groups consolidate are important determinants that influence the development of such leadership—followers' constellations. Does psychoanalytic understanding have anything to say about whether and how we can use our present day understanding to help prevent such calamitous situations in the future?

The purpose of this paper is to analyze the mutual relationships between large group regression and the emergence of a particular kind of leadership related to that regressive process, namely, leaders with the characteristics of the syndrome of malignant narcissism. The main hypothesis to be explored is that the nature of large group regression translates into the search for that

DOI: 10.4324/9781003742876-8

particular personality type—and that personalities with the syndrome of malignant narcissism are prone to aspire to leadership and are very effective in achieving leadership of the regressed large group under these conditions. In turn, the mutual influence of the culture of the regressed large group and its corresponding ideological development and the characteristic behaviors of a leader evincing malignant narcissism stimulates typical behaviors in the leader. In turn, the corresponding leadership reinforces some basic characteristics of regressed large groups. To explore that linkage, we shall review briefly the concept of regression in group processes, studying group psychology both in large groups and "mass" psychology, and in small groups, reviewing the relevant contributions by Freud, Bion, Turquet, Volkan, and others. This review will be followed by the exploration of the preferred personality structures of leadership fostered by these different group structures, and the relationship between functional leadership and pathological leadership related to the requirements expressed in group regression. I shall then summarize briefly the syndrome of malignant narcissism and its derivative leadership characteristics in social institutions and the political process at large.

Psychoanalytic Group Psychology

Freud, in his 1921 text on "Group Psychology and the Analysis of the Ego" outlined what became one of the most original and tragically relevant contributions to the study of the Dynamic Unconscious, namely, the behavior of what in German is called "Masse." It refers to mass movements, or large conglomerates of people united by a common ideal, a common sense of identity related to race, religion, nationality, or a particular ideology that unifies this enormous conglomerate of individuals in an active direction or cohesive move under the direction of a particular leader. This mass psychology has to be differentiated from the situation of crowds, that is, the accidental getting together of an enormous number of people as part of usual social interactions, without any common direction or sense of a specific mutual relationship. Freud described political mass movements, particularly of fascism and communism, years before the common characteristics of mass movements and their consequences had been experienced dramatically, as it evolved in the 20th, and now in the 21st century.

Freud pointed out that the individual who senses himself as part of such a mass movement acquires a reduced capacity for independent judgment and rational decision-making. To the contrary, what dominates the individuals within the mass movement is a sense of power by mutual identification, a sense of belonging and power derived from being part of such a large movement. It is their mutual identification that coincides with their identification with the leader of the mass movement, which provides them with a sense of shared identity, an identification with the leader who is not only powerful and idealized, but also feared. At the same time, he assumes consciously and in the mind of his followers, the responsibility for the direction of the movement, and frees all the individuals from themselves having to make decisions about that movement. More generally, mass psychology induces the projection onto the leader of the individuals' ego ideal, so that moral consciousness is projected onto the leader and the individuals in the mass feel free from moral constraints. They acquire a degree of freedom that goes together with a characteristic activation of intense affective dispositions shared by the entire mass, and is particularly of an aggressive, destructive type, the target of which is directed outside the mass movement. As part of mass psychology, the participants feel powerful and secure and united in the free, unconstrained, and personally irresponsible participation in aggression against outside, feared, hated, and depreciated groups who are perceived as threatening the mass movement. The shared sense of equality, power, and freedom from moral constraints is the counterpart to a heightened suggestibility to the commands from the leader, a suggestibility enhanced by the decrease of rational, independent judgment induced by the psychology of the mass movement.

Wilfred Bion's (1961) analysis of the relation between groups and their leadership introduced a new method of psychoanalytic exploration of group psychology. As a courageous and effective tank commander in the First World War, and in his later work as a psychiatrist in military psychiatric hospitals and War Office Selection Boards during the Second World War, he developed professional experiences with both effective task groups and regressed, demoralized ones, and their leadership. He combined his psychoanalytic training and Tavistock Clinic experience, the application of Kleinian concepts of splitting and projective identification in individual treatments with his group studies and experiences in what became a new field of psychoanalytic inquiry.

Bion's (1961) studies of small group psychology provided a complementary analysis of the intimate processes affecting the regression of individuals when they are part of a group process. He described the behavior evolving in small groups of 10 to 15 members that were exclusively engaged in observing their own experiences and behavior in limited time sessions from one to two hours. He observed typical developments that he described as the "basic assumptions groups" of "dependency," "fight-flight," and "pairing." These "basic assumptions" groups emerged typically and consistently when such a small group had no specific task that would justify its existence and link it with an environment by a concrete objective that has to be accomplished. A group that gets together with a task of learning a determined subject, developing a particular project, or constructing particular objects represents "work groups" that operate rationally and with a realistic organization of the development of the particular group task. When such a task does not exist and the only group task is the observation of the group itself and the emotional consequences of such a lack of a specific task, then the basic assumptions emerge.

The basic assumption of "dependency" is characterized by a general sense of insecurity, uncertainty, and immaturity on the part of members of the group, who look for a leader who will help them understand their situation, direct the group, provide their needs, feed them with knowledge, meaning, or security, a leader who presents self-assurance and an attitude of potency and knowledge that is supportive and reassuring, provokes his idealization by the group, and the wish to depend on him. Competition for becoming the preferred "child" of that leader, mutual jealousy for the amount of attention each member of the group gets from their idealized leader, illustrates the fact that this self-assured, knowledgeable, giving leader provides a sense of safety and security in being part of the group. In contrast, fear and insecurity develop if one falls outside the assured membership of such a group. If the leader does not provide the assurance of the gratification of the group's dependency needs, the members of the group experience strong disappointment or disillusionment, search for an alternative leader in the group who may replace him, idealize the new leader while attributing to him the attributes they had seen in the previous leader, and expect him to carry out the needed function of leadership of the dependent group.

The situation in the basic assumption group of "fight-flight" is completely different. Here there is a sense of tension and conflict, a preparedness to fight against out-groups, and a sense of group unity as part of this fighting disposition against out-groups. Sometimes, when there is no such evident adversary out-group, a division of the very group evolves into an "in-group" who stands with the leader, and an "out-group" that fights the leader and the in-group. The search here is for a strong, self-righteous, distrustful, and controlling leader, who provides leadership in the struggle with the enemy out-group or the rebellious subgroup. In contrast to the predominance, in the dependent group, of mechanisms of primitive idealization, regressive dependency, and denial of all conflicts around authority issues, here, in the fight-flight group, there is a remarkable development of splitting operations between "us" and "them," the in-group and the out-group, a sharp differentiation between the idealization of the in-group and the projection of aggression and attacks on the out-group, and a tendency to submit to the leader as part of the psychology of a shared sense of discipline required by the fight against assumed enemies. Splitting, projective identification, and denial of aggression within the internal subgroup go hand in hand with the search for a leader who will gratify the need for this organization, usually a powerful individual with paranoid features who fits the group's demand for a sharp division between the ideal inner world of the group, and a dangerous threatening external world that needs to be fought off.

In the "pairing" group, finally, a still different atmosphere prevails. Here the group selects a couple, heterosexual or homosexual, that the group perceives as united, bound together by mutual identification, love, and commitment. The group admires the couple, because it corresponds to the wish for establishing such an ideal couple love relationship, an ideal shared by all the members and expressed in this idealization but also in the related need to fight off envious feelings about this selected ideal couple. There is a sexual quality in the air, an erotized quality of relations that differs from both the regressed dependent relations of the dependent group, and from the tense, aggressive challenging and distrustful atmosphere of the fight-flight group. While the dependent group preferably selects a leader with strong narcissistic features, the fight-flight group selects a leader with paranoid features, and the pairing group a leader who tolerates the development of such a pair, helps to protect it, and conveys the assurance to the group that the erotic quality of the development of intimate relations is tolerated and welcome. The "pairing" group represents a less regressive, "Oedipal" group experience.

Within the growing interest in developing Bion's approach to groups at the Tavistock Clinic, Pierre Turquet's (1975) work stands out. With a related background in military medical services to Bion's, Turquet expanded the study of regressed group behavior to larger family groups and social institutions and, in following Bion's approach, he carried out empirical work with larger groups. He studied the behavior of large groups. These were experimental groups of 100 to 300 members, also gathered only to study the nature of their experiences and behavior over a period of an hour and a half to two hours, with the provision of a group leader. This leader, similarly to the leader provided to small groups, limits himself or herself to comment on dominant emotional experiences shared by the group, without assuming the particular leadership functions demanded by the group. The small groups establish by themselves particular expectations from the leader, once they are clearly in the dependent, fight-flight, or pairing position; the "professional" group leader will not gratify but analyze their emotional needs. Thus, the leaders that have been described for the small groups are selected and seduced into their respective leadership function in terms of the corresponding psychology of the respective small group. A similar phenomenon happens in the large group. The large group, usually, as I mentioned, composed of a membership between 100 and a maximum 300 persons, get together in concentric circles, that permit the members of still seeing each other and responding to each other—similarly as in the small group, but evidently this situation reduces enormously the possibility of the constitution of cohesive, small subgroups. All the individuals of the large group are much more isolated from each other than is the case of small group psychology.

The large group meets without any particular task except to experience and discuss its own developments. Every member has the right to speak up at any moment, and the professional group leader limits himself/herself to observing, from time to time, the dominant emotional issues affecting the group. The leader does not organize the development of any subject of the group discussions at any point. Here, again, if the large group were "structured," organized to carry out a certain task, for example, to discuss or decide about a particular subject around which it would establish an order or procedure of order and time limitations within which individuals can speak up, this would transform the group into a "work group" and become realistically focused on and occupied with such a task. The unstructured large group, to the contrary, is totally open to whatever anybody in the group may feel like saying or doing.

The typical development in such a large group situation is an enormous sense of loss of personal identity, as the individual in it cannot reliably find a commonality with anybody else. In the large group situation efforts emerge to establish subgroups on the basis of whatever members may try to find as commonalities: needs, language, religion, profession, political views, race, or appearance of any kind; but these efforts usually fail and the group develops rapidly a collective sense of intense anxiety. While people speak freely, there is a tendency not to listen to what other people are saying. Individuals who speak up obtain no feedback. Clear efforts at projective identification fail because of the difficulty to focus on and control the reactions of others to oneself. There is a general sense of impotence and fearfulness that develops in the members, and a fear of aggression to explode in the group. At times the group is able to identify a small subgroup within the large group or outside it, and gather around a joined, intense hate reaction against such a subgroup. This, temporarily, transforms the large group into a small mass that fights an external enemy, but even such efforts usually fail.

A tendency develops in the group for individuals to emerge that are trying to analyze rationally what is happening. It is characteristic for the large group that particularly intelligent, self-reflective, rational people are shut down immediately. To the contrary, naïve, cliche formulating individuals who have a simplistic statement to make tend to be supported, with a slightly derogatory, amused attitude by the group at large, but at the same time, with a shared sense of relief, and such cliché-spreading mediocrities are preferentially selected as leader of the large group. The group conveys the impression that there is a shared envy of individuals who maintain their individuality, security, rationality, and, with such a capacity, attempt to provide group leadership, while there is support of a mediocre leadership that reassures everybody and provides a calming sense of security while at the same time there is a shared subtle devaluation of that selected leader.

As an alternative development, if the intensity of anxiety and aggressive feelings is excessive, the group may veer into a paranoid direction. It selects a paranoid individual who finds a cause to fight against, a group, or an intolerable social condition, something in the external world which everybody agrees needs to be fought against and potentially destroyed. Thus, the large group, at the bottom, oscillates between the search for a narcissistic leader with a non-threatening, simplistic quality that can be depreciated and promises a tranquilizing passivity, or else, under activation of an excessive degree of aggression, a powerful paranoid leader who unifies the group into a fighting attitude that transforms the large group into a small "mass psychology" group as described by Freud.

Vamik Volkan (2004) has expanded greatly our understanding of group psychology with what he refers to as large group regression, but what has to be differentiated from the large group as originally described by Turquet (1975) and others. Both Bion and Turquet studied artificial groups, brought together for the purpose of observing group behavior. Volkan's work focuses on the study of naturally occurring groups, especially in times of crisis. Volkan, in fact, refers to mass psychology in the sense of Freud's analysis of the psychology of large conglomerates united by a sense of mutual cohesiveness, equality, and fraternity and a common set of ideas—a common ideology—that expresses their unifying disposition, including the potential relationship to an idealized, feared, and/or direction signaling leader. Volkan studied group psychological behavior in international conflicts and conflicts between nationalistic or religious opposite political groups and, particularly, the psychological developments related to the traumatic effects of the terrorist attack in New York on September 11, 2001.

In summary, Volkan proposes that, under conditions of traumatic situations, social revolutions, nature caused disasters, economic crisis, and, generally speaking, the collapse of traditional cultural structures that regulate the daily life of the individual, the strong possibility of a large group regression develops, within which the normal social structure that assures the individual of his status—role relationships—disappears. Under such conditions, there evolves a threat to normal identity that ordinarily is reinforced by the status and role conditions of every individual within this social and cultural environment. There now evolves a search for a "second skin," a new external social structure that returns the security that had protected individual identity and sense of security. Here the emergence of a large group leader becomes important in providing to the social group in crisis a voice that reconfirms their commonality, the sense of a common ideology that assures the large group of its basic existential security, historical mission, and goodness, and differentiates it from external enemies or enemy situations that had been threatening it. The leader calls for joint action to stand up and, in short, provides the large group with a new sense of identity in terms of all the individuals belonging to that mass movement.

There is a tendency of a large group in an existential social crisis to rally blindly around such a leader, who eliminates the traditional status and role relations of individuals derived mostly from their belonging to a family, to specific relations to family members, and to the social group related to it. The leader creates a new collective "family" structure in terms of the historical importance and mission of the group. The community becomes divided into a "good" segment (the large group) that obediently follows the leader, and a "bad" segment of those perceived as opposing the leader. A sharp division between "us" and "them" is established, and "them" become enemies that need to be fought off, defended against, and attacked. The large group develops a sense of shared morality of the "good" system that becomes increasingly absolutist and punitive toward those who are in conflict with it, and the group may experience periods of massive mood swings from shared depressed feelings over the nature of the critical or dramatic situation that originated the present situation, to collective paranoid projection of aggression toward outsiders. The sense of internal goodness becomes a sense of entitlement and a gradual distortion of reality, in which unpleasant and threatening aspects of reality are denied. There evolve new cultural phenomena or modified versions of traditional social customs with particular focus on joint traumas and past triumphs of the group residing in a time collapse in which past and present is confused. The leadership feeds into this collapse of the time perspective by creating a break in the actual historical continuity of the group, and filling the gap with a "new" nationalism, a new shared sentience or a "new" morality, and a transformation of the actual history of the group.

The large group members begin to experience shared symbols as "protosymbols," including shared images that depict enemy groups with symbols or protosymbols associated with bodily waste, vermin, dangerous, or toxic animal traits. The large group consolidates its unity by erecting sharp boundaries with the outside world, focusing on minor differences between itself and enemy groups, and searches powerfully for commonalities in its natural condition, origin, and convictions as part of their new "second skin" that protects its identity. The large group may initiate behaviors that symbolize its purification. It may change its attitude toward aesthetics, to what is considered beautiful and ugly, and there is a tendency for the large group to turn the physical environment into an amorphous gray–brown, (fecal or decomposing) structure. All these characteristics constitute an ideologically fundamented, consolidated, and expressively lived activation of the clear, separate "second skin" identity that provides the combination of security, power, freedom, moral superiority, and irresponsibility described by Freud for mass psychology. Volkan's analysis enriches and bridges the analysis of large group psychology by Turquet with Freud's analysis of mass psychology.

The combined analysis of group regression, from small group regression to large group regression and to mass psychology, illustrates some basic commonalities of these various processes. The motive for group regression, in all cases, is a loss of the functional relationship of individuals within a stable, small or large social, and cultural structure. This social and cultural structure is given by an ordinary living situation within a stable social environment not threatened by major political, international, or economic catastrophes or nature determined calamities. And, in the case of small groups, the loss of the functional tasks of the group by design or other circumstances replicates temporarily that loss of functional stability of the individual. This loss of the traditional social structure signifies a threat to individual identity and it signals the extent to which normal identity function is supported and assured by the individual's psychosocial environment. Massive loss of such a protective environment that simultaneously affects a selected group or an entire community leads to powerful anxiety and initiates regressive functions.

It is significant that the anxiety, in all cases, has to do with a threat of a definite experience of danger, the activation of negative, aggressive affect states, and correspondent defensive operations that we know from the study of severe psychopathology of individuals with primitive aggressive aggression dominated conflicts. These defensive operations, particularly splitting mechanisms, projective identification, denial, primitive idealization and devaluation, omnipotent control—all of them described by Melanie Klein (1946) as characteristic of the paranoid-schizoid position—emerge in the dependent and fight-flight group, where they structure the group within the given basic assumptions orientation, but they are ineffective for the individual in the large group situation. Here the only effective protection is an individual's isolating himself from the large group situation into the position of a "singleton" (Turquet, 1975), which will coincide with a sense of impotence and alienation and the loss of participation in the social process. The large majority caught up in the activation of massive paranoid-schizoid defenses of the large group will participate in a joint effort to compensate for the loss of individual identity by the collective search for leadership to replace individual identity by the "second skin" described by Volkan. In other words, it is a search for a new, shared identity linked to the dependency of a particular type of leadership. The type of leadership selected will oscillate between the narcissistic type of leader, as in the dependent group and the large narcissistic group described by Turquet, or a paranoid leader, as in the fight/flight group, in the mass movement, or in the large group described by Turquet when intense aggression overrides the reassuring search for a narcissistic, calming leader. I have described in earlier work (Kernberg, 1998) how the nature of the ideology selected by the large group, particularly in mass movements, also oscillates between a narcissistic and a paranoid type. Many political and religious ideologies contain a central, humanistic core that, under different conditions of group regression, may shift into a paranoid or a narcissistic distortion of the ideology. Moscovici (1981), in his sociological analysis of the effects of media and mass communication, has suggested that, while Marx described religion as the "opium of the people," the media and mass communication are the "Valium" of the people.

Leadership and Malignant Narcissism

In earlier analyses of the characteristics of functional leadership of social organizations, I pointed out that essential qualities of functional leadership include the following: (1) High intelligence, possibly best defined by the time span of decision-making (Jacques, 1976), that is, the capacity of leadership to foresee long time developments and orient the organization he or she leads in the light of this analysis; (2) an integrated personality structure that includes the capacity for significant self-reflection and assessment in depth of other people, essential to selecting delegate leadership and the deciding about conflicts that involve technical knowledge as well as personality features; (3) a solid, autonomous moral capacity and commitment, given the unavoidable corruptive temptations of leadership functions; (4) significant narcissistic features—in the sense of solid security and self-regard that permit leadership to tolerate the unavoidable ambivalences and aggression stemming from the internal functioning of the organization as well from external sources of challenges to it; (5) a sufficient availability of paranoid traits—in the sense of a mature distrust in contrast to naivete that would ignore aggressive and potentially threatening developments in the work relationships of the organization.

A discrete, reasonable, and controlled amount of narcissistic and paranoid features are an important aspect of leadership, in contrast to excessive dependence needs that cannot be gratified outside the leadership function and a dangerous naiveté regarding the complexity of human relations in social organizations. Precisely these two personality features, in an exaggerated and pathological way, typically characterize the leaders selected in regressive group situations, problematic organizational functioning, and mass movements. From a different perspective, Canetti (1960) described the psychological characteristics of the "feasting mass" (*Festmasse*) and the "hounding mass" (*Hetzmasse*). These refer to the predominant behavior of respectively celebrating narcissistically or aggressively persecuting large groups under the corresponding leadership of a narcissistic and potentially hypomanic leader organizing collective feasts and orgies, in contrast to the paranoid leader of an aggressive, persecutory mob. In short, an extraordinary potential for narcissistic or paranoid leadership emerges under conditions of large group regression.

At this point, we have to explore the nature of narcissistic and paranoid character traits that are characteristic, respectively, of narcissistic and paranoid personality disorders. In fact, under conditions of social disorganization, the weakening of traditional social structures, the emergence of extremist political groups and parties, individuals with these characteristics tend to become important in providing a "second skin" to the respective groups. But there is one type of particularly relevant psychopathology that combines narcissistic and paranoid traits as part of a severe type of narcissistic personality disorder, namely, the syndrome of malignant narcissism.

I have defined the syndrome of malignant narcissism in earlier studies of severe forms of pathological narcissism (Kernberg, 1984, 2018) as characterized by the presence of: (1) a narcissistic personality disorder with all its characteristic features: a pathological grandiose self, inordinate self-centeredness and a sense of superiority, strong manifestations of envy, devaluation of others, severe limitations of the capacity of emotional investment in others, and a chronic sense of emptiness that requires an ongoing search for external stimulation or the excitement derived from drugs or sexual behavior; (2) significant paranoid personality features; (3) strong egosyntonic aggression, directed against others or self; and (4) significant antisocial behavior. The basic psychopathological features of the syndrome of malignant narcissism are a dominance of unconscious conflicts around intense aggressive affect—from whatever origin, together with the development of the compensating pathology of a grandiose self. Aggressive motivation infiltrates the grandiose sense of self, leading to egosyntonic aggressivity on the one hand, and to the projection of aggression in the form of paranoid tendencies on the other. The severe deficit in the development of an internalized system of ethical values derived from the underlying basic failure in normal identity formation that affects the buildup of such an ethical structure (superego development) determines the development of antisocial behaviors.

Patients with the syndrome of malignant narcissism function along a wide spectrum of social dysfunction. The most ill patients with these characteristics suffer from a total breakdown of their capacity for social interactions, incapacity to function in work and profession, and breakdown in intimate relations, together with the development of severe affective dysregulation, and such a degree of disturbed interpersonal behavior that makes for initial confusion with borderline personality disorder. At the other extreme are patients who are able to maintain their social functions and work conditions, and only show breakdown in their personal, intimate relationships, an incapacity to significantly invest in non-exploitive behavior with others, and an extremely exaggerated concept of self and commitment to self-interests that are pursued in an aggressive way without moral restrictions. It so happens that such individuals may be perfectly adaptable to a social situation of massive group regression, in which these aspects of their personality function effectively to gratify basic needs of the regressed large group.

Under ordinary circumstances, such relatively well-functioning individuals presenting malignant narcissism possessing high intelligence, unusual technical capabilities and knowledge in some specialized area, and the capability to fulfill their ambitions to promotion within social organizations, may assume leadership of social organizations in education, health, military, and religious institutions, or industry. They usually promote the institution by identifying their personal interests with that of the institution, but, over a period of time, because of their severe incapacity to assess others, their tendency to surround themselves with adulating subordinates, and their incapacity to tolerate criticism and therefore use realistic, essential feedback for institutional operations, such institutions show a typical regression. The organization evolves a sharp differentiation of levels of emotional climates. At the top of the organization, surrounding the leadership with malignant narcissism, are individuals who also present narcissistic and antisocial features. They have learned to adjust themselves to the needs of the leader to be both loved and feared while being unaffected by his interpersonal demandingness and, at times, antisocial maneuvers, so leadership with antisocial features expands corruption at the top. At a second level of organizational functioning, including the large majority of professional and institutional staff, there develops an intensely paranoid atmosphere because of the fear of a leader who is hypersensitive to criticism, who needs to be showed love and admiration, and who cannot listen to anything running against his/her will. There is a high level of institutional "paranoiagenesis" (Jacques, 1976), with frequent turnover and breakdown of staff. At the bottom level of the institution, at the periphery of its internal emotional milieu, one finds the most capable staff members, depressed and alienated, prone to be the first ones to leave the organization, sometimes depriving an organization of the most productive and creative members of its staff. So far, I summarized what happens in organized social institutions.

Large Group Regression and Malignant Narcissistic Leadership

In contrast to the developments in well-structured social organizations, under conditions of social disorganization and large group regression, the emergence of leaders with the syndrome of malignant narcissism take further, socially dysfunctional, and threatening characteristics. The leader's narcissistic self-centeredness and grandiosity, his self-assured signaling what he believes the large group should think and do, and his promise for a brilliant future if he is followed, powerfully reassures the members of a regressed large group against the threat of the loss of individual identity, and provides them with the second skin of an idealizing mutual identity of all in identification with the leader. The reduced cognitive level of functioning characteristic of large groups (Kernberg, 1998; Turquet, 1975) responds positively to simple slogans and clichés that the leader provides them with to confirm their value, uniqueness, importance, and power. Simple slogans replace complex thinking and correspond to the large group's need to feel that they are intimately involved with the thinking of the great leader and understand him completely, and, at a deeper, unconscious level, don't need to envy him. Everybody is equal in the pursuit of simple ideals and in the proper symbolic expression of such ideas. The well-rationalized aggression against out-groups is fostered by the leader's direct, crude, and sadistic expression of animosity against such out-groups, devaluing and dehumanizing them while declaring the large group he directs to be the selected, ideal, morally justified, superior social group. Aggressive outbursts against minorities is fostered, welcome, considered heroic and morally admirable, so that freedom to express destructive behavior excites the group and creates a contaminating festive atmosphere. Bao-Lord (1990) describes how, during the Chinese Cultural Revolution, the beating up of professors by revolutionary groups in the middle of huge public gatherings contaminated the bystanders, so that massive engagement in physical attack and murder became a welcome public spectacle.

The characteristic antisocial features of the leader with malignant narcissism are reflected in practically public dishonest behavior, matched with shameless denial of that behavior. Hitler never acknowledged his clear, indirect instructions to eliminate potentially rivalrous leaders of his SA troops; he never acknowledged publicly, nor in writing, his instructions for mass murder of the Jewish population under his control, in spite of being the obvious ultimate source of these orders. Stalin would invite both privileged followers whom he wished to honor for tea at his place, and also those who already had been secretly condemned to be eliminated. This was sufficiently well known in his intimate circle to cause external anxiety in the invitees, which, apparently, greatly pleased Stalin.

The leader's evident dishonesty, the self-assured expression of lies that may be easily recognized as such by an outside observer and a broader social environment or general community is perceived by the regressed large group as a courageous standing up to conventional truth, daring to say the impossible, the leader showing courage in changing his mind at any point, and shifting over, if necessary, to declaring alternative choices of who is the selected enemy at the moment. The leader's decidedly assuming moral responsibility promotes a sense of freedom from moral constraints, excitement of moving with a powerful wave of political discontent and strife as it is manipulated from the top, and cemented by the suggestibility of the large group. Repeated attacks, ridiculing, and demeaning humiliation of selected "enemies" reinforce the group's enjoyment of sadistic behavior. It was the inhumane cruelty of ISIS that exerted an exciting attractiveness to many early international followers.

Leadership by a leader with malignant narcissism within an institutional, task-oriented organization is circumscribed by the very structure of the organization; the need to carry out its technical or professional functions, the outside world that confronts the organization with consequences of failure of leadership in carrying out ordinary boundary functions, in addition to the negative effects of decreased productivity, and deterioration of human relations in the inside of such an organization. External authorities, Board of Governors, or community oversight tends to limit, in the long run, the negative effects of deficient leadership. In an open, political field, in contrast, the negative consequences of the mutual stimulation between large group regression and the emergence of leadership with malignant narcissistic personality characteristics is much more effective in its destructive consequences.

To begin with, the crystallization of a regressed social subgroup, that is, the constitution of a large group with shared feelings of threatening insecurity related to economic, cultural, or political issues, with threats to the identity or survival of that group, is experienced and shared informally by the group. A general feeling of growing tension, anxiety, and irritability initiates the search for a "second skin," that is, a longed-for, decisive intervention by leadership to protect the well-being, security, and stability of the group's existence. The situation is open now to a self-assured, aggressive, powerful combative politician who spells out the generally shared feelings of dissatisfaction and resentment, and orients the group toward an external source of its troubles in the form of an external enemy power that needs to be fought off. A general paranoid orientation evolves and consolidates the large group in the active search, identification, and separation from the designated enemy group. The cultural availability of a preexisting ideology with strongly paranoid features, or one that can be shifted easily into a paranoid direction, may be used by a leader to establish a sense of historical continuity of this struggle with adversary forces, and include historical trauma and triumphs to provide a sense of mission in the direction of restoring such past glory or undoing historical trauma, creating a dynamic force in the pursuit of justice and right (Volkan, 2004).

The antisocial potential of the leader with malignant narcissism may manifest itself at first only in relatively discrete dishonest behaviors such as evident lies, false accusations, and circumscribed distortions of reality, all of which is expressed, however, in a courageous way that implicitly tests the extent to which the community at large may threaten the specific regressed large group with creating limits to this dishonesty or accept it. As Turquet (1975) had originally pointed out, and is also stressed by Albright (2018) and Snyder (2017), there is a "third group" constituted by the original total population that watches a combative minority—the large regressed group—enter into warfare with another social subgroup, the selected victims of the attacks by the dynamic, regressed large group possessed by an extreme, paranoid ideology. If the traditional structure of society is weakened by a present traumatic situation, an economic crisis, a lost war, a natural disaster, the initial response to the provocative dishonesty that the leadership of the regressed large group propagates may be sufficiently weak, and ordinary social reactions not sufficiently alarmed to stand up against such a distortion in social communication. Now more destructive aggressive acts, distortion of reality, open encouragement of violence may develop, with an expanding affirmation and dissemination of the certainty, self-righteousness, the sense of moral justification, and superiority emanating from the revolutionary large group under the stimulation by the leader. The aggressive, paranoid, and dishonest behavior socially fostered by malignant narcissistic leadership thus evolves into an ever-growing sense of self-confirmation and power by the group. The self-assuredness of the leader and the expansion of his paranoid, grandiose, and aggressive behavior go hand in hand with the increase of a sense of power, freedom, violent behavior, and triumphant excitement of the regressed large group.

The Dangers to Society

Jacques Semelin (2007) illustrates all these processes with the initial anti-Semitic ideology, work restrictions, and media attacks on Jews in Nazi Germany during the early stages of the Hitler regime, and their gradual escalation as initial resistance against social acts of violence was muted, and a gradual increase in physical violence, socially destructive behavior, and arbitrary legislation restricting Jewish life and robbing Jewish property was calmly accepted by the German population at large. In general, at this stage, relatively independent social structures, particularly, religious organizations, the armed forces, the financial elite, the judicial power, the media, the strength of bureaucratic organization, and tradition, become important elements that may control this regressive process or reinforce it. The combined influence of these relatively stable social structures and powers may then determine the extent to which a regressive process evolves further into the potential extreme of the development of genocidal regimes, or is controlled in the form of an ordinary dictatorship, or ends with the eventual recovery of the civilized reaction to this social regression. An independent military that traditionally rejects its identification with a particular political orientation may counteract the establishment of a totalitarian regime, that is, an effort by the malignant narcissistic leadership to establish an obligatory indoctrination of the entire population by a determined ideological doctrine.

It needs to be stressed that totalitarian systems differ from ordinary dictatorships in their imposition of an obligatory ideological system. You don't only have to fear the leader but also must love him. The totalitarian regime established by personalities with malignant narcissism will be reinforced by such an ideology centered on the idealization and fearful submission to the leader, but an ordinary dictatorship, while less effective, also tends to achieve the same submission and destructive effects on the population. The surprising reaction of the military establishment of the Soviet Union in dropping its allegiance to the communist party happened at a point when the economic failure of the communist system interfered with the effective military competition with the United States. This development contributed fundamentally to the downfall of the communist regime. To the contrary, the German military fell rapidly into place with Nazi ideology, given its crucial role in the expansionist doctrine of national-socialist ideology geared to establish the dominance of Germany over Europe.

Social media may express an identification with a dominant traditional culture that rejects the extremes that threaten a peaceful coexistence of different ideological orientations and break the expansionist power of a revolutionary extreme group. The very fact that the Internet permits the parallel diffusion, circulation, and expansion of completely contradictory ideological investments may protect a democratic political system, but it may also be used by extremist social subgroups to organize a hidden rebellion against the status quo and facilitate communication of regressed large groups, as has been illustrated by the effective recruitment tool that the Internet has signified for terrorist Islamic groups in recent times.

In general, once a totalitarian power achieves control of the media, they become an important instrument of social indoctrination. An independent judicial system may be a significant counterweight to the aggressive assault on individual's rights and invasion of individual privacy by revolutionary groups with totalitarian ideology. But when a revolutionary government is able to control ordinary judiciary power, laws and judges may easily become corrupt. An effective bureaucracy may prevent, to some extent, social disorganization and the disruption of ordinary interactions of individuals and institutions, but a highly organized bureaucracy under state control may powerfully reinforce a totalitarian system.

A dramatic overall comparative study of genocide in three very different societies carried out by Jacques Semelin (2007) illustrates the worst-case scenarios of progression of social regression of large groups with corresponding malignant narcissistic leadership into mass murder and genocide. He compares the historical developments of Rwanda, Bosnia, and Nazi Germany leading to genocidal explosion and reaches the conclusion that similar processes occurred in all three so very different societies in terms of the historical background, culture, and sociopolitical situation. In all three cases a latent animosity existed between social subgroups, Tutsi and Hutu in Rwanda, Muslims and Christians in Bosnia, the historical anti-Semitism of German culture and its rejection of the Jews. Such latent potential social splits became expressed first in all three cases, in a general ideological disposition, an extreme ideology turning one group against the other. That divisive ideology became acute at the time of social crisis derived from the complexities of decolonization in the case of Rwanda, the aftermath of the decomposition of the communist system in Yugoslavia, the consequence of the defeat of the First World War, and the later economic crisis in Germany. This led to the ascent of leadership by personalities with powerful aggressive, paranoid, and antisocial features, who started out with grandiose leadership aspirations in all three cases. The end result of this process was a totalitarian situation with a socially imposed, ideologically rationalized, leadership-supported political program called to exterminate the enemy group. We have more detailed information, at this point, of both Hitler's and Stalin's personalities that documents the pathology of malignant narcissism in both of them. It refers to their extraordinary grandiosity, the savage aggression, and personal sadistic pleasure in torturing their enemies, their dishonesty and paranoia, and the strange incapacity to evaluate the personality features of their immediate secondary leadership. It is no coincidence that Hitler felt closest to the two most similar personalities to himself in terms of grandiosity and dishonesty, Goebbels and Goering, and that Stalin ended up trusting the psychopathic Beria more than any other member of his leadership group.

When the ascent of groups with the characteristics of regressed large group psychology, and of corresponding leadership with features of malignant narcissism is socially limited in its size, effectiveness, durability, and dramatic impact on the corresponding surrounding society, such a group may emerge as a religious or political cult that ends up in self-destruction or control by the wider social community and state. Obviously, those cults leading to murder or collective suicide represent extremes of this pathology.

In earlier work (Kernberg, 2003) discussing the prevention of socially sanctioned violence, I focused on the limited tools available from a psychoanalytic viewpoint and expertise, including a focused attention on childhood neglect and violence and the corresponding interventions at the home, in early infant and child care, in the school, and the conscious effort to combat and prevent cultural bias with active, socially fostered measures against racial, political, sexual, religious, and other ideologically tinged prejudices against social subgroups. I also questioned the concept of multi-culturalism in terms of its fostering the coexistence of sharply different subcultures within the same social environment. I stressed the need that particularly immigrants from a different culture be helped to integrate into the culture of a country in which they are making their new home. So far, we have studied how we can contribute to reduce the burden of social prejudice against subgroups: concerted efforts of the educational approach in elementary and high school may be an important corrective. Regarding the selection of leadership, in social organizations as well as in political systems, I believe that we are progressing somewhat in the awareness of the psychological requirements of good leadership that may be considered in the selection not only of institutional leadership but, perhaps even more importantly, in the evaluation of potential political leadership. But this awareness does not assure the utilization and effectiveness of this knowledge.

The selection of good leadership in social organizations with clear boundaries, defined tasks, and correspondent administrative structures, is realistically feasible. Usually leaders are selected who evince appropriate technical knowledge and expertise, high intelligence, the capability to communicate with co-workers, and an appropriate background of reliable and honest work patterns. The main difficulty in the selective process lies in the area of their emotional maturity, their capacity to evaluate co-workers in depth, the presence of adequate, "paranoid" features—non-naïve critical evaluation and "narcissistic" features—the ability to stand up to criticism, and unavoidable institutional aggression. The situation is much more complex in the case of selecting political leadership. Candidates with severely paranoid and narcissistic features and even antisocial behavior may be well aware of the need to present themselves as open and friendly, attentive to others' wishes and needs, and disguise their resentful selfishness and self-absorption, and their true thinking, if the moment "is not right." Madeline Albright (2018) has described the erroneous impression Hitler conveyed in early interviews, her own experience with Chavez (Venezuela's former president), and other political leaders that did not reveal their true personality. It is regarding newly emerging, radical movements that the danger of their so well-fitting malignant narcissistic leadership be ignored—with unfortunate consequences. It is obvious that there are historical moments in which powerful social forces may operate in the direction of splitting off of social subgroups, including the unavoidable disorganizing effects of economic crises and political chaos.

Jacques Semelin (2007) recommends international action and the responsibility of the social sciences. He believes that, in the international field, individual nations, as well as the United Nations, have to adopt ethical responsibility, including the responsibility to prevent social crisis that are man-made and put populations in danger. The United Nations should react in the face of situations where the protection of human beings impress the necessity of resorting to appropriate, including coercive, measures, accepting the responsibility to intervene, facilitating receiving military rescue intervention, providing assistance to resumption of reconstruction, and reconciliation. In terms of the responsibility of the social sciences, he believes that the social researcher has at least to take on the responsibility to make known our accumulating knowledge of the causes of social crisis and particularly genocide. The study of genocide is an essential, urgent need for the field of the social sciences, and that includes psychoanalysis. Psychoanalysis can contribute with the understanding of the psychology of large group regression, the psychology of the syndrome of malignant narcissism, and, more generally, the interaction between leadership pathology and group regression. Psychoanalytic contributions to the understanding of optimal leadership in social institutions may be a helpful contribution to the evaluation of political leaders as well.

Here the contribution of the distinguished historian Timothy Snyder is relevant (*On Tyranny: Twenty Lessons from the Twentieth Century* [2017]). His 20 lessons include the call to institutions to distrust one-party states and be wary of power militias. We must remember professional ethics, believe in truth, investigate, and listen for dangerous words. He explains the importance of establishing a private life, contributing to good causes, learning from peers of other countries. He affirms that it is important to be calm when the unthinkable arrives, be a patriot, and be as courageous as one can. He thus outlines a profile of individual courage, responsibility, independence of thinking, and public action. I think these are eminently reasonable and, in fact, essential qualities that permit the individual to stand up to the dangerous imprisonment in regressive group formations and confront dishonest, corrupting, and corrupted leadership. In the political arena, malignant narcissistic leadership should not be exposed with diagnostic psychiatrist labels, but by pointing to their public, cohesively pathological, characteristic behavior. From a psychoanalytic perspective, the development of a strong personal identity, with its related capacity to evaluate oneself and others in depth, to respect the right for privacy and individual boundaries as well as boundaries for the couple in love and for the family are important contributions to the achievement of the individual stance that is described by Timothy Snyder, and so are the psychoanalytic contributions to our understanding of the psychology of small and large regressed groups and their ideological consequences. And the understanding of dangerous personality formations in social leaders may help the prevention of the toxic combination of regressed groups and malignant leaders.

References

Albright, M. (2018) *Fascism: A Warning*. New York, Harper Collins Publishing.
Bao-Lord, B. (1990) *Legacies: A Chinese Mosaic*. New York, Fawcett Columbine.
Bion, W. (1961) *Experiences in Groups*. London, Tavistock Publications.
Canetti, E. (1960) *Masse und Macht*. Frankfurt am Main, Fischer Taschenbuch Verlag.

Freud, S. (1921) 'Group Psychology and the Analysis of the Ego', in J. Strachey, A. Freud, A. Strachey, & A. Tyson (eds.) *The Standard Edition of the Complete Psychological Works of Sigmund Freud, Volume XVIII (1920–1922): Beyond the Pleasure Principle, Group Psychology and Other Works*. London, Hogarth Press, pp. 65–144.

Jacque, E. (1976) *A General Theory of Bureaucracy*. New York, Halsted.

Kernberg, O. (1984) *Severe Personality Disorders: Psychotherapeutic Strategies*. New Haven, Connecticut, Yale University Press.

Kernberg, O. (1998) *Ideology, Conflict, and Leadership in Groups and Organizations*. New Haven, Connecticut, Yale University Press.

Kernberg, O. (2003) 'Sanctioned social violence: a psychoanalytic view', *International Journal of Psychoanalysis*, 84, pp. 953–968.

Kernberg, O. (2018) *Treatment of Severe Personality Disorders: Resolution of Aggression and Recovery of Eroticism*. Washington, DC, American Psychiatric Association Publishing.

Klein, M. (1946) 'Notes on some schizoid mechanisms', *International Journal of Psychoanalysis*, 27, pp. 99–110.

Moscovici, S. (1981) *L'âge des foules*. Paris, Libraire Arthema Fayard.

Semelin J. (2007) *Purify and Destroy: The Political Uses of Massacre and Genocide*. New York, Columbia University Press.

Snyder, T. (2017) *On Tyranny: Twenty Lessons from the Twentieth Century*. New York, Tim Duggan Books.

Turquet, P. (1975) 'Threats to identity in the large group', in L. Kreeger (ed.) *The Large Group: Dynamics and Therapy*. London, Karnac Books.

Volkan, V. (2004) *Blind Trust*. Charlottesville, VA, Pitchstone Publishing.

Chapter 6

Total Belief

Delirium in the West

Jacqueline Rose

Reasons for Inclusion

Working the intersection between psyche and politics as a feminist critic with a rare poetic sensitivity, Jacqueline Rose's writings constitute an integral contribution to contemporary psychoanalytic thinking about fascism. From her consideration of Thatcherism in the late 1980s and her seminal writings on fantasy and the state, to her decades-long engagement with Israel/Palestine, Rose's work persistently demonstrates the importance of psychoanalysis within critical social theory, literary analysis, and public discourse. In this essay, which first appeared in the edited collection Psychoanalysis in the Age of Totalitarianism *(Routledge, 2016), Rose turns to Hannah Arendt in order to articulate the psychoanalytic resonances of Arendt's thought as a pioneering analyst of Nazi Germany and the origins of totalitarianism. Shifting the focus of psychoanalytic inquiry from the structure of mass identifications towards the "strange, twisted, fabric of belief" (this reader, p. 113), Rose draws on Julia Kristeva, Frank Kermode, and Freud to present the Nazis, after Arendt, as "arch-manipulators of the precarious border between lying and truth" (p. 111), violently actualizing a kind of psychic (or psychotic) delirium on the political stage. Consistent with Rose's project as an author, the essay is also a political manifesto for psychoanalysis in its "radical antagonism" (p. 123) with totalitarian belief, opposing the freedom of the mind—including its freedom to countenance the worst of what it is capable—against the colonization and banalization of thinking in Nazi Germany. But if fascism wipes out the mind, as Rose writes, "it does so by breathing life—actual, concrete life—into the unconscious (p. 118)."*

***

Was Hannah Arendt a psychoanalytic thinker? She obviously thought not. But in this chapter, I want to suggest that there is a psychoanalytic dimension to her thought, notably in relation to the dangers and perfection of totalitarian logic. One of the ways we can access that dimension most productively is through the question of how people come to invest themselves in their identifications, that is, through the category of belief. In the process I hope to show how the capacity for passionate, mind-controlling and bewildering identifications cannot be

DOI: 10.4324/9781003742876-9

assigned exclusively to 'other' cultures (identified as 'extreme'), but have also been at the heart of some of the most delirious historical moments in the West.

The category of belief is at the heart of Arendt's analysis of totalitarianism. 'It cannot be doubted', she writes in the section 'Totalitarianism' that concludes *The Origins of Totalitarianism*:

> that the Nazi leadership actually believed in, and did not merely use as propaganda, such doctrines as the following: 'The more accurately we recognize and observe the laws of nature and of life … so much more do we conform to the will of the Almighty. The more insight we have into the will of the Almighty, the greater will be our success.'
>
> (Arendt, 1973 [1958], p. 346)

As Arendt comments in a footnote, such formulations, which can be found repeatedly in the pamphlet literature issued by the SS for the ideological indoctrination of its cadets, are no more than variations on phrases from *Mein Kampf*. Hitler knew that his movement would only succeed by 'awakening a sacrosanct conviction in the heart of its followers' (Hitler, 1988, p. 339). He described the basic postulates of the movement as 'a covenant' and 'profession of faith' (1988, p. 415). He knew, that is, that Nazism had to be a total *Weltanschauung* that marshalled unconditional—passionate and visceral—allegiance: 'Experience teaches', he writes, 'that the human being fights only for something in which he believes and which he loves' (1988, p. 493).

To this end, Hitler did not hesitate, as is known, to draw on the powers of the Catholic Church: 'The mysterious artificial dimness of the Catholic churches also serves this purpose, the burning candles, the incense, the thurible, etc.' (1988, p. 430). The propositions of Nazism, writes Arendt, had the status of 'sacred untouchable truths' (1973 [1958], p. 384). If such divine blather was aimed at the youngest cadets of the party, Hitler was also clear that only a few would be equal to the psychological task. The highest echelons of the party would be composed of a type of spiritual elite. Only a minority would be willing and able to fight for their convictions. 'The more radical and exciting my propaganda was,' he wrote, 'the more did it frighten weak and wavering characters away' (1988, p. 523). You do not need to be a psychoanalyst to know that the most effective mechanism of psychic subordination is fear. Writing on what binds us to our social identities, whose germ is to be found in the merciless rule of the superego over the child's mind, Freud comments simply: 'Fear [or in the German *Angst*] is at the bottom of the whole relationship' (Freud, 1930, p. 496).[1]

It is central to Arendt's argument that the Nazis were arch-manipulators of the precarious border between lying and truth. One way of thinking about belief in relation to Nazism, therefore, would be as a set of deranged conjugations of the proposition 'I speak the truth', which always, for Lacan, contains the lie as the inverse or perverse support of any utterance. 'Please stop lying, I already believe you', is the statement by a patient which analyst Theodor Reik

(1975 [1948], p. 173) invokes in order best to capture the radically exasperated, self-defeating claim to truth-hood of any human subject (what Wallace Stevens describes as the 'nicer knowledge of/Belief, that what it believes is not true' [in Kermode, 1966, p. 34]). 'Did he believe or disbelieve?' asks Reik. 'So much lives in us—wishes and their denials, faith and mistrust, appetites and distastes' (1975 [1948], p. 173). To this extent, Nazi totalitarianism was playing on an old tune. According to Arendt (1973 [1958], p. 384), it organized itself around a strict 'graduation of cynicism expressed in a hierarchy of contempt', with sympathizers despising their fellow citizens, party members despising fellow travellers, the elite formations despising the party membership. What was above all despised was the gullibility shown by the group that was the object of contempt. Each group considered itself to be the possessor of a different, superior, level of truth. To that extent, the higher you moved up the hierarchy, the more fervent—fearless, Hitler would say—your belief, but also the closer you would get to knowing that the whole system was based on a web of deceit (this is Slavoj Žižek's [1989, pp. 28–30] version of cynicism way before its time).

Of course the leaders do not admit this to themselves. If they did the whole system would have crumbled. Right at the top are a group of men who live—who will always live and who will die—in a state of dissociation. After the war, there was not one who admitted to full knowledge of the atrocities that had taken place. As well as self-defence—legally ineffective of course—this was clearly a way of preserving an inner ideal. 'I had the highest ethics and the highest aims', Goering stated to American psychiatrist, Leon Goldensohn, who was given access to the Nuremberg defendants at the time of their trial—he had been entrusted with monitoring their mental health—'I was not to blame for these horrors ... He was a genius ... a great leader and I subscribe to his programme completely' (in Goldensohn, 2006, pp. 115, 121). (The interviews were conducted in May 1946; after being condemned to death in October, Goering committed suicide in his cell.) What of course could not be admitted was that he knew the whole system was fraudulent but went along with it regardless.

For Arendt, the consequence of the system was a type of national and international mental pandemonium which also had a strict inner logic. 'The result', she writes:

> is that the gullibility of the sympathizers makes lies credible to the outside world, while at the same time the graduated cynicism of membership and elite members eliminates the danger that the Leader will ever be forced by the weight of his own propaganda to make good his own statements.
>
> (1973 [1958], p. 384)

The main delusion of the outside world was to misread this system—to trust, on the one hand, that the enormity of its lies would be the undoing of totalitarianism, and, on the other, that the Führer could be held to his word (Neville Chamberlain's big mistake). Viewed from the outside, it was impossible that a people could be so duped, or, if they were, that their leader could not be trusted. As well as a wish-fulfilment, this is of course a type of kettle logic, as Freud famously defined the (il)logic of the unconscious (1900, pp. 119–20)—the people know and will ultimately be guided by the truth; leaders—even or perhaps especially the Leader who so misguides them—must be honourable men. That these two propositions cancel each other out does not in any sense limit their combined power. Underneath the problem of knowledge that has been so much at the forefront of discussion of Nazi Germany—who knew, who did not know?—lies a strange, twisted, fabric of belief. The question should perhaps therefore be: not who knew, but who believed and how?

If, in Arendt's account, the elites are the ultimate cynics—'not even supposed to believe in the literal truths of ideological clichés'—they nonetheless occupy in even more sinister fashion the domain of fiction (1973 [1958], p. 384). It is their role to transpose belief into evidence, to make the world conform to, mirror, fulfil, the Nazi mind. The elite do not consist of ideologists. Instead their whole education is aimed at 'abolishing their capacity for distinguishing between truth and falsehood, between reality and fiction' (1973 [1958], p. 385). Theirs is a peculiar, unique form of superiority which consists in their ability 'immediately to dissolve every statement of fact into a declaration of purpose' (1973 [1958], p. 385). Thus, while the membership need to be persuaded of the inferiority of the Jews before it can be safely asked to kill them, it is the characteristic of the elite formations to understand without question that 'the statement, all Jews are inferior, means that all Jews must be killed' (1973 [1958], p. 385). No 'mere mass phenomenon', this mentality requires a very particular form of cultivation. The whole effectiveness of the programme depends on it. Without this mentality, which was the object of the most careful indoctrination by totalitarian schools of leadership, the programme would not be able to bring itself to life. It would remain pure fiction. 'Without the elite,' writes Arendt, 'and its artificially induced inability to understand facts as facts, to distinguish between truth and falsehood, the movement could never move in the direction of realizing its fiction' (1973 [1958], p. 385).

The elite are the guardians of a hallucinatory, delirious world—Arendt does not use the word 'psychotic', although she does use the word 'borderline', which has since become a key diagnostic term in psychoanalysis (1973 [1958], p. 478).[2] Delirium always carries a risk, however. It is therefore central to this machinery that no-one must be capable of seeing the world through different eyes. For the masses to be carried, a protective wall has to be built to separate them from the outside world. Without such a wall, they would feel too acutely the discrepancy 'between the lying fictitiousness of their own and the reality of the normal world' (1973 [1958], p. 366). I am less confident than Arendt in the concept of a 'normal world', and indeed in its reality. But note how the masses are the bearers of a form of knowledge that both knows and doesn't know itself. If the system never stops working, it is because the masses must be endlessly protected from the spectre of disbelief. Disbelief haunts the system, the other side of the delirium to which it is inextricably wed. This goes beyond the dimension of complicity, but it is not covered either by the idea of false consciousness or indeed by that of bad faith. It is as if Nazism constructed itself with the most painstaking attention to an order of belief that it knew only too well was beyond belief—'*incroyable*', as Julia Kristeva (2007) has put it (she argues that it is Freud's forays into this domain of belief that is at the core of the hostility against him). Provided we add that the element of unbelievability is not a threat to belief, but one way that belief operates, how—clearly at historic moments such as this one—it most effectively protects itself. For Kristeva we are touching on an order of necessity or compulsion—hence the title of her book: *This* Unbelievable *Need to Believe* (my emphasis).

It is not therefore simply the divine grandiosity of Nazism that is at issue, but the way the propositions of Nazism moved into the realm of incontrovertible, sacred fact and thereupon were immediately bound to fulfil themselves. The difference between a statement and a programme, Arendt observes, is that only the former can be contested—it is because the gap between the two was abolished that the Nazis could believe themselves to be the agents of a divine will. To say that the belief is delusional (which of course it was) is not therefore enough. What matters is how the form of the delirium—its mental enactment—turns the Nazi, and above all Hitler, into the agent of God. Remember this quotation:

> It cannot be doubted … that the Nazi leadership actually believed in, and did not merely use as propaganda, such doctrines as the following: 'The more accurately we recognize and observe the laws of nature and of life … so much more do we conform to the will of the Almighty. The more insight we have into the will of the Almighty, the greater will be our success.'
>
> (1973 [1958], pp. 345–46)

This is why Hitler announced his political intentions in the form of prophecy, of which the most famous example is his announcement to the Reichstag in January 1939: 'I want today once again to make a prophecy: In case the Jewish financiers … succeed once more in hurling the peoples into a world war, the result will be … the annihilation of the Jewish race in Europe' (1973 [1958], pp. 349).[3] This sounds like speculation—'in case the Jewish financiers'—but it is in fact prediction, or rather two predictions bound by a hidden relation of causality: the Jews *will* succeed in precipitating world war, the Jews *will* be killed. It is a type of double apocalypse: the Jews are already guilty of the end of the world, from which the world must, and will, be saved.

Belief in the system therefore hangs on a strict order of time. The movement produced a mentality which 'thought in continents and felt in centuries'—Himmler described it as working 'for a great task which occurs but once in 2,000 years' (speech on 'Organization and Obligation of the SS and the Police', in Arendt, 1973 [1958], p. 316). 'There is hardly a better way to avoid discussion,' Arendt wryly noted, 'than by releasing an argument from the control of the present and by saying that only the future will fulfil its merits' (1973 [1958], p. 346). You cannot argue with a form of belief that has already secured its own future (this is not belief *in* the future, but belief *as* the future). 'All debate about the truth or falsity of a totalitarian dictator's prediction', she comments, 'is as weird as arguing with a potential murderer whether his future victim is dead or alive—since by killing the person in question the murderer can promptly provide proof of the correctness of his statement' (1973 [1958], p. 350). As well as being a declaration of intent, Hitler's prophecy abolishes the distance between today and all the potential tomorrows of the world. It seizes the future according to a law or chain of fatality whose latent, sometimes explicit, nature is divine. 'Man only does or suffers,' wrote Arendt, 'what, according to immutable laws, is bound to happen anyway' (1973 [1958], p. 349). It was de Toqueville, she reminds us, who wrote of the appeal of 'absolutist systems which represent all the events of history as depending on the first great causes linked by the chain of fatality, and which, as it were, suppress men from the history of the human race' (de Toqueville in Arendt, 1973 [1958], p. 345).

Working on this subject, I found myself rereading *The Sense of an Ending* (1966) by Frank Kermode. I was struck by how central the question of belief, and indeed apocalypse—hence the title of the book—is to his deservedly famous study of fiction and time. The lines already cited from Wallace Stevens—'the nicer knowledge of/Belief, that what it believes is not true'—form one of the epigraphs to Kermode's second chapter on 'Fictions'. For Stevens, 'the last and greatest fiction' is 'the fiction of an Absolute' (1966, p. 41). Kermode tracks this fiction throughout the book but he is also concerned—indeed at moments he struggles—to wrest the domain of literary fiction, whose only validity is its inventiveness or effective force, from what he calls its other 'dangerous relations' (1966, p. 37). In this discussion, totalitarianism is central precisely because of its power to bend the world to the mind. Nietzsche's argument that the only relevant question is how far an opinion is 'life-furthering, life-preserving, species-preserving' (in Kermode, 1966, p. 37) might be seen as in danger of encouraging people who believe that death on a large scale can also be a way—is in fact the only way—of preserving a species, of preserving life. This is not, as I read it, a bland critique of relativism (nor the even blander suggestion that Nietzsche has some affinity with, or in its strong version, responsibility for, Nazi atrocity). It is far more precisely an attempt to come to grips with what fiction can do, its internal grip or authority, and, specifically in relation to Nazism, the brutality and unseemly haste with which fiction tipped into the register of fact—the problem with delirium being not that the belief is false but instead that it becomes real so fast: 'If the value of an opinion is to be tested only by its success in the world', writes Kermode echoing Arendt, 'the validity of one's opinion of the Jews can be proved by killing six million Jews' (1966, p. 38).

'There might even be a relation', Kermode writes, 'between certain kinds of effectiveness in literature and totalitarianism in politics' (1966, p. 39).

Thus, 'the consciously false apocalypse of both *King Lear* and the Third Reich force us to recognize that "it is ourselves we are encountering whenever we invent fictions"', fabrications *in extremis* both (1966, pp. 38–9). There is, however, a crucial difference. Unlike *Lear*, Nazism tells us 'nothing about death' as universal, shared experience, but instead projects it onto, enacts it by means of, others. We could say that perversely Nazism never really countenances the death it performs (belonging rather, committing the other, to the realm of 'non-existence'; in Arendt's words, it knows 'neither birth nor death' [1973 (1958), p. 473]). And Nazism, as we have seen Arendt describe it, abolishes the distinction between fiction and reality, or statement and programme—Kermode calls it a 'degenerate fiction'—by presupposing, as he puts it, 'a total and adequate explanation of things as they are' (an irony given Nazism's preoccupation with what it termed degenerate art) (1966, p. 39; see also Peters, 2014). Kermode's is not therefore a positivist account of reality but reality as the endless capacity and openness of words. It is precisely because it loses its sense of belonging in time that Nazism starts its climb back up to the world of the gods. In literature, uncertainty hovers over time. Unlike the 'equivocally offered' futures of Shakespearean tragedy, the Third Reich was the disastrous consequence of trying 'to impose limited designs on the time of the world' (1966, p. 88). In tragedy, on the other hand, 'the great crises and ends of human life do not stop time' (1966, p. 89).

I had forgotten how important Arendt was to Kermode's argument, as well as how central Jewish thought was to his vision of the critic. What prevents apocalyptic grandiosity—the means of the world careering to its end—is the ceaseless interpretability of things which it is the task of the critic to cultivate. The sole 'myth' of Jewish thought is that there are as many interpretations of the text 'as may be found in the created world with which the book is coextensive' (Kermode, 1985, p. 90). Insisting that the world is a book that 'can be exfoliated into the universe', and that this process is endless, becomes then a, if not the, key counter-myth to the belief that time can be halted, world and word perfectly aligned, that 'the validity of one's opinions of the Jews can be proved by killing six million Jews' (Kermode, 1966, p. 38; 1985, p. 90). In this light, Nazism is an anti-hermeneutic. The aggressiveness of totalitarianism, Arendt insists, does not spring from lust for power but simply from the ideological drive 'to make the world consistent' (1973 [1958], p. 458). On this too Hitler was explicit: 'The essentials of a teaching', he wrote in *Mein Kampf*, 'must never be looked for in its external formulas, but in its inner meaning. And this meaning is unchangeable' (1988, p. 416).

I want now to push this a little further in psychoanalytic terms. Although it is rarely explicit, whenever I read Arendt, I am struck by this aspect of her writing. To her surprise, she was awarded the Sigmund Freud Preis of the Deutsche Akademie für Sprache und Dichtung in 1967 (her biographer, Elizabeth Young-Bruehl, who herself went on to become a psychoanalyst, comments that Arendt would have won no prizes for sympathy with Freud). It is, however, central to her understanding of totalitarianism that it involves the inner domination of the human spirit, an 'inner coercion whose only content is the avoidance of contradictions' (Arendt, 1973 [1958], p. 478) (the 'inner meaning' in Hitler's terms). What distinguishes totalitarianism from all other political movements is its demand for the 'total, unconditional, and unalterable loyalty of the individual member' (in Hitler's words, the problem of 'influencing the freedom of the human will') (Arendt, 1973 [1958], p. 323; Hitler, 1988, p. 430). It achieves this deathly allegiance because it has discovered 'a means of dominating and terrorizing human beings from within' (1973 [1958], p. 325). Everything outside the movement is dying (1973 [1958], p. 381). This, one could say, is why Frau Goebbels murders her five children in the last days of the regime (a moment shockingly rendered in Oliver Hirschbiegel's 2004 film *Downfall*, based on Hitler's final ten days in his Berlin bunker). In all of this there seems to be, for the participants themselves, something inexplicable involved. Looking back on his life, Albert Speer describes the inner compulsion that drew him to Hitler before he knew, but when, as he acknowledges in his interviews with journalist Gitta Sereny, he already should have known: 'The truth is that for a reason I still cannot explain to myself, perhaps like the thief who feels impelled to return to the scene of his crime, something very deep inside myself drew me towards the Chancellery' (Sereny, 1995, p. 526).

Totalitarianism is external coercion but it works above all through the inner life, relying, in Arendt's words, 'on the compulsion with which we can compel ourselves' (1973 [1958], p. 473). It relies, that is, on our inner attraction to force—to what Freud will describe in his analysis of the superego as the cruelty which regulates the traffic between the different agencies of the mind. (As Arendt also remarks, cruelty can also feel like a liberation from a society's liberal and humanitarian hypocrisy—a warning first the 2010–15 coalition, and now Conservative, governments in the UK, with their mixture of social liberalism and economic cruelty, might do well to heed.) Cruelty, as Freud describes it, is the last resort of the humiliated (the superego wreaks on the defenceless ego all the subjugated child's wrath against its parents). The law of ruthless expansion, Arendt writes, was therefore a 'psychological necessity before it [was] a political device' (1973 [1958], p. 330). The front generation which emerged from the humiliation and violence of the First World War, she suggests, 'read not Darwin but the Marquis de Sade' (1973 [1958], p. 330). As we know, there were then strictly no limits to what could take place. Faced with the mentality of the SS, it would become the almost impossible task of the next generation to take the measure of the psychically destructive powers of a form of conviction so intense that it seems to have the power to destroy the mind itself, to grasp that 'the psyche can be destroyed even without the destruction of the physical man; that indeed, psyche, character, and individuality seem under certain circumstances to express themselves only through the rapidity or slowness with which they can disintegrate' (1973 [1958], p. 441).

If totalitarianism wipes out the mind, however, it does so only by plunging its roots so effectively into the worst of what the mind is capable of. The reality of the camps was unbelievable precisely because the image of that reality could be found in the hidden echo chambers of the human heart. 'Everything that was done in the camps', Arendt writes, 'is known to us from the world of perverse, malignant fantasies' (1973 [1958], p. 445). At moments like this, as I see it, Arendt raises the psychological stakes of her discussion of the lies, deceit, and false actualization of the Nazi world. Nazism made its dreams come true (one definition of the psychotic is that their dreams come true). If it colonizes, destroys, the mind, it does so by breathing life—actual, concrete life—into the unconscious. We should then be sceptical about the Nazi claim that the only private individual in Germany was someone who was asleep (1973 [1958], p. 339). Under such forms of coercion, nobody was ever free, not even—I would add especially—when they were asleep.

As I read this account, what it evokes most powerfully for me is the world of Daniel Paul Schreber, the Leipzig High Court Presiding Judge, whose deranged 1903 memoirs were the object of one of Freud's few forays into the realm of psychosis. In her 2004 study of the meta-psychology of belief, *Le Besoin de croire—métapsychologie du fait religieux*, French psychoanalyst Sophie de Mijolla-Mellor gives central place to Schreber (in a chapter called 'Ivresses Sacrées' or 'Sacred Intoxications'). Schreber believed that he was to be inseminated by God, in order to repopulate the earth with a new race. This makes him the carnal embodiment of God's will and futurity whose more abstract version—although abstract is not quite the right word—we have already seen at the heart of Nazism. His solution to the problem of suffering (and we should never underestimate the extent to which Nazism presented itself as a solution to the suffering of the German people) is to try to think, as Mijolla-Mellor puts it, 'from the point of view of God' (2004, p. 157). For Mijolla-Mellor, belief always contains this potentially delirious element, as it tries to counter the collapse of the child's faith in her or his own narcissistic omnipotence and in the parental capacity to restore the child's lost infantile ideal. Belief rises out of that melancholy recognition, as its most fervent denial (which is why, for Kristeva, belief is the privileged domain of the adolescent). If psychoanalysis then inspires its adherents to a type of faith in turn, it is at least in part because it allows the analyst, not just a new creed, but to make her or his way back to the mainspring of belief in the infantile mind, to play in the psychic forecourts of conviction (much of Mijolla-Mellor's book is devoted to analysing this dimension of belief in Freud's early psychoanalytic movement).

Freud was contemptuous of religious passion from which, as we know, he did all he could to distance himself (although, as I have written elsewhere, and as others have more fully documented, his relationship to his own Jewishness was complex—see, for example, Said, 1993; Yerushalmi, 1991). In doing so he also underestimated the wider social force of delusional systems, like Schreber's, which elevate the subject to an ecstatic, albeit tortured, relation to God. And by brushing aside longing for paternal protection as the regressive component of faith, he also sidestepped the potentially delirious tie that binds man to the divine. This is to make of Schreber—as Mijolla-Mellor does—a demonstration or test case of the unconscious element of belief. What Schreber then allows us to see so graphically is how this whole system relies on a systematic and interminable invasion of the realm of thought. Although Mijolla-Mellor does not make the link, the similarities to Arendt's account of totalitarianism is striking. That link is also historical—Schreber's father, as we now know, was at the heart of the new late nineteenth-century Gymnasium project, unsurpassed in its physical exactions, that laid down some of the educational foundations for Hitler (the cruelty of these exactions—the belts, chin, head and backstraps to which Schreber was subjected—is well known).[4] This is from Schreber's *Memoirs*. He is describing his penetration by the divine rays:

> This influence showed itself relatively early in the form of *compulsive thinking*—an expression which I received from the inner voices themselves and which will hardly be known to other human beings, because the whole phenomenon lies outside human experience. The nature of compulsive thinking lies in a human being having to think incessantly; in other words, man's natural right to give the nerves of his mind their necessary rest from time to time by thinking nothing (as occurs most markedly during sleep) was from the beginning denied me by the rays in contact with me; they continually wanted to know what I was thinking about. For instance I was asked in these very words: 'What are you thinking of now?'; because this question is in itself complete nonsense, as a human being can at certain times as well think of *nothing* as of *thousands of things at the same time*, and because my nerves did not react to this absurd question, one was soon driven to take refuge in *falsifying my thoughts*. For instance the above question was answered spontaneously: 'He should' scilicet think 'about the Order of the World'; that is to say the influence of the rays forced my nerves to perform the movements corresponding to the use of these words.
>
> (Schreber, 1988, p. 70, italics original)

Compulsive thinking obliges you to falsify your thoughts. Real mental freedom consists in the freedom to think nothing (to drift off), or to think a thousand things at the same time (another kind of drifting). This is the opposite of thinking about the 'Order of the World', which requires above all that the mind be self-present and consistent (an 'unchangeable inner meaning' in Hitler's [1988, p. 416] terms). Under totalitarianism, Arendt writes, 'the self-coercive force of logicality is mobilized lest anybody ever start thinking'—by which she means, not compulsively but on their own terms (1973 [1958], p. 473). Unlike authoritarianism, total domination does not aim to restrict freedom but to abolish it completely, including that of 'spontaneity in general', including, we might say, the capacity of the mind to drift and roam (1973 [1958], p. 405).

There must be no secrets. Schreber's instructions are precise. As if his tormentors had understood only too well that the human mind makes its best bid for freedom simply by losing itself, by changing tack, by being open to the confused bits and pieces of mental life. This could be a definition of the unconscious—which consists in the ability of the mind to double and escape itself.

Arendt then comes very close to suggesting—after Lacan we might say—that deception is the very kernel of human thought. 'Simply because of their capacity to think', she writes, 'human beings are suspects by definition, and this suspicion cannot be diverted by exemplary behaviour, for the human capacity to think is also a capacity to change one's mind' (1973 [1958], p. 430). It is impossible 'to know beyond doubt another man's heart'—psychoanalysis would add that it is no less impossible fully to know one's own. Torture then becomes a 'desperate and eternally futile attempt' to enter completely the mind of another, 'to achieve what cannot be achieved' (the idea of knowing another's mind is already a form of invasion which torture elevates to a craft) (1973 [1958], p. 430). It is then Schreber's dubious privilege—as a form of childhood memory that anticipated the brutality of totalitarianism to come—to lay bare the nerve mechanism of torture at its core (he belongs at the tortuous, rather than ecstatic, extremity of belief). Torture is the inverse image of mental freedom. It is the state's rejoinder to, as well as recognition of, the fact that we are all suspects. (The common official argument that it is an exceptional measure, reluctantly embraced, is therefore as psychologically as it is politically evasive.) Hence the mutual suspicion that pervades all social relationships under totalitarian rule.

Taking my cue from Schreber, I am tempted to say that Arendt is describing the deep, violent, psychic coercion of totalitarian rule. Schreber's vulnerability to such coercion is acute—it is precisely his paranoia to live it so literally, body and soul—but the structure of such coercion has its germ in the origins of mental life (the argument, made first by Morton Schatzman [1973], that Schreber is remembering his childhood, takes on an added meaning here). All children, writes Mijolla-Mellor, believe in the capacity of their parents to read their thoughts. The delirium of the paranoid repeats this belief ad infinitum. In his famous 1919 essay 'On the Origin of the "Influencing Machine" in Schizophrenia', Victor Tausk—one of Freud's most important and troubled interlocutors—writes:

> We are familiar with this infantile stage of thinking, in which a strong belief exists that others know of the child's thoughts. Until the child has been successful in its first lie, the parents are supposed to know everything, even its most secret thoughts [...] The striving for the right to have secrets from which the parents are excluded is one of the most powerful factors in the formation of the ego, especially in establishing and carrying out one's own will.[5]
>
> (in Fliess, 1969 [1948], p. 45)

If there is no secrecy, there is no mind. Underneath the totalitarian aim to control, as Hitler put it, 'the freedom of the human will', lies the delusion that everything, everyone, can be fully known. When Arendt writes of total domination, what she is describing therefore is the destruction of the unconscious.

In the final pages of *The Origins of Totalitarianism*, Arendt describes the ultimate freedom as being identical with the capacity to begin, just as freedom as a political reality is identical with the space of movement between men (her definition of democracy). Over such beginnings, 'no logic, no cogent deduction can have any power because the chain presupposes, in the form of a premise, the beginning' (1973 [1958], p. 473). The beginning is the supreme creative capacity of man. It is therefore each new birth that totalitarianism hates, a hatred that is wholly compatible of course with forced eugenics, because each new birth might 'raise its voice in the world', threatening a multiplicity of possible futures that are uncontrollable and unknown (1973 [1958], p. 473). Once again we can turn to Kermode's (1985) 'equivocally offered futures' of Shakespearean tragedy as the antidote. Political freedom and psychic freedom are therefore inseparable. Only if the child is allowed its secrets and lies, only if language can circulate in the head and in the city space, will there ever be freedom for mankind.

Of course I am pushing Arendt further than she would probably wish to go. Arendt may be against the tyranny of logic, she may at moments come close to a psychoanalytic vision of the mind, but she is also cautious. In these final pages 'duality and equivocality and doubt'—what we might call the core of the Freudian subject—reappear as something which the citizen must be protected against (1973 [1958]: 476). But this is because they are the attributes of the bereft, lonely man in the crowd, whose uncertainty makes him vulnerable to totalitarian coercion. The lonely man is surrounded by a hostile world (Schreber would then be the loneliest man on earth), whereas the solitary man is alone but 'together with himself' since men have the capacity 'of talking with themselves' (she is citing Cicero; 1973 [1958], p. 476). In solitude, I am '"by myself", together with myself, and therefore two-in-one, whereas in loneliness I am actually one, deserted by all the others' (1973 [1958], p. 476). Once again Arendt is talking about the innermost life—here it is the resonances with D.W. Winnicott's capacity to be alone in the presence of the other that are striking. It is by means of thought, as I see it—myself alone with myself, alone with a thousand thoughts or none—that Arendt strives to deliver the modern subject from the crowd (the subject mass of totalitarian coercion) in order to restore his civic and psychic dignity.

'Work and the free play of the imagination', Freud writes to Swiss pastor, Oskar Pfister in 1910, 'are for me the same thing, I take no pleasure in anything else' (6 March 1910, in Freud and Pfister, 1964, p. 35). For Freud, such freedom requires a full reckoning with the horrors of the world which, even by the 1930s, Pfister can only with the greatest reluctance be brought to contemplate. Freedom consists in freedom from idealization and, with it, from any form of sacred belief. Pfister himself suggests that the point in ethical matters is to be 'free thinkers without being heroes' (18 February 1909, in Freud and Pfister, 1964, p. 18). No false gods. Freud was less immune to their powers than it might seem from his later writings on religion. In 1899 he wrote a poem to Fliess extolling him as 'the valiant son who at the behest of his father appeared at the right time,/ To be his assistant and fellow worker in fathoming the divine order' (29 December 1899, in Freud, 1985, pp. 393–4). By the time he starts his correspondence with Pfister ten years later, something has happened to place any such appeal to the divine order under erasure. Psychoanalysis will henceforth join the ranks of the disbelievers. Of *The Future of an Illusion*, he writes to Pfister somewhat mercilessly, 'I wanted to strike a blow at superstition, stupidity and goggle-eyed self-abasement' (1 April 1926, in Freud and Pfister, 1964, p. 102). Even in the poem, Freud had called on the 'higher powers to claim as his right, conclusion, belief and doubt'—something of an odd mix (as if one could appeal to the higher powers for the right to doubt them). But by 1909, probably because he has started to father his own movement, Freud has become acutely aware of the danger to psychoanalysis of its demanding any such allegiance, of its becoming its own form of faith. 'The value of what we write must depend', he insists, 'on its containing nothing accepted on authority ... I do not call for any act of faith on your part' (30 March 1909, in Freud and Pfister, 1964, p. 22). 'I have deliberately set myself up only as an example, but never as a model, let alone an object of veneration' (10 May 1909, in 1964, p. 23). More defensively, when an acquaintance of Pfister's, sympathetic to psychoanalysis, demurs from being considered a member of its 'school', Freud retorts: 'Has our "school" secret signs or rites, does it swear by my words, or worship me with incense?' (12 July 1909, in 1964, p. 27).

Freud's disclaimers, his rhetorical question, of course neatly sidestep the place of belief inside his own movement (a key strand of Mijolla-Mellor's book). But whether or not history will bear Freud out on this question, it is crucial to psychoanalysis, crucial to Freud, that psychoanalysis dissolves belief in the crucible of transference where—at least this is the risk and challenge—it most strongly germinates and spreads. To this extent, as if in anticipation of Arendt and indeed of his own later work on mass psychology, Freud is offering psychoanalysis as its own antidote to idealization, to the sacred perversity of the group—starting with the group of two that is the analytic pair (just one reason why it is such a mistake to argue that there is no social being on the analytic couch). To call Freud a sceptic, as indeed he might call himself, is therefore not quite right, since he immerses himself, and indeed the whole practice of psychoanalysis, so firmly inside the register of belief. We could say that psychoanalysis is one of the few places in the culture where belief is given its full weight (this is also the starting premise of Mijolla-Mellor and Kristeva).

What one finds in reading Freud's correspondence with Pfister, is that it is out of the transference, a concept slow to emerge in Freud's thought, that psychoanalysis draws its understanding of belief. Thus, Freud writes to Pfister, failure to acknowledge the power of transference in the early days of psychoanalysis meant that it remained untouchable, divine. In the early cathartic method, the transference was taken for granted, 'rather like the omnipresence of the divine being' who is assumed to be the onlooker, but is unmentioned (19 July 1910, in Freud and Pfister, 1964, p. 42). This meant that the negative transference— hostility to the analyst 'as it is in the case of most decent neurotics'— was overlooked (there can be no negative transference to a God whose existence, whose name, remains unspoken) (19 July 1910, in 1964, p. 23). If psychoanalysis fails to tolerate the unconscious hostility of the patient, it will find itself in the position of Christ who pronounces 'Thy sins are forgiven thee; arise and walk' (25 November 1928, in 1964, p. 125). It is a startling analogy and Freud does not let it go. 'Besides', he writes,

> the above statement calls for analysis. If the sick man had asked: "How knowest thou that my sins are forgiven?" the answer could only have been: "I, the Son of God, forgive thee." In other words, a call for unlimited transference.
>
> (25 November 1928, in 1964, p. 125)

Perhaps there is no other place in Freud's writing where he so unequivocally links the issue of belief to that of transference, and of both of these to the question of freedom (nor, indeed, where he so unambiguously divorces psychoanalysis from the order of Christian forgiveness). Freud has brought the issue of belief into the consulting room. This seems to me to be a far more important intervention into the question than *The Future of an Illusion*, in which belief is no more than an illusion to be dissipated by the reason of the mind (for me Freud's most un-Freudian work). And, again, more interesting than the *Papers on Technique*, where love is the daemon of the cure. Instead what counts is how the analytic process responds to the potentially sacred powers of conviction. To preserve his mental freedom and move on, the analysand must retain his right to be suspicious even of a forgiving God.

Freud does not therefore want the world to be either forgiven or saved. Like the patient, he wants it to know itself. As the correspondence progresses, it becomes clearer and clearer that the free play of the imagination—the only thing, apart from work, that gives Freud true pleasure—is the freedom to countenance the worst of what human nature has to offer (the death instinct, he states in 1930 in another revealing moment, is not 'a requirement of my heart' but a requirement of the way things are; Freud to Pfister 7 February 1930, in Freud and Pfister, 1964, p. 133). Freud's own negative transference, we could say, reaches to the gods. In this he is true to his historical moment. What he wants is for the world to take the measure of what it is—or will be, since he does not live to see the worst—capable of. This, I suggest finally, might help us take the true measure of the distance, or radical antagonism, between psychoanalysis and totalitarian belief.

Notes

1 In German in Das Unbehagen in der Kultur, Gesammelte Werke, vol. 14, p. 496.
2 The term 'borderline', coined in 1938 by Adolf Stern, started to acquire more general psychoanalytic currency in the 1950s, at the time Arendt was writing the book, although she may well not have taken cognisance of it.
3 The full text is: 'I want today once again to make a prophecy: In case the international Jewish financiers within and outside Europe succeed once more in hurling the peoples into a world war, the result will be, not the Bolshevization of the world and with it a victory of Jewry, but the annihilation of the Jewish race in Europe' (Goebbels, 1948, cited in Arendt, 1973 [1958], p. 349).
4 Although his reading is controversial, Morton Schatzman was the first to discuss this aspect of Schreber's history in *Soul Murder: Persecution in the Family* (1973).
5 Tausk's essay was first published in German in 1919 and in English in 1933.

References

Arendt, H. (1973 [1958]) *The Origins of Totalitarianism*. New York and London: Harcourt Brace Jovanovich.

Fliess, R., ed. (1969 [1948]) *The Psychoanalytic Reader*. New York: International Universities Press.

Freud, S. (1900) *The Interpretation of Dreams*. In *The Standard Edition of the Complete Psychological Works of Sigmund Freud [SE], volume IV: The Interpretation of Dreams (First Part)*. Translated from the German under the General Editorship of James Strachey in collaboration with Anna Freud, assisted by Alix Strachey and Alan Tyson. London: Hogarth.

Freud, S. (1930) *Civilization and Its Discontents*. SE vol. XXI: 57–146.

Freud, S. (1985) *The Complete Letters of Sigmund Freud to Wilhelm Fliess 1887–1904*, trans. and ed. J. Moussaieff Masson. Cambridge, MA: Harvard University Press.

Freud, S. and Pfister, O. (1964) *Psycho-Analysis and Faith*, ed. H. Meng and E.L. Freud. New York: Basic Books.

Goldensohn, L. (2006) *The Nuremberg Interviews*, ed. R. Gellately. London: Pimlico.

Hitler, A. (1988) *Mein Kampf*. Mumbai: Jaico.

Kermode, F. (1966) *The Sense of an Ending: Studies in the Theory of Fiction*. Oxford: Oxford University Press.

Kermode, F. (1985) *Forms of Attention: Botticelli and Hamlet*. Chicago: University of Chicago Press.

Kristeva, J. (2007) *Cet incroyable besoin de croire*. Paris: Bayard.

de Mijolla-Mellor, S. (2004) *Le Besoin de croire: metapsychologie du fait religieux*. Paris: Dunod.

Peters, O., ed. (2014) *Degenerate Art: The Attack on Modern Art in Nazi Germany*. Exhibition at the Neue Gallerie, New York. Munich: Prestel.

Reik, T. (1975 [1948]) *'Who Am I?' Listening with the Third Ear*. New York: Farrar, Straus and Giroux.

Said, E. (1993) *Freud and the Non-European, Response by Jacqueline Rose, introduced by Christopher Bollas*. London: Verso.

Schatzman, M. (1973) *Soul Murder: Persecution in the Family*. New York: New American Library.

Schreber, D.P. (1988) *Memoirs of My Nervous Illness*, trans. and ed. by I. Macalpine and R.A. Hunter, new introduction by S. Weber. Cambridge, MA: Harvard University Press.
Sereny, G. (1995) *Albert Speer: His Battle with the Truth*. London: Picador.
Yerushalmi, Y.H. (1991) *Freud's Moses: Judaism Terminable and Interminable*. New Haven, CT: Yale University Press.
Žižek, S. (1989) *The Sublime Object of Ideology*. London: Verso.

Part III

Masculinity and Perversion

Chapter 7

Masculinity and the Fascist State of Mind

Christina Wieland

Reasons for Inclusion

This chapter provides a short introduction to Wieland's important work, spanning multiple articles (e.g., Wieland, 2017, 2023) and her book, The Fascist State of Mind and the Manufacturing of Masculinity: A Psychoanalytic Approach *(2014), that uses psychoanalytic theory, from Freud, Klein, and Bion, to consider the links between masculine identity, social crisis, and fascist mindstates and political movements. Excerpted from Wieland's 2014 book, this chapter draws on a wide variety of works—Nancy Chodorow's work on masculine identity and Klaus Theweleit's classic psychoanalytic work on fascism,* Male Fantasies, *as well as texts by Sebastian Langer, Eric Santner, and Alexander Mitscherlich—to establish a connection between mass social crises and masculine humiliation, feminization, and castration, which inspire psychic defences, including regression, narcissism, and paranoia. The fascist group, Wieland argues, provides a solution to the specific, traumatic humiliations experienced by the fragile male ego in times of widespread crisis. Wieland's contributions are essential for anyone who wishes to understand fascism from a feminist, psychosocial perspective.*

***

> War is to man what maternity is to woman.
>
> (Benito Mussolini quoted in Bollas, 1993)

In Part I of this book (i.e., Wieland, 2014) I examined the boy's struggle to establish his masculine identity at a time when his differentiation from mother is difficult due to the excessive use of projective identification. Mourning for the loss of the breast and, of accepting his difference from mother are the twin demands made on him as he grows up and differentiates himself from mother. Having a good relationship to father helps him in this difficult negotiation of separateness, attachment and loss.

However, differentiation brings with it separation, loss, responsibility and guilt. A deep wish for non-differentiation and merging with the object remains in all human beings men or women. This wish is symbolically satisfied in religion, art and in loving and sexual relationships.

However, the wish for non-differentiation in boys can easily become a dangerous feminine wish to be one with mother which spells the death of his

DOI: 10.4324/9781003742876-11

masculinity. In the previous chapters I have looked at the deeply repressed wishes for non-differentiation within the male individual and the delusional internal world that can be created (in *Bacchae* and in Schreber for instance) when these wishes become dominant. One way that these wishes can be satisfied without a loss of masculinity is within certain male homogeneous types of groups. The fascist group with its stress on the sameness of its members and its stress on the extermination of the outsider, is an extreme type of a homogeneous group and follows the extreme traumatic circumstances of the First World War and the traumatic effects of the Depression of the 1930s in Germany.

I have argued that traumatic circumstances often undo precarious solutions both within the individual and within society, in this way plunging the individual into feelings of helplessness and fears of annihilation. Feelings of humiliation have the same traumatic effect on the individual leaving him feeling helpless as his ordinary defences collapse and a kind of 'death' is threatening the ego. In this case the individual may become a small helpless child wanting a mother to retreat to as Michael Roper reports examining the stories of many traumatised men in First World War (Roper, 2009); or he might turn this trauma into a new retreat that both endorses and denies his wish for an undifferentiated state. This new retreat is fascism.

I shall examine these issues in what follows.

Masculinity, Humiliation and Violence

As we have seen fascism uses violence not only as a way of defeating its opponents but, more importantly, as a way of creating the new virile man. I have examined this issue in my clinical example in Chapter 1 but I shall look at this once again here.

On the use of violence by men Anthony Clare writes:

> Government think-tanks, international and national commissions, local task forces and clinical workshops sit and solemnly deliberate on the origins of human violence and often the most obvious feature—that it is the activity engaged almost exclusively by men—receives no attention.
>
> (Clare, 2000, p. 38)

He comments that across cultures a man is more than 20 times 'likely to kill a man than a woman is to kill a woman, and a man is even more likely to kill a woman than a woman is to kill a man' (2000, p. 38). Clare also considers rape and sexual abuse as 'the commonest and often the most severe forms of physical abuse by men on women' (2000, p. 43). He goes on to examine organized violence such as wars, genocides and ethnic violence and atrocities. Clare rejects the biological explanations and comes down on the side of socialization and gender stereotypes (2000, p. 68).

However, we do not have to go down the route of either the biological or the socialization thesis to explain male violence. Psychoanalysis, although it has retreated from this thorny subject can, nevertheless, give us some explanations. As we have seen in Chapter 4, Klein talks about the boy's 'excessive protestations of masculinity' and the use he makes of his aggression to assert his threatened masculinity and his sense of humiliation as he is faced with his feelings of inferiority towards the mother (Klein, 1928).

In this sense, aggression and violence can be seen as masculine defences against feelings of humiliation and dissolution of identity. We would expect therefore to find that males who are insecure in their sense of self and in their masculinity would feel easily humiliated and, under certain circumstances, use violence to bolster their masculinity (the patient in Chapter 2 is an example of this). It is as if violence makes the insecure or humiliated male respectable.

Studies on violent fundamentalist groups cite shame, humiliation and feeling disrespected as the most consistently present feature in the development of terrorism (Alderdice, 2002; Varvin, 2003; Chodorow, 2003). National or group trauma and humiliation is closely related to this loss of identity and narcissistic investment (Volkan, 2003). Another characteristic mentioned in studies on terrorism is that most terrorists are overwhelmingly young dissatisfied men (Varvin, 2003; Akhtar, 2002, 2003; Alderdice, 2002).

Salman Akhtar writes: 'The leader is usually a traumatized and charismatic individual … The followers are usually *single, sexually inhibited young men*, equally traumatised themselves and struggling to achieve a sense of selfhood and a cohesive identity' (Akhtar, 2002, p. 91; italics mine). Paxton mentions that the leader is always male and refers to fascism as a 'masculine fraternity' (Paxton, 2004).

One author who linked masculinity, humiliation and violence is Nancy Chodorow. In her paper 'Hate, humiliation and masculinity' she connects masculine vulnerability to terrorism, nationalism and fundamentalism (Chodorow, 2003, p. 102). As I have looked at this paper in Chapter 5 I shall only remind the reader of Chodorow's description of the 'fault-lines' of masculinity. She defines these as:

> 1. masculinity defined by a negative statement—as *not-female*, that is the male as defensively separating from, and warding off, the female 'other' and defining himself as not-female; and
> 2. maleness as adult man rather than boy-child, not humiliated, shamed or defeated by another man.
>
> (Chodorow, 2003, p. 103)

The first component which is part of the defensive separation from mother—male as not-female—constitutes a main part of most contemporary authors understanding of the vulnerability of masculinity (see Wieland, 2014, ch. 5). The second component is the main dynamic of the positive Oedipus complex and constitutes Freud's main understanding of the 'repudiation of femininity', that is femininity as submission to another man which equals femininity and castration (Freud, 1937).

For Chodorow any threat or humiliation that the individual or the ethnic or religious community or nation endures, becomes also a threat to masculinity. Humiliations—which include defeat in war and occupation of a country as well as the helplessness that accompany them—have the unconscious meaning of feminization and of loss of selfhood. The humiliation of the group with which one identifies becomes a personal humiliation. This is true for ordinary warfare and ethnic and nationalist violence as well as for childhood fist-fights. But she sees the extreme violence of the holocaust and of other genocides as involving both components of masculinity—the fear of humiliation by a man *and* the 'regressive pull' and fear of the fusion with mother. In this sense her analysis helps us to link phenomena at different levels—the level of individual identity, the level of group identity (cultural, religious) and the level of national identity. We can also differentiate phenomena at the oedipal level that include a traumatic defeat by a father or brother on the one hand; and the wish to delete and erase the trauma by a merging experience with mother on the other. In this sense there are two ways in which a man can become feminised: (1) by merging with mother—an omnipotent wish and (2) by being belittled by father or other males—which threatens to render him helpless and throw him back to being mother's baby and expose his wish for a merging experience with her.

In this sense we can follow the chain from humiliation to helplessness to a merge with mother, feminisation and the reaction through violence. Violence now defines the male.

The wish to go back to mother following a traumatic event is movingly explored by Michael Roper in his study of soldiers' response to trauma in the First World War (Roper, 2009). Roper found that very often, under extreme stress or trauma, a return to a state of infantile dependence occurred and often the word 'mother' was the last word the soldiers uttered as they lay dying. It is as if trauma had the power to dissolve the myth of heroic masculinity. What was left was a vulnerable human being feeling like a little child wanting to be taken into mother's arms. Roper quotes Wilfred Bion's description of his own regressed fears and longings at a moment of extreme anxiety:

> The strain had a very curious effect; I felt that all anxiety had become too much; I felt like a small child that has had a tearful day and wants to be put to bed by its mother; I felt curiously eased by lying down on the bank by the side of the road, just as if I was lying peacefully in someone's arms.
>
> (Quoted in Roper, 2009, p. 1)

And a German soldier crashed by a tank and being delirious moaning 'Mutter, Mutter, Mutter' and approached by an English soldier who held his hand and whispered 'All right son, it's all right. Mother's here with you' (Roper, 2009, p. 2).

The clash here with ideas of heroic masculinity could not be stronger. The little boy wanting to be enveloped in mother's arms is hardly a model of the hero 'standing alone'. For men secure in their sense of self these experiences may strengthen their understanding of themselves and their own vulnerability. However, for others these experiences may be a source of utter humiliation and 'unmanning' at a time when masculinity was seen as a capacity to fight and die 'like a man'.

However, this less than heroic masculinity finds a container within the army and the camaraderie of fellow soldiers. Going back to civilian life many men declared that they missed the intimacy of comradeship and of shared experience. Adjusting to civilian life after a time at the front is notoriously difficult. The army with its shared experience acts as a container not only for extreme anxiety but also for male anxieties.

At the time of writing the shocking statistics about ex US soldiers who fought in Afghanistan taking their own lives dominate the headlines. The fact that more US soldiers died by their own hands after they had been discharged from the army than in battle, speaks volumes about traumatic experiences not contained within a group (or in any other way). The army that had caused their trauma was also the container for their trauma. The loss of this container drives many men to suicide or mental illness.

Men, Groups and Homogenisation

We can begin to understand why male groups are so important for men, so much so that as we have seen Lionel Tiger attributed a genetic wiring to the male drive towards group formation. Tiger, like Robert Bly (Bly, 1990) has been very influential in the USA triggering more male groups to be formed where men searched for their 'lost' masculinity (Parker, 1997).

But how can we explain this attraction of males to groups in a psychoanalytic way? I suggest that the answer can be sought in the realm of narcissism. An explanation of group phenomena in terms of narcissism has been offered by many theorists and examined in Chapters 6 and 7 (Freud, 1921; Bion, 1961; Anzieu, 2001; Kernberg, 2003a, 2003b; Hinshelwood, 2006, 2007). In this sense individual narcissism becomes invested in the group and in the leader with whom they identify. To answer the aforementioned question of how masculinity can be 'lost' we can say that it is male narcissism (phallic narcissism) that has been lost or wounded and seeks its re-instatement within a male group led by a male leader.

We can say that individuals with wounded narcissism seek groups to restore their narcissistic integrity. If we take into account the boy's primary narcissistic wound *vis-à-vis* the mother (Wieland, 2014, chs. 4 & 5) we can see why insecure men, that is men who have not worked through this early narcissistic trauma, are attracted to groups or ideologies, and why very insecure men are more likely to join groups as a way of bolstering their masculinity as well as their fragmenting personality. Religious and political fundamentalism thrives on group narcissism (Hinshelwood, 2006, 2007; Kernberg, 2003a) which seems to restore the early narcissistic illusions of wholeness and omnipotence. National and group humiliations re-kindle the narcissistic trauma and drive some men towards extreme military groups where masculinity is underwritten by violence.

The restoration of narcissistic omnipotence is part of the function of religion. The combination of religious elements with the worship of violence is the terrain of fascism.

According to Klaus Theweleit, Hitler basically offered a new religion. He writes:

> It seems to me misleading to see the Führer as a demagogue—or his speeches as theatrical. Both terms deny not only the needs of the participating crowd but above all the undeniable fact that the Führer is bestowing a gift on his people. He offers them a religion—not a substitute, but a real one.
>
> (Theweleit, 1989, p. 413)

In relation to this Theweleit quotes from Albert Speer's diaries:

> But it was when the ritual was finally agreed upon—indeed it was almost canonized—that I first became aware that the whole thing was meant to be taken literally. I had always believed all these parades, processions, and initiation ceremonies to be part of a virtuoso propagandistic review. It was now clear that for Hitler it was a matter of founding a church
>
> (Speer, quoted in Theweleit, 1989, footnote 53, p. 475)

The fascist religion that Hitler offered had to do with the fusion of males together and the fusion of the group with the Führer. In this fusion the worship of purity coupled with the worship of violence and war became the 'making of the man'.

Theweleit examined the drive for fusion as a main characteristic of fascist groups. In his book *Male Fantasies* (1987, 1989) he looks at the novels of some men from the Freikorps[1] and examines the main themes that emerge out of these novels. In relation to the key themes of these texts he writes: '… I described the impulse towards fusion as a key dynamic of fascist organization formation and fascist propaganda …' (1989, p. 213). In relation to this Theweleit sees the basic dynamic as a longing for a 'unification with maternal bodies, within which it can become "whole", born to completion' (1989, p. 213). However, he goes on to say that this kind of fusion is 'marked by revenge, which, as we have seen, cannot fail to transform the artificial and violent symbiosis that is to follow into a relationship of domination' (1989, p. 213).

In another passage he writes: 'Almost all authors discussed in this study provide similarly celebratory accounts of the sameness of the soldier males' (1989, p. 350).

This kind of mass identity that is created through the 'sameness of soldier males' uses aggression, violence, militarist language and militarist paraphernalia to make sure that we make no mistake that these are real men—hard, military and ready to die. But even death is not a quiet affair but has to happen in an explosion, with a bang, and with the violent dissolution of body and mind. Theweleit dwells on this characteristic of the fascist mind—the wish for an explosion, which becomes a moment of violent fusion, a moment of an anti-erotic dissolution of the ego. He quotes one of the formulations favoured by the Freikorps: 'To smash the world to pieces, and then perish' (1989, p. 350). In another place he puts it like this:

> The texts of the soldier males perpetually revolve around the same central axes: The communality of the male society, non-female creation, rebirth, the rise upwards to hardness and tension; the phallus rising to a higher level. The man is released from a world that is rotten and sinking (from the morass of femaleness); he finally dissolves in battle.
>
> (1989, p. 361)

Although Theweleit's study has been criticised on many grounds (for instance that the Freikorps were not fascists and not everybody who belonged to the Freikorps went on to join Hitler's NSDAP and that Hitler himself never joined the Freikorps) I think that his analysis of the fusion sought in the pre-fascist and fascist groups is very insightful and revealing of the underlying forces and contradictions involved in the fascist state of mind.

Masculinity and Feminisation

The fear of feminisation and of not being proved to be a man seems to have been a widespread masculine fear in Wilhelmine Germany (Santner, 2000), and probably in the whole of nineteenth-century Europe and can be linked to what Alexander Mitscherlich has called the 'fatherless society' (Mitscherlich, 1973). Mitscherlich linked this to the fact that fathers in modern society are, on the whole, absent from the household as work has progressively moved from the home to the workplace. In this sense children grow up without a personal engagement with a father who sets boundaries and creates frustration but who is present to work this through with his own children. In the place of the personal father a series of rules and severe discipline stepped in to fill the gap. In this way the obedient individual is created who lacks strong emotional ties and who is ready to substitute the group for the family as a place of emotional fulfilment. This leads inevitably to a mass society yearning for an authority figure.

This seems to support my argument that male group phenomena are used, not only to bond men together as Lionel Tiger has suggested (Tiger, 1969), but more importantly to supply a ready-made male identity for the fatherless sons. Mitscherlich does not refer to the development of masculinity but his analysis of the mass society and the 'sibling society' or 'fatherless society' touches on the father vacuum in the development of masculinity within modern society and therefore on the development of systems which promote the homogenisation of men as one big organism larger than life. This bigger-than-life masculinity is always in fear of contamination by women and those representatives of the feminised man—the Jews.

The Jew as the feminised man was a stereotype of nineteenth-century Germany, and more widely, Europe, and was connected with the fact of circumcision which was seen to be feminising the male. This led to the Jew being seen not only as feminised and degenerate but also as diseased, or more than that, as the disease itself (Santner, 2000; Gilman, 1993; Geller, 1992).

Eric Santner talking about Gilman's work writes: 'According to Gilman florid fantasies about the consequences of circumcision abounded in nineteenth century European culture in general and in medical discourse in particular' (Santner, 2000, p. 110).

And:

> In the medical discourse of the nineteenth century ... circumcision was as evil as it was inescapable for the Jew because it led to the specific diseases that corrupted the individual and eventually the body politic ... The linked dangers of sexuality, syphilis, and madness were constantly associated with the figure of the male Jew. [...] Central to the definition of the Jew was the image of the male Jew's circumcised penis as impaired, damaged, or incomplete, and therefore threatening to the wholeness and health of the male Aryan.
>
> (Gilman, cited in Santner, 2000, p. 111)

But Gilman's work also talks about the link between 'circumcision, feminisation, and antisemitism' in European culture (Santner, 2000, p. 110).

We can now see the chain of associations Hitler used in *Mein Kampf* between Jews, disease, degeneracy, Germany's defeat in First World War, and the contamination and weakening of German blood. We are now in a position to complete the last link which links the Jew to the feminized male and the feminine part of the self. In this chain of associations the fear of feminisation is projected onto a minority which is then seen not only as abject, but also as contaminating and as threatening the health of the nation. The discourse was now one of disease and contamination versus health and purity of blood.

In an article entitled 'What does man want?, or the political meaning of the phallus' Daniel Boyarin examines the masculinity problems in colonised territories. In this article Boyarin quotes Frantz Fanon:

What does a man want?
What does the black man want?
At the risk of arousing the resentment of my coloured brothers, I will say that the black is not a man.

(Fanon, 1967, quoted in Adams and Savran, 2002, p. 280)

This citation by Frantz Fanon exploring the influence of colonialism on the colonised male expresses this influence as unmanning. Boyarin comments: 'The racial other lacks the phallus; "he" is always castrated' (Boyarin, quoted in Adams and Savran, 2002, p. 280). He continues by comparing the colonised male with the European Jews and the perception in both cases that they were 'castrated'.

I shall not go into the Fanon thesis of the divided colonised subject and the self-contempt that this engenders as he tries to emulate the master country's culture. What is important for my argument here is how much humiliation in males is linked to being feminised, unmanned or castrated.

However, Boyarin also looks at the original intention behind the custom of circumcision. Commenting on rabbinic literature he comments: 'Circumcision was understood somehow as rendering the male somewhat feminine, thus making it possible for the male Israelite to have communion with a male deity' (Boyarin, quoted in Santner, 2000, p. 118).

We now begin to understand that the loathing of the Jew in European culture is not a straight forward affair and that envy has a great part to play. If the Jew by the virtue of being feminised comes closer to God, he is obviously to be envied and all the sacrifices that the European male has had to make—such as being removed from mother prematurely and undergoing a series of harsh training to toughen up—may look rather futile. The envy of the Jew, and of woman, can only be counteracted by hatred and loathing.

A look at the protagonist of National Socialism, Adolf Hitler, may throw some more light on the relationship between insecure masculinity and the fascist state of mind. In his book *The Mind of Adolf Hitler* (1973)[2] the psychoanalyst Walter Langer examines, among other things, Hitler's sexuality and gender identity. Contrary to most people's expectations he sees Hitler as having a 'strong feminine component in his physical makeup' (Langer, 1973, p. 172). Langer continues:

> There is every reason to suppose that during his early years, instead of identifying himself with his father as most boys do, he identified himself with his mother … Many writers and informants have commented on his feminine characteristics—his gait, his hands, his mannerisms, and his way of thinking. Hanfstaengl reports that when he showed Dr Jung a specimen of Hitler's handwriting, the latter immediately exclaimed that it was a typically feminine hand.
>
> (Langer, 1973, p. 172)

Langer comments on his 'over submissiveness' in the army, his 'extreme sentimentality, his emotionality, his occasional softness, and his weeping' and suggests that his fear of cancer is also an indication of his identification with his mother as his mother died of cancer.

Ian Kershaw reporting on the impression Hitler made on those who knew him quotes Helene Hanfstaengl's remark to her husband 'believe me he is an absolute neuter, not a man' (Kershaw, 1998, p. 187). Kershaw also adds that her husband Putzi Hanfstaengl who was a close friend and supporter was convinced that Hitler was impotent (Kershaw, 1998, p. 187). Hitler's avoidance of intimate relationships and his fear of women are well documented (Kershaw, 1998; Hayman, 1997; Fromm, 1974).

His disgust and repugnance of sexual activity but also his fascination with the subjects of sex, homosexuality, and prostitution is also well documented (Kershaw, 1998, pp. 45–46). But Kershaw insists that the rumours about Hitler's sexual perversions and 'sordid sado-masochistic practices' are based on 'dubious evidence' and that there is no solid evidence to corroborate this (1998, p. 46).

After examining the scarce evidence that exists about Hitler's sexual life Erich Fromm concludes:

> Whatever the nature of Hitler's perversion, the details hardly matter, nor does his sexual life explain anything more about him than what we know already. In fact, the credibility of the scarce data we have on his sexual life rests mainly on our knowledge of his character.
>
> (Fromm, 1974, p. 548)

'It is remarkable', Erich Fromm writes, 'that quite a few women who had been close to Hitler committed—or tried to commit—suicide: Geli Raubal, Eva Braun (twice), Renee Muller, Unity Mitford, and a few, more doubtful cases quoted by Maser' (Fromm, 1974, p. 548).

His relationship with Geli Raubal his 18-year-old niece, is perhaps the only one that resembled a normal human relationship. (We can deduce the incestuous theme here.) People around him reported that he looked like a man in love. The absolute control he attempted to exercise over her reminds one of the young Hitler as described by his friend Kubizek (see Chapter 6). The relationship lasted for 4 years until Geli's controversial death—suicide or murder. After her death Hitler looked like a broken man and as far as we know he never loved another woman again. On the subject of intimacy Langer writes about Hitler:

> He has cut himself off from the world in which love plays any part for fear of being hurt, and what love he can experience is fixated on the abstract entity—Germany, which, as we have seen, is a symbol of his ideal mother.
>
> (Langer, 1973, p. 167)

Langer's book *The Mind of Adolf Hitler* has been severely criticised by historians when it was finally published in 1973 for its historical shortcomings (Pick, 2012). But the book seemed to have survived the criticism and became an unexpected best seller in the 1970s. From the psychoanalytic viewpoint, however, we can only admire the insightfulness with which Langer understood Hitler's internal world in its contradictions and deadly denials.

Conclusion

In this chapter I have brought together several components of both masculinity and fascism. My argument is that insecure masculinity and humiliation and, therefore, violence, are linked, and they are linked via the same route that makes masculinity insecure and vulnerable in the first place. This is the wish for merging and the wish to erase the reality of difference, separateness and loss. These wishes, and the fears attached to them, are evoked especially in times of individual or social and political crisis as the traumatised self seeks refuge in mother's protective body.

As I hope to have shown, the wish for merging activates the death instinct and in the male activates the castration complex as a buffer against the death instinct (Jones, 1932). Merging with mother becomes now a matter of castrated masculinity. In the fascist state of mind the state of merging, which is a state of narcissistic elation, takes place within a wholly masculine container—the male violent or militaristic group. This homogenised militarist group is a compromise formation that allows males to have a narcissistic, merging experience without being feminised. This homogenised group is necessarily paranoid and touches on a psychotic state of mind. Plurality itself is experienced as contaminating because it contains femininity not only as the 'other', but as a desirable and therefore threatening state. Fragments of expelled femininity are everywhere and have to be exterminated. Hence, the metaphor for the 'enemy within', the Jew is not one of whole objects but of millions of parasites or viruses as Hitler's *Mein Kampf* exemplifies (I shall examine this in Chapter 9).

My exploration of the fascist state of mind brings together two different modes of functioning in a malignant way, that is in a way that destructiveness becomes dominant and assumes perverse qualities: (1) a sado-masochistic mode and (2) a delusional/homogenised mode. Both are ways the male tries to deal with the femininity inside.

The sado-masochistic mode is a surrender of the ego to a harsh superego Freud named this kind of superego a 'pure culture of the death instinct' (Freud, 1923, p. 53) and Bion called it an 'ego-destructive superego', or a 'super' ego devoid of any morality (Bion, 1962, p. 97).

We can say that this functioning has been in evidence in the 'normal' cultural personality structure in Germany during the last decades of the nineteenth century and until the end of the First World War and has been described as the 'authoritarian character' or the 'authoritarian personality' (Horkheimer, 1936; Fromm, 1941; Adorno et al., 1950; Reich, 1933; Mitscherlich, 1973; Money-Kyrle, 1978).

It is necessary to say that the authoritarian state of mind is not, in my opinion, a fascist state of mind. However, I suggest that the totalitarian state of mind presents itself as a seduction to liberate the individual from this slavery of the superego present in the authoritarian state of mind. In this sense, the authoritarian personality predisposes the subject towards a totalitarian, homogenised state of mind where the slavery of the superego is abolished. The fusion with the Führer abolishes, however, if only momentarily, the sado-masochistic mode, together with the object itself, and establishes omnipotence as the predominant personality trait. The Fuehrer himself has undergone the same kind of fusion—first with the omnipotent part of himself—the 'Great Mother', Nature, History—and then with his followers. Any relation to reality can now be relinquished as the ego is merged with the superego and the superego with the ego-ideal and with the id in the delusional mother/baby union. Any ego functioning is hijacked by the totalitarian 'Fuehrer' and can exist only in relation to totalitarian aims. However, since fascism, as we have seen, cannot exist in a pure state an oscillation between a sado-masochistic state and a homogenised state characterises the fascist state of mind. Submission and homogenisation co-exist and give the fascist state a different dynamic from that of an authoritarian dictatorship both within the psyche and in society.

I suggest that the authoritarian personality acted as a kind of 'psychic retreat' (Steiner, 1993) for the German people to contain aggression and guilt and the terrors of the core complex from the mid-nineteenth century up to the end of First World War. Under conditions of extreme trauma and humiliation psychic retreats can be destroyed and the individual is thrust into a confusing world. Such a national trauma was, for Germany, the defeat in the First World War and the humiliating terms that were imposed on her by the allies. Added to these, the Crash in 1929 and the Depression that followed acted as further traumatic situations.

The dissolution of the ego's defences in traumatic circumstances means that the individual is exposed to primitive anxieties of annihilation and loss of identity including the loss of a secure gender identity. The masochistic surrender of the ego to the superego which had been up to the end of the war the normal 'cultural type' (Dicks, 1972) meant that the ego remained weak and unable to face traumatic changes in the environment, especially the loss of a strong, non-humiliated authority. The new retreat was to embrace fascism and a charismatic leader with whom one was invited to merge, and who promised the destruction of the traumatic reality and the rebirth and regeneration of the nation. The surrender to a leader who promised his followers a part of himself and participation to a new rebirth, spelled the creation of a different kind of retreat which had all the hallmarks of a pathological organization with psychotic traits (Segal, 1972; Steiner, 1993). This surrender is different from the submission to the superego. This kind of surrender does away with the superego and with any differentiation within the self. The omnipotence that it creates claims to be liberation.

What I am describing could be any cult or religion as well as extreme political ideologies. However, what distinguishes fascism, and other extreme fundamentalist/terrorist ideologies, from a peaceful religious cult is the use of organized violence and militarism, not as a means to an end but *as an ideal in itself*. It is simultaneously a religion and a gang.

The fact that my emphasis has been on masculinity and the ego-syntonic use of violence in masculine identity does not preclude women from this state of mind. However, violence in women is not, on the whole, ego-syntonic and does not enhance their feminine identity. Of course, as supporters of violence or of violent parties like the Nazi Party women vicariously experienced their own aggression and their own sense of omnipotence. Claudia Koonz shows how as supporters of the National Socialist Party in Germany women have been ardent campaigners and contributed a great deal to the success of the Party. I shall examine her contribution to the understanding of women's part in National Socialism in Chapter 9.

Here I offer a tentative hypothesis about the relation between the fascist state of mind and masculinity. I suggest that the fascist state of mind is a 'compromise' solution between a wish to merge (which is experienced as a feminine wish) and a wish to bolster masculinity. It is a compromise solution in the sense that a symptom according to Freud is a compromise solution.[3] In this sense the wish is not given up but appears in a disguised form: The child's wish to merge with mother is not given up as impossible. Instead it appears in its disguised form as a delusional 'male merge' within an all-male omnipotent group led by an omnipotent Fuehrer. Instead of dealing with reality the group is now taken up by several basic assumptions[4] at the same time—the messianic delusion co-existing with the fighting mode and the dependence mode creates the mixture of ideas that is fascism. The persecution of those seen as weak, soft or feminine is now inevitable.

In the next chapter I shall expand on the fraudulent identity of the fascist based on this hotchpotch of delusional ideas.

Notes

1 The Freikorps were right-wing private armies or warlords that roamed Germany after the First World War and attacked socialists, communists, and trade unionists. Eventually, they were disbanded or absorbed into the Nazi movement. Hitler did not belong to the Freikorps. Klaus Theweleit uses their writings to understand proto-fascist and fascist emotions and ideas.

2 Walter Langer, a psychiatrist and a psychoanalyst, was approached in 1941 by the USA Intelligence Services and was given the task of providing a psychological profile of Adolf Hitler which could predict his likely moves and development. The result was a secret report which later became the book *The Mind of Adolf Hitler* (1973).

3 For Freud, a symptom was a compromise between the gratification of a wish and its denunciation.
4 Bion distinguished three basic assumptions as best describing a regressed group: dependence, fight-flight and pairing.

References

Adams, R., & Savran, D. (eds.) (2002) *The Masculinity Studies Reader*. Malden, MA, Blackwell.
Adorno, T.W., Frenkel-Brunswik, E., Levinson, D. J., & Nevitt Sanford, R. (1950) *The Authoritarian Personality*. New York, The Norton Library.
Akhtar, S. (2002) 'The psychodynamic dimension of terrorism', in C. Covington, P. Williams, J. Arundale, & J. Knox (eds.) *Terrorism and War: Unconscious Dynamics of Political Violence*. London, Karnac.
Akhtar, S. (2003) 'Dehumanization: origins, manifestation, and remedies', in S. Varvin, & V. Volkan (eds.) *Violence or Dialogue: Psychoanalytic Insights on Terror and Terrorism*. London, International Psychoanalytical Association.
Alderdice, L. (2002) 'Introduction', in C. Covington, P. Williams, J. Arundale, & J. Knox (eds.) *Terrorism and War: Unconscious Dynamics of Political Violence*. London, Karnac.
Anzieu, D. (2001) 'Freud's group psychology: background, significance, and influence', in D. Anzieu (ed.) *On Freud's 'Group Psychology and the Analysis of the Ego'*. London, The Analytic Press.
Bion, W. R. (1961) *Experiences in Groups*. London, Karnac.
Bion, W. R. (1962) *Learning from Experience*. London, Karnac.
Bly, R. (1990) *Iron John: A Book About Men*. Shaftesbury, Dorset, Element Books.
Chodorow, N. (2003) 'Hate, humiliation and masculinity', in S. Varvin, & V. Volkan (eds.) *Violence or Dialogue: Psychoanalytic Insights on Terror and Terrorism*. London, International Psychoanalytical Association.
Clare, A. (2000) *On Men: Masculinity in Crisis*. London, Chatto & Windus.
Dicks, H. (1972) *Licensed Mass Murder: A Socio-psychological Study of Some SS-Killers*. London, Sussex University Press in association with Heineman.
Freud, S. (1921) 'Group psychology and the analysis of the ego', in J. Strachey, A. Freud, A. Strachey, & A. Tyson (eds.) *The Standard Edition of the Complete Psychological Works of Sigmund Freud, Volume XVIII (1920–1922): Beyond the Pleasure Principle, Group Psychology and Other Works*. London, Hogarth Press, pp. 65–144.
Freud, S. (1923) 'The ego and the id', in J. Strachey, A. Freud, A. Strachey, & A. Tyson (eds.) *The Standard Edition of the Complete Psychological Works of Sigmund Freud, Volume XIX (1923–1925): The Ego and the Id and Other Works*. London, Hogarth Press, pp. 3–68.
Freud, S. (1937) 'Analysis terminable and interminable', in J. Strachey, A. Freud, A. Strachey, & A. Tyson (eds.) *The Standard Edition of the Complete Psychological Works of Sigmund Freud, Volume XXIII (1923–1925): Moses and Monotheism, An Outline of Psycho-Analysis and Other Works*. London, Hogarth Press, pp. 209–254.
Fromm, E. (1941) *Escape from Freedom*. New York, Holt, Rinehart and Winston.
Fromm, E. (1974) *The Anatomy of Human Destructiveness*. Harmondsworth, Penguin Books
Geller, J. (1992) 'The unmanning of the wandering Jew', *American Imago*, 49, pp. 227–262.
Gilman, S. (1993) *Freud, Race and Gender*. Princeton, NJ, Princeton University Press.
Hayman, R. (1997) *Hitler and Geli*. London, Bloomsbury.

Hinshelwood, R. D. (2006) 'Racism: being ideal', *Psychoanalytic Psychotherapy*, 20, pp. 84–96.
Hinshelwood, R. D. (2007) 'Intolerance and intolerable: The case of racism'. *Psychoanalysis Culture and Society*, 12, pp. 1–20.
Horkheimer, M. (ed.) (1936) *Autorität und Familie*. Paris, Librairie Félix Alcan.
Jones, E. (1932) 'The phallic phase', in Ernest Jones (ed.) *Papers on Psychoanalysis*. London, Maresfield Reprints.
Kernberg, O. (2003a) 'Sanctioned social violence: a psychoanalytic view – Part I', *International Journal of Psychoanalysis*, 84, pp. 683–698.
Kernberg, O. (2003b) 'Sanctioned social violence: a psychoanalytic view – Part II', *International Journal of Psychoanalysis*, 84, pp. 953–968.
Kershaw, I. (1998) *Hitler 1889–1936: Hubris*. London, Penguin Books.
Klein, M. (1928) 'The early stages of the Oedipus complex', in M. Klein (ed.) *Love, Guilt and Reparation and Other Works*. London, Hogarth Press.
Langer, W. (1973) *The Mind of Adolf Hitler*. London, Secker & Warburg.
Mitscherlich, A. (1973) *Society without the Father*. New York, Jason Aronson
Money-Kyrle, R. (1978) *The Collected Papers of R.E. Money-Kyrle*. Perth, Clunie Press.
Parker, I. (1997) *Psychoanalytic Culture*. London, Sage.
Paxton, R. (2004) *The Anatomy of Fascism*. London, Penguin Books.
Pick, D. (2012) *The Pursuit of the Nazi Mind*. Oxford, Oxford University Press.
Reich, W. (1933) *The Mass Psychology of Fascism*. Harmondsworth, Penguin Books.
Roper, M. (2009) *The Secret Battle: Emotional Survival in the Great War*. Manchester, Manchester University Press.
Santner, E. (2000) *My Own Private Germany: Daniel Paul Schreber's Secret History of Modernity*. Princeton, NJ, Princeton University Press
Segal, H. (1972) 'A delusional system as a defence against the re-emergence of a catastrophic situation', *International Journal of Psychoanalysis*, 53, pp. 393–401.
Steiner, J. (1993) *Psychic Retreats*. London, Routledge
Theweleit, K. (1987) *Male Fantasies, Vol. 1*. Oxford, Polity Press.
Theweleit, K. (1989) *Male Fantasies, Vol. 2*. Oxford, Polity Press.
Tiger, L. (1969) *Men in Groups*. Melbourne, Nelson.
Varvin, S. (2003) 'Trauma and its after effects', in S. Varvin, & V. Volkan (eds.) *Violence or Dialogue: Psychoanalytic Insights on Terror and Terrorism*. London, International Psychoanalytical Association.
Volkan, V.D. (2003) 'Traumatized societies', in S. Varvin, & V. Volkan (eds.) *Violence or Dialogue: Psychoanalytic Insights on Terror and Terrorism*. London, International Psychoanalytical Association.
Wieland, C. (2014) *The Fascist State of Mind and the Manufacturing of Masculinity: A Psychoanalytic Approach* (1st ed.). Routledge.
Wieland, C. (2017) 'The primitive container of fascism: Masculine anxieties and defences in times of trauma and uncertainty', in N. Mintchev, R. Hinshelwood (eds.) *The Feeling of Certainty. Studies in the Psychosocial*. Cham, Palgrave Macmillan. https://doi.org/10.1007/978-3-319-57717-3_8
Wieland, C. (2023) 'Trauma and the fascist state of mind: The emptying of the self and the road to perdition', *Psychoanalytic Inquiry*, 43(2), pp. 84–95. https://doi.org/10.1080/07351690.2023.2163145

Chapter 8

Fascism and the Web of Perversion

Sue Grand

Reasons for Inclusion

Grand's excellent paper on the eroticised bonds that sustain fascist groups is an important intervention in contemporary psychoanalytic studies on fascism. Fascism has been theorised as a form of perversion by Lacanian theorists like Slavoj Žižek, Juliet Flower MacCannel (1993), and Antonios Vadolas (2009). This rich line of theorising, however, tends to be neglected by those using object relational psychoanalysis to understand fascism, who emphasise defences like splitting and projection over the erotic and sexualised aspects of fascist politics. Focusing on the United States and its history of Black slavery and fascistic political movements from the KKK onwards, Grand explores the interplay between narcissism, masculinity, racism, erotic relations between leaders and followers, and the violent othering of non-conforming bodies. The result is a rich and nuanced picture of the relational, psychosexual lives of people involved in fascist movements, and an essential contribution to psychoanalytic studies in fascism.

***

As a young boy growing up in Mussolini's Italy, Umberto Eco only knew Fascism. In 1942, at the age of ten, he writes an essay for the Italian Fascists. The essay must address the rhetorical question, "Should we die for the glory of Mussolini and the immortal destiny of Italy?" (Eco, 1995, p. 1). Eco is smart, and he knows the 'right' answer. He wins that competition, receiving what may have been his first award. By 1943, Mussolini is deposed. In 1945, Milan is liberated by partisans, and DUCE is executed. Once, he was all powerful and idealized. Now, his body is kicked and spat upon. Eco's mother sends him out to buy the newspaper. Each newspaper was now endorsed by one of five or six different political parties. In a system of one party, absolute rule, these parties had previously had a clandestine, subversive existence. Suddenly emergent in a public cacophony of difference, they all cheered the end of dictatorship, and the return of freedom. For the first time, Eco learns that "freedom of speech is freedom from rhetoric" (1995, p. 1). Looking back, Eco says he was reborn as a free man.

Many years pass, and Eco writes another essay, this one is an antidote to the first. In 1995, he publishes *Ur-Fascism*, because fascism is reemergent. In this

DOI: 10.4324/9781003742876-12

essay, he revisits his early memories, and asks, "Is there still another ghost stalking Europe?" (1995, p. 2). He warns his reader that a neo-fascist turn is surfacing. Illuminating this ghost, Eco argues that fascism has no particular ideological essence. The *content* of its ideologies differ, but its *structure* re-occurs. He lists 14 features that characterize what he calls Ur-fascism or Eternal Fascism. Many of these characteristics co-exist in unquestioning contradiction, because fascism disdains thought and reflectivity. The result is what Loewenstein describes as "epistemological insanity" (2023, p. 133). As Eco puts it, "Thinking is perceived as a form of emasculation. Therefore, culture is suspect insofar as it is identified with critical attitudes." Thinking is considered passive, effete, and it is feminized. Fascism is a muscular "cult of action for action's sake;" in which "*life is permanent warfare*" (Eco, 1995, p. 7, italics in text). As Fromm ([1941] 1970) suggested, the demagog offers an "escape from freedom," a reprieve from isolation, ambiguity, and doubt. Martial combat, heroic violence; a sanctified past; a call for supremacy; moral indignation and a moral void; a collectivized self; threats from without and within: This is fascism's structure.

From the perspective of 2025, the characteristics described by Eco are disturbingly familiar. In 1995, when Eco wrote this essay, this stalking ghost was being resurrected throughout Europe. Where once there was Hitler, Mussolini, Franco, and Salazar, now—in 2025—we have Putin, Orban, Modi, and Trump. Democracy is at risk. As Salberg suggests [Chapter 12 in this reader] the world seems to have forgotten fascism's menace. Instead, the world is falling prey to its phallic enticements. In the United States, that enticement is manifest in MAGA fever. But fascism is not new to the United States (see Rachel Maddow, 2023). As Spector and Venkatasubramanian suggest (2023), there has always been a "living core" of fascism in this country. The characteristics of Ur-Fascism reoccur throughout our history. In the United States, White democracy was always rooted in a totalitarian regime of racialized persecution. As Singh puts it, "white liberal democracy has continually imagined fascism as its monstrous Other (but) fascism might be better understood as its doppelganger or double" (Singh, 2017 p. 26). It is the racial violence and oppression inherent in White liberal democracies that causes Toscano (2023) to argue that liberal democracies exist on *continuum* with fascism. Paxton (2004) identifies the KKK as the first fascist movement, well before Mussolini formalized Fascism. As Toni Morrison (1995) put it, fascism is the succubus twin of racism. What many White people are just discovering, African Americans have always known: They were the first to recognize the threat emerging in Europe during the 1920s (Baldwin, 1962; Duensing, 2023). The KKK fed into White Christian Nationalism in the 1930s. These were pro-Nazi movements, infected with the virulent antisemitism (Hochschild, 2022) that characterizes the alt-right today.

Persecutory Practices and Hard Bodies

War is to man what maternity is to the woman.

(Mussolini, *The Doctrine of Fascism*, 1932; italics in text)

> Anything relating to sexuality is not a private matter, but signifies the life or death of a people; world power or insignificance.
>
> (Heinrich Himmler, wedding speech, cited in Toscano, 2023, p. 133)

For Mussolini and Hitler, for Putin and Trump, the call to fascism seems like a call to repair the collective unmanning of men. In the United States, and in Europe, nationalism is seen as the antidote to aggrieved White male supremacy (see Brown, 2019; Wieland, 2015). This phallic restitution has contempt for the weak, the 'deviant,' and the feminine. In these regimes, Real Men fight, and Good Women Mother. The righteous are sanctified, they are 'pure' and they are ascendant. Homosexuals, the Black and the Jew: these are considered sub-human. These systems promise communal protection and rescue through submission to an all-powerful Father. But the price of this rescue is the persecutory control of the body politic. These controls are often infused with erotic texts and subtexts that deify cruelty (see Theweleit, 1987, 1989). Mobilized by the demagog, lit up by the crowd, these subtexts involve contradictory enticements, prescriptions, and prohibitions. The 'righteous' often have lurid projections about the degenerate and the 'deviant'. In these movements, fascists issue moralistic edicts; they seek and attack transgressors, *and* they engage in the unholy acts that they have forbidden. At other times, they perform machismo, dread sexuality, and repudiate the women whom they sexualize (Theweleit, 1987). In both positions, they praise a pure and fungible Mother-Wife, who is without sexual subjectivity. All of this is infused with racism and antisemitism. All of this draws on fiery tropes of Christianity: Hell awaits 'natural' 'carnal man' and only the 'pure' will be saved (Edwards, [1741]2020; see also Richards, 2023).

These themes are traced in Wieland (2015) psycho-historical work on fascist masculinity. And they are evident in Theweleit's (1987, 1989) examination of interwar narratives and memoirs written by male German fascists. The sheer pleasure of violence, the link to erotic paranoia and erotic hatred: This link is *not* mere psychoanalytic speculation. And this link is *not* unconscious in the fascist mind. In Theweleit's masterwork, *Male Fantasies*, he traces this explicit language and imagery in the narratives and memoirs written by male German fascists in the interwar period. In this meticulous study, fascist men are witch hunters for whom female sexuality is evil incarnate. These are the narrative descriptors for the proletarian women who wanted socialism in Germany after WWI: they are a 'bloody mass'; they are 'whores,' 'knife women,' they are 'hiding weapons under their skirts.' The communism of Rosa Luxenberg signified indiscriminate fornication (Ehrenreich, 1987, p. xiv). In these memoirs, sexed and gendered paranoia seemed to ignite the "mobilizing passions" (Paxton, 2004) that infuse fascism. There are manly ecstasies in blowing these women apart and penetrating them with bullets.

This celebration of violence—the preoccupation with a repellant, menacing sexuality—is operating now, in the White Christian Nationalism that sees homosexuals and transsexuals multiplying everywhere. Ostensibly, they are 'groomers,' they are 'pedophiles,' they will rape your daughter and turn your sons into girls. To MAGA, Black and Brown hordes are fornicating with whiteness and polluting that whiteness. To White Christian Nationalists, liberalism permits the pregnant woman to double as murderer: She might abort *her baby the day before she gives birth*. Only the 'righteous' can purge these 'deviants' and the democracy that birthed them. Theweleit (1987) finds that the befouled vagina was projected onto the brief democratic republic in interwar Germany. To these fascist men, "The morass that called itself the German republic is only the vagina of a giant whore" (1987, p. 392). When democracy itself is the whore spawning all these deviants, violence becomes the sacred duty of the crowd.

These sexed and gendered fixations gestate in cults of phallic supremacy (see Ben-Ghiat, 2020; Wieland, 2015, 2023). In articulating Ur Fascism, Eco highlights this culture of machismo, with its fusion of Eros and violence:

> Since both permanent war and heroism are difficult games to play, the Ur-Fascist transfers his will to power to sexual matters. This is the origin of *machismo* (which implies both disdain for women and intolerance and condemnation of nonstandard sexual habits from chastity to homosexuality). Since even sex is a difficult game to play, the Ur-Fascist hero tends to play with weapons.
>
> (Eco, 1995, p. 10)

Exploring authoritarian and fascist movements, Ben-Ghiat (2020) and Wieland (2015, 2023) trace this fixation with phallic hardness and phallic dominance, with its associated dread of everything 'female.' In particular, Wieland suggests that certain epochs evoke a male urge toward maternal fusion; this urge is experienced as the annihilation of masculinity. The fascist solution repudiates dependency on mother and substitutes martial dependency on, and fusion with, the fascist leader. A similar emphasis on the 'erotic politics of fascism emerges in the work of Reich ([1933]1970), Barratt (2020a, 2020b), and Diamond (2021, 2023).

In this article, I want to join with all of these authors, and probe the nexus of sex/gender/violence that is foundational to fascist movements. I want to highlight fascism's category of 'deviance,' and suggest that this 'deviance' is a site of hope even as it is a site of persecution. To pursue this inquiry, I explore intersecting phenomenon: fascism's hetero-hyper-masculinity; its sexed and gendered splitting; its moral sanctimony; and its projective web of perversion. Lastly, I will delve into the absolute control exerted over women, their bodies, and their sexuality. I agree with Barratt that "libidinality is implicated in the allure of authoritarianism and fascism" (2020a, p. 123). As Barratt suggests, we will not be able to understand or resist fascism without excavating what S. Hartmann (2022) has called, "the erotics of terror".

We need to look at the erotic fever ignited by dictators. But we also need to decenter these dictators and their minions. It is important to foreground the 'deviant'[1] and 'vaginal'[2] bodies who do not conform with fascism's dictates. I will suggest, with Charlap (2019), that these non-conforming 'unregulated' bodies question—and endanger—the phallic arrangements of the State. As Marasco (2021) suggests, we need to understand that trans liberation is not just a feminist project, it is an *anti-fascist* project. It is for this reason that trans-persons are the object of persecution in most authoritarian regimes.

All of this is evident in our contemporary alternative right. Just as Wieland (2015) would have predicted, Trumpism offers a grandiose, manic reparation for the perceived psychic and cultural wounds of White masculinity. MAGA draws its force from turning White male shame into rage. To transmute shame into rage, MAGA inflames racism, antisemitism, sexism, and the hatred of invading hordes. This is organized along strict gender binaries: male/female, dominance/submission, phallic/faggot, Mother/slut, purity/befoulment. This binary hierarchy, "forces a split between the self and relationships so that in effect men have selves, whereas women ideally are selfless" (Gilligan & Snider, 2018, p. 6). This strategy is reminiscent of the rise of Nazism in Germany. As Ben-Ghiat (2020), Fromm ([1941]1970), and Wieland (2015) note, Nazism was an antidote for cultural humiliation, defeat, rage, and deprivation after WWI. It was also a reaction against the sexual license and gender fluidity of interwar Berlin. In mimicry of Hitler's exhortations, Trump casts a halo over the White, 'traditional life' of the past. In the United States, that past was one of White masters and Black and indigenous slaves; it was 'pure' White women and 'lascivious' Blacks; criminalized homosexuality; and dominating men and subjugated women. To MAGA's followers, that memory seems idyllic. To restore its entitled position, whiteness is writing Jesus onto guns, so that Christ jettisons 'feminine' gentleness and compassion, becoming the right's phallic warrior (see Heschel, 2020). This violent inversion of Jesus is not peculiar to the contemporary alt-right. The Argentinian Junta praised Catholicism. But the Junta was a "nexus of religious, sexual and violent impulses" that moved to "repress human sexuality and to divert its insistent resurgence into religious violence" (Graziano, 1992, p. 55). The result: disappeared women were raped before they were killed.

Phallic Seductions and Phallic Mirrors

> In fascism, sexuality like wealth belongs to a powerful oligarchy. The masses are disposed of both.
>
> (Macchiocchi, cited in Toscano, 2023, p. 144)

As we examine this history, fascism certainly seems like an extreme form of Ruti's "gender obsession disorder" (2018). To legitimate its quest for power, MAGA is inscribing deviance onto trans, lesbian, and homosexual bodies; on immigrant bodies; on Black, Brown and indigenous bodies; and onto the bodies of women who seek abortion. In MAGA, there is only one legitimate form of sexuality: heterosexuality. There are only two biological genders. Women are either sluts or mothers. There are the White well-regulated bodies who conform to MAGA's sexed and gendered edicts. They are sanctified, and they seem entitled to power. Those who lack these identity markers, who do not (cannot) mirror this White phallic dominance: These will be purged through a conflagration.[3]

Fascist movements own women's sexuality. And while fascist movements dictate conformity and sexual repression, they do not merely prohibit desire. As Toscano (2023) points out, fascist movements have a thin veneer of moral purity and sexual repression. But the erotic arrangements of fascism are much more complex. As Fromm ([1941]1970), Reich ([1933]1970), and Barratt (2020a, 2020b) observe, fascist regimes *arouse and activate* the desires that expand their powers. Describing fascist rallies, Lowenthal and Guterman describe the agitated link between leader and crowd as a "striptease without end" (2021, p. 17). These regimes *also* awaken forbidden homoerotic desires. At Hitler rallies, at Trump's rallies, an electric current seems to run through the crowd. The crowd seems lit up in ecstasy, in desire for the Father. Trump excites his crowd with his aggression, his shameless White supremacy. His followers bask in his love, delighting in his proud, wanton, misogynist heterosexuality. At its surface, authoritarian and fascist movements extol moral sanctimony and sexual repression. But its rituals are phallic displays of enticement. The crowd's arousal occludes thought, evokes unthinking loyalty, and fuses individual lust with the martial lust of the State. We can see this operating in Mussolini's performance of machismo:

> Mussolini cut an incredible figure in the 1930s. Strutting on the balcony of the Palazzo Venezia in comic opera style in front of 100,000s of people chanting 'DUCE! DUCE!'. He built up an elaborate cult of personality around himself. News photos regularly showed him in a position of command, riding on horseback, flying an airplane, or driving a high performance car. He would strip to the waist to address farmers in the hot sun, or pose wresting with a lion cub.
>
> (From: *The Death of the Duce*, Benito Mussolini, April 28, 2020, WWII National Museum website)

This display is reminiscent of the video of Trump, face bloodied, fist pumped, yelling 'fight, fight,' at his assassination attempt. This video has gone viral. Twinning violence with the phallic ideal, posturing as the Great Father, Mussolini signified erotic prowess in a cult of Thanatos. Godlike, Hitler and Mussolini had a hypnotic effect on their crowds. Trump has that effect as well. These Leaders are "obscene fathers" (Toscano, 2023); they arouse ecstatic hope and passionate surrender. Like Putin, they perform virility and violence for the masses. To maintain absolute power, these Leaders must become the masses' object of desire. For the crowd to partake of his narcissism, he must be loved without the capacity for loving (Toscano, 2023). At his rallies, the Leader speaks to his sanctified followers: the righteous, the Christian, the heterosexual, the White. The cis man who wants to *be* him. The cis woman who wants to *have* him. The woman who praises her own subordination and domesticity. But Trump is also speaking to cis men in another forbidden, dissociated register: He seduces and then mortifies their *homoerotic desire*. We can imagine the moral savagery of this repressed homoerotic desire. Disavowed lust and shame, the fervor of rage, the fear and envy of the women who get to desire Trump: These readily convert into sadistic violence. There have been increased attacks on democratic leaders and institutions, election workers, librarians, the FBI, the raced and gendered other. All of this feeds on itself, in an escalating cycle of arousal, persecution, and violence.

To achieve absolute power, the demagog requires a perfect mirror for his hetero-hyper-masculine prowess. This requires a third female figure in the fascist narrative. This figure is neither the lascivious whore nor the desexualized wife/Mother. This is a woman whose sexuality is owned, not repressed (see Moshtagh, 2023). This is a woman whose passion is for him, and only for him. Her desire never deviates from its role as a mirror. In Michela C, the dictator meets his perfect subject:

> "DUCE, I saw you yesterday during your tumultuous visit to our city" wrote Michela C. of Siena in December, 1925. "Our eyes met. I told you of my admiration, devotion … I feared I would never know love in my life. Now I know that I love you … I understood that I had touched your heart from the heated way you looked at me just before I fainted."
>
> (quoted in Ben-Ghiat, 2020, p. 119)

While Michela C turns her adoring gaze on Mussolini, let's turn our gaze toward Mussolini's *other* witnesses. Think about this: what if a woman *laughs* at Mussolini's posturing? What if this woman is looking at another woman, instead of admiring his muscles? Imagine the cracks in his narcissism. In fascistic movements, this narcissistic rage is channeled into another embodied category, the Othered body. This is the category of the unregulated and the reviled. The hetero woman who laughs, the lesbian woman, the unwanted, the Black, the Jew, the 'vermin.' The woman who wants sex not babies. The non-binary. The cis man who wants another cis man. The cis man who looks at this Leader and *doesn't want him, and doesn't want to be him*. The trans woman and the trans man. The drag queens. The biological man who *wants* to be divested of his penis, so that he can call himself woman. Asian, Black, Brown and White people engaged in 'racial mixing.' All of these embodiments pose an existential threat. They are watching; they are looking *at* him and *through him*. What they see is not what the dictator wants to be seen. They are watching and they do *not* mirror his phallic narcissism. In MAGA's state of fragile narcissism, these eyes seem to be everywhere. This is a shaming panopticon that evokes volcanic rage. This gaze must be excised from Good White Christian existence. Nontraditional families, racial/ethnic 'mixing,' sexed and gendered fluidity: As Reich ([1933] 1970) suggested, these forms of love and sex do not pay obeisance to the Father. Their freedom defies phallic dominion; if this gets out of hand there will be *no* phallic dominion.

The Web of Perversion

Reading fascist narratives along with Theweleit (1987, 1989), we are exposed to a foul, projective psychosis that sees a web of perversion in the *Other*. But it is apparent that the web of perversion is fascism *itself*. Toscano (2023) refers to this as a "cathedral of erotic misery." As Barratt (2020b), Reich ([1933]1970), Hofstadter (1964), and Young-Bruehl (1996) suggest, fascism's response to 'unregulated bodies' is to demonize, persecute, and over-sexualize these enemies within. To maintain its claim to purity and dominance, reactionary regimes create this locus of subhuman, repellant objects. These objects are always paradoxical. They are vast and dangerous. They are contemptible for their weakness, but their seductive powers are almost overwhelming. Regardless of whether the regime is religious or secular, as Theweleit (1987, 1989) suggests, these subhuman objects are figured as agents of unholy lust. Reich traced this form of antisemitism in *Mein Kampf* (Hitler, [1925]2004). In *Mein Kampf*, the Jewish male is feminized. But he is *also* an incubus, penetrating innocent Aryan women, depositing his foul seed,

> With satanic joy in his face, the black-haired Jewish youth lurks in wait for the unsuspecting girl whom he defiles with his blood, thus stealing her from her people. … Just as he himself systematically ruins women and girls, he does not shrink back from pulling down the blood barriers for others, even on a large scale. It was and it is Jews who bring the Negroes into the Rhineland, always with the same secret thought and clear aim of ruining the hated white race by the necessarily resulting bastardization, throwing it down from its cultural and political height, and himself rising to be its master.
>
> (Hitler, [1925]2013, *Aryan and Jew*, p. 187)

According to Hitler, the Jewish woman is a malignant seductress. She births mongrel babies, spreads syphilis, weakness, and idiocy. To Hitler, sex between Aryans and Jews was 'inter-breeding;' it "was nothing else but to sin against the will of the eternal creator" (Reich [1933]1970, quoting Hitler, p. 76).

In fascism, these psychotic phantasms write destruction on the real body of the Other.

One might think, naively, that the 'pure' would avoid the repellant 'contaminating' object. But authoritarian minions tend to enact their prohibited lusts on the 'contaminating' body, and then, they purge contagion through sadism. Hartmann is one of the most eloquent explicators of this web of perversion. Studying African-American slavery, she illuminates an 'erotics of terror.' Here the female slave is categorized as primitive and always willing; she cannot be raped because, supposedly, she always 'wants it,' that is, she wants the White master who tortures her, and rapes her, and castrates/kills the father/husband who tries to save her. In this narrative, the predatory White master can never be a 'rapist.' African-American slavery was a totalitarian regime; it did not meet Eco's criteria for fascism. But, as I have noted, the KKK was the first fascist movement (see Paxton, 2004). The same 'erotics of terror' were at the core of the KKK's racist passions: the paranoia about Black male rape of the 'pure' White woman, the real White rape of the ostensibly 'impure' Black woman, the castration and lynching of innocent Black men. West also describes this 'psychosexual logic of racism.' To West (1982), the White man has a disavowed lust for the black penis that he castrates; the White man neutralizes the White woman's desire because he dreads her desire for this Black man. Caine (2023) finds the same dynamic in South African Apartheid: the white expulsion of blackness, and the libidinal attraction to the blackness which whiteness categorizes as repellant. All of this is enacted through the rape, torture, and murder of Black men and women.

This irresistible pull toward that which it extrudes as contaminating and repellant also appears in S. Heschel's description of antisemitism:

> Women and men play different roles in anti-Semitic heteronormative economy … male Jews are sexually abnormal in the anti-Semitic script, whereas Jewish women are portrayed as perfidiously seductive objects of dangerous desire … As an eroticized object, Jews are enemies and lovers, hated and yet desired as the mysterious object of hate … antisemitism associates Jews with carnal impurity, gender inversion, and sexual perversion … that was intended to portray Jews as undermining a 'decent society.'
>
> (Heschel, 2020, pp. 76–77)

Fixated on the projective perversion of the Other, lit up by racism and antisemitism, fascist regimes define erotic law and savage punishment. Then, fascist agents violate their own law because they are so compelled by that which they persecute and kill. In the Nazi concentration camps, guards held Jewish women in rape camps. In their eroticized death cult, the guards raped the Jewish women, whom they considered a contaminant to their Aryan powers (Hedgepeth & Saidal, 2010). Then contagion was purged: Many of these women were killed. All of this began in interwar Germany. In the same era, the German American Bund and the KKK were extolling their holy war, their White purity and supremacy, and spreading terror about lascivious Black and Jewish bodies. In White Nationalist movements, there always seems to be this contradiction between the surface of moral sanctimony and the web of perversion that fuels its persecutory passions. As Heschel points out, in the United States, lynching often occurred right after Sunday church services. To borrow Jackson-Sow's condemnation of White racism, authoritarian and fascist regimes seem to "want the pleasures of guilt and the appearance of innocence" (2022, p. 113).

The War on the Family

In the West, we are all suffering from the effects of neo-liberalism (see Friedman & Nakash, 2023; Hollander, 2017). To Reich, when capitalism begins to disintegrate under its own weight, "the conflict between sexuality and compulsive morality will of necessity reach its peak" (Reich, 1933/1970, p. 91). Ask Trump: Supposedly, Mexican rapists are invading America. Ask QAnon: Hillary Clinton ostensibly ran a vast network of pedophilia out of a pizza parlor in Florida. Meanwhile, Jeffrey Epstein got a pass and got rich running a REAL pedophile ring. Reich's perspective suggests that, in this shift from flawed democracy to neo fascism, the law of "divine violence" (Graziano, 1992) will be activated. The virgin/whore split intensifies, male sadism is cast as purification, and 'pure' women are increasingly enlisted to police 'wanton' women.

As citizens, we know the decay wrought by neo-liberalism. As psychoanalysts, we can understand cultural swells of paranoid-schizoid anxiety. We can feel the urge toward splitting, with its incorporation of goodness and its projection of badness (see Grand, 2023). We are familiar with the fragmentation that occurs with the return of the repressed. When splitting and projection falter, the repressed threatens to breach the protective barrier. In this neo-fascist era, the arousal ignited by the phallic leader will spill outside of its acceptable form. This fills fascism with dread. The only solution is projection; the raced/gendered category of deviance will keep expanding. But these paranoid-schizoid systems are inherently unstable. To keep the repressed from rebounding to the fascist collective, 'deviance' must be hunted down, brought under control, or annihilated. But what would happen if all that killing was effective? 'Deviance' would become a meaningless repository for extruded 'perversions'; fascist agents would suffer the return of the repressed. The paranoid state seems to know this: It is the sexed and gendered outliers who can return and destabilize the traditional family. This dread inspires the endless purges described by Arendt (1959).[4]

In the context of Trumpism, we can imagine Trump caught in this contradiction. Trump evokes, extrudes, and attacks the homoerotics that he ignites. He struts around with gorgeous women; these women are ciphers, mere tools in the competition with men. As long as his homoerotic desires are split off into those 'trans' and 'faggots,' we might not notice how much he seems to lust for Putin. We might not recall that he bragged about his love letters from Kim Jong Un of North Korea. Trump seems to be right: He could shoot someone on Fifth Avenue in NYC and not lose a single follower. In the eyes of his followers, he can do anything *except have sex with a man*. If the category of deviance was emptied out, there would be no projective container for Trump's homoerotics.[5] If Trump's homoerotic desires really became visible to his followers, American fascism might start to lose its grip. For this reason, the category of deviance must be persecuted, but it must never be entirely vanquished. This category must remain as the split off repository of fascisms' disavowed lusts. But if 'deviance' is not vanquished, the shaming panopticon goes on *looking at*, and through, the phallic leader. Collective anxiety escalates as cracks appear in phallic myths.

As Eco notes, these regimes have many defenses against this threat. In particular, nationalism spreads terror about the destruction of the family. As Reich suggested, the patriarchal family indoctrinates deference to phallic dominance; it is foundational to fascism. Witnessing the rise of Nazism in 1933, Wilhelm Reich makes this argument in *The Mass Psychology of Fascism*. Employing a Marxist/Freudian lens, Reich analyzes *Mein Kampf* and the social/historical context of post WWI Germany. In Reich's view, the patriarchal family is the essential building block of the capitalist/authoritarian state. It maintains its control and its structure through moralism and sexual/economic constraints, so that woman cannot even *imagine* resisting male dominance. The Father expects unquestioning submission from his wife and children, much as he unthinkingly submits to the layers of authority above him. For Reich, the reactionary turn is:

> More than anything else, it is a fear of 'sexual freedom' conceived of as sexual chaos and sexual dissipation in the mind of the reactionary thinker. ... In this interplay between economic and structural factors, it is the authoritarian family that represents the foremost and most essential source of reproduction of every kind of reactionary thinking; it is a factory where reactionary ideology and reactionary structures are produced. Hence, the 'safeguarding of the family,' i.e., of the authoritarian and large family, is the first cultural precept of every reactionary policy. This is what is essentially concealed behind the phrase, 'safeguarding of the state, culture and civilization'
>
> (Reich, [1933]1970, p. 60)

Reich emphasizes the centrality of cis female Eros to this project: This is inherently problematic, because it overlooks all of the sexed and gender outliers who *also* endanger the patriarchal family. But Reich's point is that, to achieve—and stabilize—capitalism, women's sexuality had to be repressed. With this repression, women could be conscripted into unpaid domestic labor, into the reproduction of phallic narcissism. Unthinking, she would keep producing the next laborers, the next conscripts for war. She would be prepared for submission to the State, in a seamless transition to fascism.

What Reich understood in 1933, we are clearly witnessing in 2024/2025: the fascist preoccupation with the traditional family. No wonder White Christian Nationalism enlists women in their own oppression. No wonder neo-fascism is obsessed with transsexuality, and with women who want sex but not babies. The sexually agentic woman who doesn't *mother*, the biological man who is a trans woman: They blow up the patriarchal family. If a biological man *voluntarily* gives up his masculine status, maybe that status is not the absolute guarantor of power. What if a biological woman can have surgery and take hormones and acquire masculinity? When that happens, the phallus is not wholly owned by the Father. Girls can just come and take it. Even Black and Brown girls can come and take it. No wonder MAGA is howling about the destruction of the traditional family.

Vanishing Vaginas

As Wieland (2015) notes, fascism certainly seems terrified of any embodiment that threatens its phallic narcissism. To stop fascism, we need to listen to these embodiments and protect them. To do this, I think we need to re-center vaginal bodies[6] in our conversations about fascism. Most literature on this subject appropriately places masculine trouble in the foreground. This is necessary. But this centering of masculinity can replicate fascism's erasure of women and the 'deviant' body. In examining fascism's hetero-hyper-masculinity, it seems clear that this masculinity requires the "vanished vagina" described by Theweleit (1987) and by Horney ([1967]1973). This vanished vagina is the desexualized Mother, the vacant Wife, the Virgin who awaits marriage *without* desire. To Theweleit, the very medium for the male fascist's power is the sexually untouched, dissolving/exploding body of the woman. For Trump, 'grabbing their pussies' confers this power. Either way: sexual avoidance or sexual assault, the subjective desiring vagina *vanishes*.

In authoritarian and fascist regimes, the oppression of women is a feature, not a bug. Here in the USA, Roe is overturned, a national ban on abortion is possible, miscarrying women have been incarcerated, and the right to contraception is at risk. Pregnant women risk death if they can't get a medical abortion. In Texas, vigilantes can receive a $10,000 bounty for hunting down anyone who aids a woman seeking an abortion after 6 weeks. Fetal cells are elevated as 'persons,' while women's personhood is eviscerated (see for example, Gentile, 2023). The surveillance and control of vaginal bodies is evident to anyone who identifies with she, her, hers.

This reflects the archaic "dread of woman," described by Horney ([1967]1973). To Horney, men deny this dread in themselves, by alternately idealizing *and* disparaging women. As part of this defense, he may also

> withdraw his libido from her and to concentrate it on himself and his genital. This … restores his masculine self-respect by reactively strengthening

> his phallic narcissism. The female genital no longer exists for him; the 'undiscovered vagina is a denied vagina'.
>
> (Horney, [1967]1973, p. 144)

This is an apt description of the alt-right. In that vein, Diamond posits fascism's unconscious fantasy: "a male dread of being swallowed up and absorbed into the dark hole of the mother's body, ultimately to be devoured by her" (2023, p. 97). This dread points to what Winnicott describes as the dread of dependence. Women's monthly blood, female agency, and desire (and desirability): In many patriarchal cultures, signs of female sexuality/subjectivity seem both mysterious and menacing.

Woman-Not-Woman: Guns and Fascist Women

In the United States, women are being stripped of autonomy and agency. And yet, we must hold limitless accountability for the enticement and the unmanning of men. We must be concealed AND we must be surveilled. We are sexually objectified AND we must signify purity and innocence. In every neo-fascist iteration, we are prisoners to sanctified, maternal mythologies: the edict to stay home, make the babies who will become the warriors and laborers of the state. If we are *not* domesticated, we are Sirens, we are Delilah, we are Medusa; our gaze will turn you to stone. Our passions are seen as murderous, we are Medea, we want birth control, we abort our own babies. Patriarchy always seems to be at risk from our 'perverse' unregulated couplings, from lesbians, bi-sexual, and trans women, from all those Black, Brown and Jewish women who are gestating the 'Great Replacement.' Ask the "incels": feminists should be raped. Ask the alt-right: only White women merit paternalistic protections from rape. Those protections are incendiary racist propaganda and pretense. I don't have much sympathy for alt-right women, but I hardly think their bodies are being treated with tender respect by their alt-right men. It is really just a question of *which* men are permitted to rape and batter *which* women.

The more authoritarian the world gets, the more our bodies are violated. Women can be forced to birth babies conceived in incest and rape, and, simultaneously, condemned as the *not-Mother, the not-entitled-to-mother*. In the United States, Black and Brown women have been forcibly sterilized. Around the world, children have been removed from their indigenous mothers, stolen from the Magdalene laundries, sold in African-American slavery, kidnapped by the Argentine Junta, and separated from their asylum-seeking mothers at the US–Mexican border. The rupture of the Other Mother's maternal bond: In these regimes this is sanctioned by the anointed cis woman/Mother. Forced birth and the destruction of the Other Mother's attachment: These are the salvation of White supremacy, just punishments for women's unregulated sexuality (see Richards, 2023).

At the center of fascism, we find a male demagog. But women often find fascism alluring, with its promise of supremacy, of borrowing phallic powers. These women legislate female domesticity and oppression, borrow phallic power, and police, betray, and sacrifice their sisters. In the United States, their names are, among others, Gini Thomas and Amy Comey Barrett. In Italy, her name is Giorgia Meloni. Fascism may be a cult of hetero-hyper-masculinity, but that trope can be written on female bodies. As Marasco (2021), Macciocchi (1979), and Theweleit (1989) point out, these movements would be ineffective without the support of fascist wives and mothers. And so fascism praises a 'martyred and baneful, necrophiliac femininity', to paraphrase Marasco (2021), that obscures its own oppression. Fascist narratives insist that women stay home and mother, but *this* motherhood is cast as a heroic battle against those who would undermine the State. In Hitler's speech to the National Socialist Women's Organization (1933, pp. 309–311), he writes martial contest onto women's child-bearing, and onto their domesticity. The result is a proud female anti-feminism (see Marasco, 2021).

While these movements assail any form of gender fluidity in the Other, they create an exemption for cruelty: e.g., an alt-right woman with gender fluidity. This is fascism's sanctified version of trans. This woman stays home and births the babies *and* she wears combat boots and carries a gun. For Marasco (2021), this figure is Ashli Babbitt, the armed alt-right woman who was killed and 'martyred' while assaulting the United States Congress on January 6th, 2021. In *Hitler's Furies*, Lower (2013) examines the role of these women-not-women in Nazism. Lower estimates that, in Eastern Europe, 500,000 women were facilitators, or perpetrators, of genocide. Some SS wives were sent, with their husbands, to the Ukraine. There they performed domesticity *and* they were vicious perpetrators. Lower describes how these perpetrator selves assumed the cloak of violent hyper-masculinity. Johanna Alvater Zelle was one of the most sadistic Nazis in the Ukraine. Her specialty was luring Jewish children with poisoned candy. According to Lower, when Alvater became violent, she wore male clothes and took on a masculine appearance. To Lower, "such mutations were … illustrative of the malleable roles that women in the East slipped into and out of" (2013, p. 130). Alvater was described as the 'she-man' lover/agent of her murderous superior. Lower's research argues that she was not alone. Other SS wives

> Slipped into another role—a hybrid character that embodied the stiff Nazi patriot, brazen cowgirl, and cold-blooded antisemite. They carried whips, they brandished pistols and rifles, they wore riding pants and they rode horses.
>
> (2013, p. 241)

Raimo (2024) sees the same neo-fascist gender fluidity in the far-right Italian Prime Minister, Giorgia Meloni. As Raimo notes, Meloni assails the right to abortion; she uses the masculine term 'il presidente,' and her motto is 'I'm Giorgia, I'm a woman, I'm a mother, I'm a Christian.'

Once, I naively imagined some gendered solidarity with women. Now I know that having a vagina does not make you a woman, a sister. I have more in common with a trans sister without a cis vagina, than I do with alt-right women.

Conclusion

Meanwhile, the patriarchy accrues capital and power and keeps committing atrocities. It seems that in every regime of fascism, state terror, racism, or genocide, this heteronormative, homophobic Virgin/Whore split seems particularly lit up and sorted according to classed/racialized categories of 'them' and 'us.' Too many are oblivious agents; we are servicing the regime and repudiating the 'deviant.' In the United States, these sexed and gendered tropes have fed indentured servitude, chattel slavery, convict labor, indigenous genocide, the extra-judicial killings of Black and Brown people, American First, the German-American Bund, and now, MAGA. In the United States, we have defeated fascism before (see Maddow, 2023), but it has never been so menacing.

In so many ways, Trumpism mirrors the sex/economic/racial ideology of Nazism. And so, as I draw to an end here, I want to return, again, to Reich's analysis (1933/1970). To reprise: for Reich, the bedrock of capitalism is the heteronormative patriarchal family, in which women are kept economically dependent, restricted to the domestic sphere, dominated and controlled by an authoritarian husband/father. Reich anticipated a woman's predicament in MAGA. He underlined that, in these systems,

> *the wife must not figure as a sexual being but solely as a child-bearer.* Essentially, the idealization and deification of motherhood, which is so flagrantly at variance with the brutality with which mothers of the toiling masses are actually treated, serve as a means of preventing women from gaining a sexual consciousness ... and of preventing sexual anxiety and sexual guilt feelings from losing their hold. *Sexually awakened women, affirmed and recognized as such, would mean the complete collapse of the authoritarian ideology.*
>
> (Reich, [1933]1970, p. 105; italics in the original)

Although he certainly overstates the anti-fascist power of women's sexual liberation, Reich ([1933]1970) is getting at something that I have tried to illuminate in this article. I hear him suggesting that sexed and gendered outliers can rock the ship of State. To Reich, the awakening of female sexuality would de-stabilize capital and undermine totalitarian structures, because women would seek unregulated sex for their own pleasure *not* for reproduction. Her body would no longer be an instrument to produce the next workers and the next soldiers. Pursuing her own desires, given access to birth control and abortion, she would have enough free time to *think* about her condition. She would see her own exploitation, and secede from the patriarchal, authoritarian family. Her body would no longer be an agent of the State. Of course, I don't think that is enough to subvert fascism. But what if we joined with *all* the sexed and gendered outliers, with the whole category of racialized 'deviance'? Reich is onto something. We would be formidable.

Notes

1 Authoritarian and fascist movements construct opposing categories of the 'pure' and the 'deviant.' This is used to justify dominance and subjugation.
2 'Vagina' will refer to cis gender women and to other bodies who are identified with being female, or who have been feminized by the state due to their 'deviance.'
3 Recently, Kevin Roberts, the president of the Heritage Foundation, said that the United States is "in the midst of a second American Revolution, which will remain bloodless if the left allows it to be" (cited in podcast, 'Heritage Foundation Head refers to "second American Revolution," July 3, 2024, NY Times).
4 For another example of these escalating attacks on internal enemies see the Cambodian genocide (see https://cla.umn.edu/chgs/holocaust-genocide-education/resource-guides/cambodia or https://hmh.org/library/research/genocide-in-cambodia-guide/.)
5 Sometimes this is more visible. Trump described the love letters he exchanged with the leader of North Korea, saying they 'fell in love.'
6 I use vaginal bodies to refer to cis women and also as a metaphor for those who are feminized and subordinated in the fascist regime.

References

Arendt, H. (1959). *The origins of totalitarianism*. Harper Collins Publisher.
Baldwin, J. (1962, November 10). Letter from a Region of my Mind. *The New Yorker*.
Barratt, B. (2020a). Psychoanalytic notes on the erotic politics of fascism and authoritarianism. *Psychoanalysis, Culture & Society*, 26(1), 118–128. https://doi.org/10.1057/s41282-020-00181-6
Barratt, B. (2020b). *Reassessing Wilhelm Reich's mass psychology: Libidinality, authoritarianism, and the rise of fascism*. Parkmore Institute.
Ben-Ghiat, R. (2020). *Strongmen: Mussolini to the present*. W.W. Norton and Company.
Brown, W. (2019). *In the ruins of neoliberalism: The rise of antidemocratic politics in the west*. Columbia University Press.
Caine, D. (2023). Apartheid's paradox: Impossible borders, unspeakable intimacy. *Psychoanalysis, Culture and Society*, 28(3), 103–121. https://doi.org/10.1057/s41282-022-00358-1
Charlap, L. (2019). The locker room. *Studies in Gender and Sexuality*, 20(4), 263–273. https://doi.org/10.1080/15240657.2019.1673983
Diamond, M. J. (2021). *Masculinity and Its Discontents: The Male Psyche and the Inherent Tensions of Maturing Manhood*. London and New York: Routledge.
Diamond, M. J. (2023). Perverted containment: Trumpism, cult creation and the rise of destructive American populism. *Psychoanalytic Inquiry*, 43(2), 96–109. https://doi.org/10.1080/07351690.2023.2163147

Duensing, A. F. (2023). "A heritage of fascists without labels": Black antifascism and the productive politics of analogy. In G. D. Rosenfeld & J. Ward (Eds.), *Fascism in America: Past and present* (pp. 247–277) Cambridge University Press.
Eco, U. (1995). Ur-fascism. *The New York Review of Books*. June 22, 1995 Issue.
Edwards, J. (2020). Sinner in the hands of an angry god. In P. Lopate (Ed.), *The glorious American essay: One hundred essays from colonial times to the present* (pp. 9–22). Pantheon Books. (Original work published in 1741).
Ehrenreich, B. (1987). Foreward. In K. Theweleit (Ed.), *Male fantasies: Women, floods, bodies, history* (Vol. 1, pp. IX–XIX). University of Minnesota Press.
Friedman, A., & Nakash, O. (2023). Repetition compulsion and sociopolitical trauma: A neoliberal artifact. *Psychoanalytic Dialogues*, 33(2), 200–213. https://doi.org/10.1080/10481885.2023.2173969
Fromm, E. (1970). *Escape from freedom*. Henry Holt. (Original work published 1941).
Gentile, K. (2023). The magic of a fetal fetish in the face of climate crisis and the expanse of dense temporalities. *Contemporary Psychoanalysis*, 59(1–2), 43–63. https://doi.org/10.1080/00107530.2023.2247797
Gilligan, C., & Snider, N. (2018). *Why does patriarchy persist?* Polity Press.
Grand, S. (2023). On hatred: Perpetrator fragments and totalitarian objects. *Psychoanalytic Dialogues*, 33(4), 543–650. https://doi.org/10.1080/10481885.2023.2220764
Graziano, F. (1992). *Divine violence: Spectacle, psychosexuality, and radical Christianity in the Argentine dirty war*. Westview Press.
Hartmann, S. (2022). *Scenes of subjection: Terror, slavery, and self-making in nineteenth century America*. W.W. Norton and Co.
Hedgepeth, S. M., & Saidal, R. G. (2010). *Sexual violence against Jewish women during the Holocaust*. Brandeis University Press.
Heschel, S. (2020). Erotohistoriography: Sensory and emotional dimensions of anti-semitism. In S. Ury & G. Miron (Eds.), *Antisemitism and the politics of history* (pp. 65–87). Brandeis University Press.
Hitler, A. (2004). Mein Kampf. (R. Manheim, Trans.). *Free Thought Books*. (Original work published in 1925).
Hitler, A. (2013). Aryan and Jew. In A. Rabinbach & S. L. Gilmman (Eds.), *The third Reich sourcebook, volume 47*. University of California Press. (Original work published in 1925).
Hochschild, A. (2022). *American midnight: The great war, a violent peace, and democracy's forgotten crisis*. Mariner Books.
Hofstadter, R. (1964, November). The paranoid style in American politics. *Harper's Magazine*.
Hollander, N. (2017). Who is the sufferer and what is being suffered? Subjectivity in a time of social malaise. *Psychoanalytic Dialogues*, 27(6), 635–650. https://doi.org/10.1080/10481885.2017.1379318
Horney, K. (1973). *Feminine psychology*. W.W. Norton and Co. (Original work published in 1967).
Jackson-Sow, M. (2022) Whiteness as Guilt. *UCLA Law Review*, 69, pp. 100–116. https://doi.org/10.2139/ssrn.3761432
Loewenstein, E. A. (2023). In dark times: Psychoanalytic praxis as a form of resistance to fascist propaganda. *Psychoanalytic Inquiry*, 43(2), 130–144. https://doi.org/10.1080/07351690.2023.2163150
Lowenthal, L., & Guterman, N. (2021). *Prophets of deceit*. Verso.
Lower, W. (2013). *Hitler's furies: German women in the nazi killing field*. Houghton Mifflin Harcourt Publishing.

Macciocchi, M. A. (1979). Female sexuality in fascist ideology. *Feminist Review*, 1(1), 67–82. https://doi.org/10.1057/fr.1979.6
Maddow, R. (2023). *Prequel: An American fight against fascism*. Crown Publishing.
Marasco, R. (2021). Reconsidering the sexual politics of fascism. *Blog* June 25, 2021.
Morrison, T. (1995). Racism and fascism. *The Journal of Negro Education* 64(3), 384–385. https://doi.org/10.2307/2967217
Moshtagh, N. (2023). The abject, the silence and the crime: Intricacies of abortion in Iran. *Contemporary Psychoanalysis*, 59(1–2), 99–111. https://doi.org/10.1080/00107530.2023.2236508
Mussolini, B. (1932). The doctrine of fascism. https://sjsu.edu/faculty/wooda/2B-HUM/Readings/The-Doctrine-of-Fascism.pdf
Paxton, R. (2004). *The anatomy of fascism*. Penguin Books.
Raimo, V. (2024, August 4). Why a black and white feminist film was bigger than 'Barbie' in Italy. *New York Times*. https://www.nytimes.com/2024/08/04/opinion/theres-still-tomorrow-paola-cortellesi.html
Reich, W. (1970). *The mass psychology of fascism*. The Noonday Press. (Original work published in 1933).
Richards, D. A. J. (2023). Patriarchal religion in U.S. Constitutional Law: Originalism as 'political religion' unmasked. *Contemporary Psychoanalysis*, 59(1–2), 23–42. https://doi.org/10.1080/00107530.2023.2239683
Ruti, M. (2018). *Penis envy and other bad feelings*. Columbia University Press.
Singh, M. P. (2017). *Race and America's long war*. University of California Press.
Theweleit, K. (1987). *Male fantasies (volume one): Women, floods, bodies, history*. University of Minnesota Press.
Theweleit, K. (1989). *Male fantasies (volume two): Male bodies, psychoanalyzing the white terror*. University of Minnesota Press.
Toscano, A. (2023). *Late fascism*. Verso.
Wieland, C. (2015). *The fascist state of mind and the manufacturing of masculinity*. Routledge.
Wieland, C. (2023). Trauma and the fascist state of mind: The emptying of the self and the road to perdition. *Psychoanalytic Inquiry*, 43(2), 84–95.
West, C. (1982). *Prophecy, deliverance: An Afro-American revolutionary Christianity*. Westminster Press.
Young-Bruehl, E. (1996). *The anatomy of prejudice*. Harvard University Press.

Part IV

Psychosocial Approaches

Chapter 9

Authoritarian Family Ideology and the Mass Psychology of Fascism

Wilhelm Reich

Reasons for Inclusion

With the generous permission of the Wilhelm Reich Museum, who are currently in the process of reissuing the original English translation by Theodore P. Wolfe, we are delighted to include below the second chapter of Reich's The Mass Psychology of Fascism. *Initially published in German in 1933, while he was still one of the foremost psychoanalysts of his generation, Reich's path-breaking investigation of Hitler's "mass-psychological success" (this reader, p. 166) inspired writers such as Fromm, Adorno, Theweleit, Deleuze and Guattari, and Kernberg. Following the recommendation of the Wilhelm Reich Museum, we have chosen to include the second chapter of Reich's book, which was reviewed and updated by Reich for the 1946 edition as translated by Wolfe. In this chapter, Reich asks about the historical and sociological situation which shaped the mass psychological structure of the middle class, making them vulnerable to demagogy, obfuscation and emotional manipulation. "We shall limit ourselves", he writes, "to the problems of sexual ideology" (p. 167). We include Reich's investigation of authoritarian family ideology in the psychosocial section of our reader, in conversation with papers exploring the ideological environment which facilitates fascist movements.*

***

Führer and Mass Structure

Future historians will be likely to conclude from Hitler's success that only the great man makes history, by firing the masses with "his idea." National Socialist propaganda was indeed built upon this "Führer ideology." The mechanism of their success was unknown to the propagandists of National Socialism, nor did they dare to comprehend the historical soil of the National Socialist movement. Quite in keeping with this, the National Socialist, Wilhelm Stapel, wrote in his CHRISTENTUM UND NATIONALSOZIALISMUS: "Because National Socialism is an *elementary* movement, it cannot be countered with arguments. Arguments could only be effective if the movement had grown by arguments." Speeches in National Socialist meetings were indeed characterized by very clever

DOI: 10.4324/9781003742876-14

manipulations of the *emotions* of the mass individuals and by *strict avoidance of objective argumentation*. Hitler, in MEIN KAMPF, emphasized repeatedly that the only correct mass-psychological technique was that of avoiding arguments and of keeping the "big final goal" before the masses. The true nature of the "final goal" *after* the seizure of power is demonstrated by Italian fascism. Similarly, Göring's edicts against middle-class economic organizations, the failure of the "second revolution" to materialize, the failure to keep the promises of Socialist measures, etc., all these clearly showed the reactionary function of fascism. How little Hitler himself knew the mechanism of his successes is shown by the following statement:

> This broadness of outline from which we must never depart, in combination with steady, consistent emphasis, allows our final success to mature. And then, to our amazement, we shall see what tremendous results such perseverance leads to—results that are almost beyond our understanding.[1]
>
> (1943, p. 185)

Thus, Hitler's success could by no means be explained by his reactionary role in the history of capitalism, for had this role been openly admitted in the propaganda, it would have had the opposite effect from that which was intended. Investigation of Hitler's mass-psychological success must start from the fact that a Führer or the advocate of an idea can succeed *only if his ideology or program is concordant with the average structure of the mass individual*. This leads to the further question, *What historical and sociological situation created this mass structure?* With that, the problem of mass-psychology is no longer one of metaphysics but of actual social life. *Only if a Führer structure is concordant with the structure of the average mass individual can a "Führer" make history*. Whether he makes history in a *lasting* sense or merely *temporarily* depends only on whether his program is in the direction of the progressive social process or against it. It is misleading to explain Hitler's success by National Socialist demagogy, the "obfuscation of the masses" or such meaningless terms as "Nazi psychosis." For the question is precisely *why the masses were accessible to demagogy, obfuscation and a psychotic situation*. The answer to this question requires an exact knowledge of *what goes on in the masses*. To say that the Hitler movement had a reactionary function is insufficient. For the mass success of the NSDAP seems to be at variance with this reactionary function. Millions of people affirmed their own subjugation. This contradiction cannot be explained on a political or economic basis, but only mass-psychologically.

National Socialism used different means with different classes and made different promises according to the class it wished to win over at a given moment. In the spring of 1933, for example, the *revolutionary* character of the Nazi movement was emphasized, in an attempt to win the industrial workers. The Nazis proceeded to "celebrate" May Day after having first placated the aristocracy in Potsdam. To conclude from this that the success was due only to political swindle would mean denying the possibility of social revolution. The question is: *why do the masses fall for political swindle?* They had every possibility of evaluating the propaganda of various parties. Why did they fail to discover that Hitler promised to the workers the expropriation of the private means of production while at the same time he promised the capitalists protection against expropriation?

Hitler's personal structure and life history are irrelevant for an understanding of National Socialism. True, it is interesting that the middle-class origin of his ideas fits the mass structure which readily accepted these ideas.

Like any other reactionary movement, Hitlerism gained its support from the various strata of the middle class. National Socialism laid bare all the contradictions which characterize the mass-psychology of the middle class. We will have to comprehend these contradictions and their common origin in the imperialist conditions of production. We shall limit ourselves to the problems of *sexual* ideology.

Hitler's Origin

The leader of the rebelling German middle classes was himself the son of a minor official. He relates how he had to go through that conflict which characterizes the mass structure of the middle classes. His father wanted to make an official of him, but the son rebelled and decided "under no circumstances" to give in; he became a painter and with that, poor. But alongside this rebellion against the father there remained the respect for his authority. This ambivalent attitude—*rebellion against authority with simultaneous respect and submission*—characterizes any middle-class structure at the period of transition from adolescence to maturity and is accentuated by straitened circumstances.

Of his mother, Hitler speaks with a great deal of sentimentality. He assures us that only once in his life did he cry: when his mother died. His theory of race and syphilis (*vide infra*) shows clearly his sexual defense and his neurotic idealization of motherhood.

As a young Nationalist, Hitler, who lived in Austria, decided to take up the fight against the Hapsburgs who, as he said, "delivered the German fatherland to Slavization." In his controversy with the Hapsburgs, the reproach that there were a few syphilitics among them assumes an important place. This would not seem important were it not for the fact that the idea of the "poisoning of the people" and the problem of syphilis came up again and again and formed, after the seizure of power, a central part of internal politics.

Originally, Hitler had sympathized with Social Democracy because it fought for universal suffrage by ballot which might have led to a weakening of the hated "Hapsburg regime." But he was repulsed by the Social-Democratic emphasis on classes, the negation of the nation and its authority, of the right to the ownership of social means of production, of religion and morals. What finally turned him definitely against Social Democracy was the demand that he join the union, which he refused to do.

His ideal became Bismarck, because he had unified the German nation and because he fought the Austrian throne. His further development was decisively influenced by the antisemitist Lueger and the German Nationalist Schönerer. He now formulated nationalistic *imperialist* goals which he intended to reach by better means than the old "bourgeois" nationalism. What determined the choice of these means was the *realization of the power of organized Marxism, and the realization of the significance of the masses for any political movement.*

> Not until the international world view—politically led by organized Marxism—is confronted by a folk world view, organized and led with equal unity, will success, supposing the fighting energy to be equal on both sides, fall to the side of eternal truth. What gave the international world view success was its representation by a political party organized into storm troops; what caused the defeat of the opposite world view was its lack up to now of a unified body to represent it. Not by unlimited freedom to interpret a general view, but only in the limited and hence integrating form of a political organization can a world view fight and conquer.
>
> (1943, p. 384f.)

Hitler soon realized the inconsistency of Social-Democratic politics and the impotence of the old bourgeois parties, including the German National party.

> All this was only the necessary consequence of the absence of a basic new anti-Marxist philosophy endowed with a stormy will to conquer.
>
> The more I occupied myself with the idea of a necessary change in the government's attitude toward Social Democracy as the momentary embodiment of Marxism, the more I recognized the lack of a serviceable substitute for this doctrine. What would be given the masses, if, just supposing, Social Democracy had been broken? There was not one movement in existence which could have been expected to succeed in drawing into its sphere of influence the great multitudes of workers grown more or less leaderless. It is senseless and more than stupid to believe that the international fanatic who had left the class party would now at once join a bourgeois party, in other words, a new class organization.
>
> The "bourgeois" parties, as they designate themselves, will never be able to attach the "proletarian" masses to their camp, for here two worlds oppose each other, in part naturally and in part artificially divided, whose mutual relation can only be struggle. The younger will be victorious—and this is Marxism.
>
> (1943, p. 173f.)

The basic anti-Soviet tendency of National Socialism became apparent at an early stage:

> If land was desired in Europe, it could be obtained by and large only at the expense of Russia, and this meant that the new Reich must again set itself on the march along the road of the Teutonic Knights of old, to obtain by the German sword sod for the German plow and daily bread for the nation.
>
> (1943, p. 140)

Thus Hitler saw himself confronted with the following questions: How can the National Socialist idea be carried to victory? How can Marxism be fought effectively? How can one gain influence over the masses?

To this end, Hitler appealed to the *nationalist* emotions of the masses, at the same time resolving to organize on a mass basis like Marxism, and to develop a propaganda technique of his own and to use it consistently.

As he openly admitted, he proposed to achieve nationalist imperialism by methods borrowed from Marxism and its technique of mass organization. *The reason for the success of this mass organization lies in the masses and not in Hitler.* His propaganda could take root because of the authoritarian freedom-fearing structure of the people. Thus Hitler's sociological importance does not lie in his personality but in the significance which he is given *by the masses*. The problem is made all the more acute by the fact that Hitler held the masses, with the aid of which he was to accomplish imperialism, in thorough contempt. He stated candidly that "the mood of the people was always a mere discharge of what was funneled into public opinion from above."

What was the structure of the masses that it made them absorb Hitler's propaganda in spite of everything?

On the Mass Psychology of The Lower Middle Classes

We stated that Hitler's success was due neither to his "personality" nor to the objective role of his ideology in capitalism, nor to a mere "obfuscation" of the masses who followed him. We focussed attention on the question, *What was it in the masses that caused them to follow a party the aims of which were, objectively and subjectively, strictly at variance with their own interests?*

To begin with, the fact has to be remembered that the National Socialist movement, in its initial success, leaned on the so-called middle classes, that is, the millions of private and public officials, small business people and farmers. *With regard to its social basis, National Socialism was originally a middle-class movement*. This was the case wherever it developed, be it in Italy, Hungary, Argentine or Norway. It follows that this middle class, which had previously belonged to the bourgeois Democratic parties, had undergone a change, that it had changed its political standpoint. The social position and the corresponding psychological structure of the middle class explain the basic differences, as well as the similarities, between the bourgeois-liberal and the fascist ideologies. The fascist middle class is the same as the Democratic-Liberal, only in a different epoch of capitalism. In the election years of 1930–32, the growth of National Socialism derived almost exclusively from the German Nationalist party, the Wirtschafts partei and the various minor parties of the Reich. Only the Catholic Center Party maintained its position even in the Prussian election of 1932. Only at that time did National Socialism succeed in making an inroad into the masses of the industrial workers. But the mainstay of the Swastika was always the middle class. During these years of 1929–32, the period of the severest economic disruption of the capitalist system, the middle class entered the political arena in the form of National Socialism and put the brakes on a revolutionary reorganization of society. Political reaction well knew the decisive importance of the middle class. "The middle class is of decisive significance for the existence of the State," said a handbill of the German Nationalists of April 8, 1932.

After January 30, 1933, the social significance of the middle class played an important role in the discussion of the Left. Up to that time, the question had been neglected, partly because attention was focussed on the development of political reaction, partly because the politicians did not think in *mass-psychological* terms. In these discussions of the "rebellion of the middle class" two main opinions were expressed. One group maintained that fascism was "nothing but" the guard of big business. The other, while not overlooking this aspect, emphasized the "rebellion of the middle class." The advocates of this standpoint were blamed for minimizing the reactionary function of fascism, they were reminded of Thyssen's nomination as economic dictator, of the abolition of the middle class economic organizations, the retreat of the "second revolution," in brief, of the reactionary character of fascism which, in the summer of 1933, became increasingly manifest.

In these violent discussions, something important was overlooked, which led to a good deal of confusion: the fact that National Socialism revealed itself more and more as imperialistic nationalism which tried to eliminate anything "Socialist" from the movement and which prepared for war on all sides, did not contradict the other fact that fascism, *seen from its mass basis, was in fact a middle-class movement*. Without his promise to fight big business, Hitler never would have won over the middle-class strata. They carried him to victory because they were *against* big business. Under their pressure, the Nazis had to institute *anti*-capitalistic measures, just as under the pressure of big business they had to scrap them again. One must distinguish the subjective interests resting in the mass basis of a reactionary movement from the objective reactionary function. These contradict each other, although they were at first united in the *totality* of the Nazi movement. Unless one makes this distinction one cannot have a common understanding because in speaking of "fascism," some will be referring to the objective role of fascism, and others to the subjective interests of the fascist masses. The antithesis of these two aspects of fascism is the basis of all its contradictions just as their unification in the *one* form, "National Socialism," characterizes the Hitler movement. Insofar as National Socialism had to emphasize its middle-class character (*before* the seizure of power and immediately afterwards) it was in fact *anti-capitalistic and revolutionary*. Insofar as (for the solidification and maintenance of its regime) it shed its anticapitalistic character more and more and showed its capitalistic function more and more exclusively, it became the extreme defender of imperialism and the capitalist economic order. It is entirely irrelevant how many of its leaders had an honest or dishonest "Socialist" attitude or how many were out to deceive the people and to grab power for themselves. Such considerations are no basis for effective anti-fascist politics. One could have learned to understand German fascism from Italian fascism, for Italian fascism also showed these two strictly contradictory functions and their fusion into one concept.

Those who deny or underestimate the function of the mass basis of fascism claim that the middle class—because it neither possesses the essential means of production nor works with them—cannot really make history and thus oscillates between capital and the industrial workers. They overlook the fact that, while the middle class cannot make *lasting* history, it can make *temporary* history. That it can do so is demonstrated by Italian and German fascism. We mean here not only the smashing of the labor unions, the untold victims of barbarism, but, more than anything else, the blocking of the development of the economic crisis into social revolution. It is clear that the greater in size and influence the middle-class strata are in a nation, the more decisive is their role as a social factor. Between 1933 and 1942 we witnessed the paradox that fascism, in the form of an *international* movement, was able to outstrip revolutionary internationalism. The Socialists and Communists nurtured illusions with regard to the progress of the revolutionary movement compared with the progress of reaction. This meant political suicide, the best motives notwithstanding. This question deserves careful attention. The process which has taken place during the past decade in the middle classes of all countries deserves far more attention than the trivial and well-known observation that fascism means extreme economic and political reaction. With the latter, nothing can be done politically, as the history of the years from 1928 to 1942 has amply proven.

The middle class made its entrance as a social force in the form of fascism. What is relevant is not the reactionary intentions of a Hitler or a Göring but the social interests of the middle-class strata. The middle class, as a result of its character structure, is an enormous social power, a power far beyond its economic importance. It is that stratum which keeps alive several thousand years of patriarchy with all its contradictions.

That a fascist movement exists at all is undoubtedly a sociological expression of nationalist imperialism. But the fact that this fascist movement was able to become a mass movement and could thus attain the power to fulfil the imperialistic function—that is the effect of the mass movement of the middle class. Only out of these contradictions can the contradictory phenomena of fascism be comprehended.

The social position of the middle class is determined by three factors:

a) its position in the capitalist production process;
b) its position in the authoritarian state machinery; and
c) its specific family situation, which is directly determined by its position in the production process and which determines its ideology. While the economic situation of the small farmers, the officials and small businessmen is different, their family situation is essentially *the same*.

The rapid development of capitalistic economy during the 19th century, the progressive mechanization of production, the development of monopolistic syndicates and trusts all led to a progressive pauperization of the lower middle-class business and tradespeople. Unable to compete with big business, small enterprises inevitably failed.

> The middle class can expect nothing from this system but ruthless destruction. The alternative is: whether all will become a large gray mass of proletarians where all have equally much, that is, nothing, or whether the individual will be able again by his own strength and industry to create his own property. Middle class or proletarian: that is the question.

Thus speaks the Deutschnationale Partei before the Reichs-presidential elections in 1932. The National Socialists were not clumsy enough to create a wide gap between middle class and industrial workers and were therefore more successful.

In the propaganda of the NSDAP the fight against the large department stores played a large role. But the conflict between the role which National Socialism played for heavy industry on the one hand and the interests of the middle class on which National Socialism depended was expressed, e.g., in Hitler's talk with Knickerbocker:

> We shall not make German–American relationships dependent on a shop (he was referring to the fate of Woolworth in Berlin) … the existence of such enterprises means furthering bolshevism … It destroys many small enterprises. For that reason, we shall not tolerate them. But you can rest assured that your enterprises of this kind in Germany will be treated no differently from similar German enterprises.[2]

The debts of private business to foreign countries were a heavy burden on the middle class. But while Hitler favored their payment because his foreign policy was dependent on it, his followers demanded that they be scrapped. The middle class rebelled "against the system" by which it meant the "Marxist regime" of Social Democracy.

The economic crisis made a solid organization of the middle-class strata necessary, but equally strong factors militated against it. The competition between the small enterprises had always prevented the development of a feeling of solidarity such as the industrial workers had developed. Because of his social position alone, the middle class individual cannot develop solidarity either with his own social stratum or that of the industrial workers; with his own stratum because there competition prevails, and with the industrial worker because he fears nothing more than proletarianization. Yet, in spite of this, the fascist movement brought about a unification of the middle classes. The question is, on what mass-psychological basis did this take place?

The answer lies in the social position of the minor officials, government and private. The economic position of the average official is inferior to that of the average specialized industrial worker; this is partly compensated by certain—or uncertain—prospects of advancement, and in the case of the government official, that of a lifelong pension. The official, thus dependent on government authority, develops an attitude of competition toward his colleagues which prevents the development of solidarity. The social consciousness of the official is not characterized by the fate he has in common with his colleagues, but by his attitude toward government authority and the "nation." This attitude is one of complete *identification with state authority* in the case of the government official, with the business enterprise in the case of the private official. He is a subject no less than the industrial worker. Why, then, does he not develop a feeling of solidarity like the industrial worker? Because of his position in between authority and industrial workers. On the one hand he is a subject of this authority and on the other hand its representative; as such he enjoys a privileged position morally even if not economically. The most clear-cut embodiment of this mass-psychological type is the top sergeant.

The power of this identification with the master is seen in a gross form in the servants of aristocratic homes, in butlers, valets, etc., who change completely by taking over the thinking and demeanor of the ruling class and often, in order to hide their modest origins, even exaggerate them.

This identification with the authorities, the firm, the state, the nation, etc., which can be expressed by the formula, "*I* am the authority, the firm, the state, the nation," is a potent psychological reality and one of the best illustrations of an ideology which has become a material force. At first the employee or official only has the ideal of becoming like his boss, but gradually, under the influence of the chronic material dependence, his being actually changes in the direction of the ruling stratum. Always looking above himself, the middle-class individual develops a *divergence between his economic position and his ideology.* He lives in straitened circumstances but keeps up appearances, often to a ridiculous degree. He feeds himself poorly but invests in "decent clothing." The silk hat and the Prince Albert coat became the material symbol of this character structure. Few things are, at first glance, more characteristic of a population than its clothing. The attitude of "Keeping up with the Joneses" specifically distinguishes the middle-class structure from that of the industrial worker.[3]

How deep is this identification with authority? That such an identification exists has long been a well-known fact. The question is, however, in what manner emotional factors—superimposed on the immediate economic conditions—give a solid basis to this middle-class structure to such an extent that it stands firm even in times of crisis, at a time when unemployment destroys the immediate economic base.

We have said that the economic position of the various strata of the middle classes varies, while their family situation is essentially the same. *This family situation* is the emotional foundation of the structure just described.

Family Fixation and Nationalistic Feeling

The family situation of the various strata of the middle classes is, to begin with, not separated from their economic position. The family is—except for the employees and officials—identical with the small economic enterprise. The family members work in the small business; this saves the hiring of expensive help. On the farm, the identity of family and mode of production is even more complete. The close interweaving of family and economy is the reason why the agricultural population is "bound to the soil," why it is "traditional" and thus so accessible to the influence of political reaction. It is not merely the economic situation which creates these "ties to the soil" and this traditionalism; rather, the mode of production requires a strict familial attachment of all family members to one another, and this attachment presupposes a far-reaching sexual suppression and repression. Only the combination of these two factors creates the typical peasant thinking the center of which is patriarchal sexual morality. The difficulties which the Soviet government encountered in the collectivization of agriculture were due not to the "love of the soil" but essentially to the authoritarian family ties which result from the agricultural mode of production.

> For one thing, the possibility of preserving a healthy peasant class as a foundation for a whole nation can never be valued highly enough. Many of our present-day sufferings are only the consequence of the unhealthy relationship between rural and city population. A solid stock of small and middle peasants has at all times been the best defense against social ills such as we possess today. And, moreover, this is the only solution which enables a nation to earn its daily bread within the inner circuit of its economy. Industry and commerce recede from their unhealthy leading position and adjust themselves to the general framework of a national economy of balanced supply and demand.
>
> (1943, p. 138)

This was Hitler's point of view. It does not matter that it is nonsensical from the standpoint of economics or that the political reaction will never succeed in stopping the development of mechanized farming, with its danger to the small farmer. Its mass-psychological propaganda value is, nevertheless, enormous because of its appeal to the compulsive familial structure of the middle class.

The close relationship between family attachment and agricultural mode of production inevitably found its expression in National Socialist measures. Since the Hitler movement was basically a middle-class movement, one of its first steps to win over the middle strata was the edict concerning the *New Order of Agricultural Ownership* of May 12, 1933. This edict went back to age-old forms and concepts such as the "inexorable tie of blood and soil." A few typical excerpts will make this clear:

> The inexorable tie between blood and soil is the indispensable pre-requisite of the healthy life of a people. The agricultural legislation of past centuries in Germany safeguarded this tie which exists in the natural feeling for life of the people. The farmstead was the *unsaleable* heritage of the ancestral farm family. Later, foreign laws came in and destroyed the legal basis of this custom. Most German farmers, with their healthy feeling for the basis of their country's life, nevertheless retained the custom of handing down their farm, intact, from generation to generation.
>
> It is the imperative duty of the government of an awakening nation to secure the inexorable tie between blood and soil by the institution of a law regulating the right of succession.
>
> The inheritance of a hereditary farm (*Erbhof*) which is registered in the local district court takes place according to the *Anerbenrecht*. The owner of an Erbhof is called farmer. A farmer has only one Erbhof. He has only one child which can take over the Erbhof. This child is the *Anerbe*. The other heirs are supported by the farm until such time as they reach economic independence. If they become needy through no fault of their own, they still can take refuge on the farm. If the farm is not registered, the right of succession takes place according to the Anerbenrecht.
>
> An Erbhof can be owned only by a farmer who is a *German citizen* and of *German blood*. Nobody is of German blood who has among his male ancestors, or among his other ancestors for four generations back, a person of Jewish or colored origin. It goes without saying, however, that every Teuton is, in the sense of this law, a German. Marriage with a person not of German blood will deprive the children of such marriage of the right to own an Erbhof.
>
> The purpose of this law is that of protecting the farms against heavy indebtedness and harmful splitting up through inheritance, and of maintaining them enduringly as the heritage of free farm families. At the same time, it intends to effect a healthy distribution of agricultural property. A great number of well-functioning small and medium farms, distributed as equally as possible over the whole nation, is necessary to maintain the health of the people and the state.

What tendencies are expressed in this law? It was in conflict with the interests of the large landowners whose aim was the absorption of the small and medium-sized farms. This conflict, however, was more than outweighed by a second potent interest of the large landowners, that of maintaining the agricultural middle class which was the mass basis of their power. Not only does the small farmer identify himself with the large landowner in the sense of being a *private owner* of land. What is more important is that the continued existence of small and medium-size farms guarantees the continued existence of the typical patriarchal atmosphere of the family which is identical with the economic unit. This type of family produces the best Nationalist fighters and changes the women structurally in the direction of the Nationalist ideology. This is the basis of the famous "moral value of a healthy peasantry." The problem is, however, a sex-economic problem.

The interweaving of individualistic production and authoritarian family in the middle classes is one of the sources of the fascist ideology of the "family with many children." We shall meet this problem again in another connection.

The alignment of the small economic units one against the other is reflected in the alignment of the families against one another and the competition between them. These phenomena are characteristic of the lower middle classes, in spite of the fascist slogans of the "corporate idea." The basic elements of fascist ideology are individualistic principles, such as the "Führer principle," family politics, etc. What is collectivistic in fascism derives from the socialist tendencies in its mass basis, while the individualistic elements derive from the interests of high finance and the fascist leadership.

In view of the natural organization of humanity, such an economic and familial situation could not continue to exist unless its existence were safeguarded by other basic elements. One of the most important among them is the patriarchal relationship between man and wife and a specific kind of sexual living.

In trying to distinguish himself from the manual worker, the lower middle-class individual can do so only in the forms of his sexual and family life, since his economic position is no better than that of the industrial worker. He compensates for what he lacks economically by way of sexual morality. This is the official's strongest motive for his identification with state authority. Since one does not enjoy the economic position of the upper middle classes but at the same time identifies oneself ideologically with them, the sexual moral ideologies must make up for the economic deprivations. The forms of sexual and, with that, of cultural living, serve mainly the purpose of snobbish distinction from the "lower" strata.

The sum total of these moralistic attitudes—the core of which is the attitude toward sexuality—expresses itself in *ideas*—ideas, not behavior—of *honor* and *duty*. The effect of these two words on the lower middle class is enormous and deserves the closest attention. They also constantly recur in the fascist ideology of dictatorship and race. In practice, everyday middle-class existence and middle-class business produce precisely the opposite behavior. In private trading, a bit of dishonesty is part of existence. When a peasant buys a horse, he will depreciate it in every way possible. When he sells the same horse a year later, it has become younger and better. "Duty" is based on business interest and not on national character. One's own wares will always be the best, that of the other fellow always inferior. Depreciation of the competitor, rarely an honest act, is an essential tool of "business." The overpoliteness and deference to the customer on the part of small business people show the brutal compulsion of economic existence which in the long run must warp even the best of characters. In spite of this, the concepts of "honor" and "duty" play a dominant role in the lower middle classes. This cannot be explained on purely economic grounds. For in spite of all hypocrisy, the depth of feeling connected with these concepts is genuine. The question is its source. The analysis of the lower middle class individual leaves no doubt about the connection between his sexual life and his ideology of "honor" and "duty."

The father's economic position as well as his position in the state are reflected in his patriarchal relationship with the other members of the family. The authoritarian state has a representative in every family, the father; in this way he becomes the state's most valuable tool.

The father's authoritarian position reflects his political role and discloses the relationship of family and authoritarian state. The same position which the boss holds in the production process, the father maintains in the family. He in turn reproduces submissiveness to authority in his children, especially his sons. This is the basis of the passive, submissive attitude of middle-class individuals toward Führer figures. Without really knowing it, Hitler built upon this attitude of the lower middle classes:

> The people in their overwhelming majority are so feminine by nature and attitude that sober reasoning determines their thoughts and actions far less than emotion and feeling.
>
> And this sentiment is not complicated, but very simple and all of a piece. It does not have multiple shadings; it has a positive and a negative; love or hate, right or wrong, truth or lie, never half this way and half that way, never partially, or that kind of thing.
>
> (1943, p. 183)

It is not a matter of being that way "by nature" but of being a typical example of the reproduction of an authoritarian social system in the structures of its members.

For the patriarchal position of the father requires the strictest sexual inhibition on the part of the women and children. Under lower middle class influence, the women develop an attitude of resignation which covers up repressed sexual rebellion; the sons develop, in addition to a submissive attitude toward authority, a strong identification with the father which later becomes identification with any kind of authority. It will remain a mystery for some time to come as to how the psychic structures of the decisive stratum of society fit the economic system and the purposes of the powers that be like the parts of a watch. What we are describing as the mass-psychological structural reproduction of the economic system is the basic mechanism of the formation of political ideologies.

The attitude of economic and social competition becomes a factor in the development of middle-class structure only at a very late stage. The reactionary ideologies which are then formed are built up secondarily on psychological processes which take place in the infant when it is growing up in the authoritarian family atmosphere. There we find, to begin with, competition between the children and the adults, and between the children among themselves in relation to the parents. This competition, which in adults and in extrafamilial life is predominantly economic, takes place in the framework of the highly emotional family relationships of love and hatred. This is not the place to discuss these in detail. What is important here is the following: the sexual inhibitions which constitute the prerequisite of the continued existence of the authoritarian family and the essential basis of the structure of the lower middle class individual are brought about with the aid of religious fears which thus become sexual guilt feelings and deeply anchored. This leads to the problem of the connection between religion and denial of sexual pleasure. Sexual weakness undermines self-confidence; compensation is effected by rigid character traits or brutal sexual behavior. The necessity for sexual self-control, for maintenance of sexual repression, leads to the development of compulsive, emotionally highly charged ideas of honor, duty, courage and self-control.[4] The compulsiveness and emotional charge of these ideas, however, is in strange contrast to the actual behavior. The genitally gratified individual is honest, conscientious, courageous and self-controlled, without making any fuss about it. These attitudes are organic parts of his personality. The individual with a weakened genitality and a contradictory sexual structure, on the other hand, must incessantly remind himself to control his sexuality, to preserve his sexual honor, to fight temptations courageously, etc. Every child and adolescent goes through the struggle against the temptation to masturbate. In this struggle, all elements of the reactionary human structure develop. In the lower middle classes, this structure is most strongly developed and most deeply anchored. This compulsive suppression of sexuality provides mysticism, of whatever kind, with its energy and also with some of its contents. To the extent to which the industrial workers are under the same social influences, they also develop the corresponding attitudes; due to their different way of living, however, they develop opposite, sex-affirmative attitudes to a far higher degree. The emotional anchoring of these structures by means of unconscious anxiety and their masking by apparently asexual character traits make it impossible for one to reach these deep layers of the personality with intellectual arguments. The importance of this fact for a practical sex policy will be discussed in Chapter VIII.[5]

We cannot discuss here in detail the significance of the *unconscious* fight against the individual sexual demands for the breeding of metaphysical and mystical thinking. We shall only mention one aspect which is characteristic of National Socialist ideology. Again and again one finds the series, *personal honor, family honor, race honor, national honor*. This series is consistent with the series of stages in individual structure formation. But it should include the socio-economic background *patriarchy, compulsive marriage, sexual aggression, personal fight against one's sexuality, compensatory idea of honor, etc.* The last in the series is the ideology of "national honor." It is the irrational core of National Socialism. Its comprehension requires a further preliminary consideration.

The fight of authoritarian society against the sexuality of children and adolescents takes place in the framework of the authoritarian family which thus far has proven the best institution for this fight. By their very nature, sexual needs impel contacts of various kinds in the world. If they are suppressed, they can express themselves only within the narrow framework of the family. Sexual inhibition is the basis of the familial incapsulation of the individuals as well as the basis of an individualistic ideology. Metaphysical, individualistic and familial sentimental behavior are only different aspects of one and the same process, sex negation. Realistic, non-mystical thinking on the other hand, go with loose family ties and, to say the least, indifference toward ascetic sexual ideologies. The important point is that sexual inhibition is a means of producing a fixation to the authoritarian family; that it turns an original biological tie of the child to the mother—and of the mother to the child—into an indissoluble sexual fixation and thus creates the inability to establish new relationships.[6] The core of the family tie is the mother fixation. The subjective, emotional core of the ideas of *homeland* and *nation are ideas of mother and family*. The mother is the homeland of the child, as the family is its "nation in miniature." Thus one understands why the National Socialist, Goebbels, took the following as a motto for his Ten Commandments, in the National Socialist Volkskalender for 1932: "The homeland is the mother of your life, don't ever forget it." The *Angriff* wrote on the occasion of Mother's Day in 1933:

> MOTHER'S DAY. The national revolution has blown away everything that is petty. Ideas are leading again and are leading us together, family, society, nation. The idea of Mother's Day will honor that which signifies the German idea: The German Mother! Nowhere has the woman and mother as important a role as in the new Germany. It is she who preserves the family life from which spring the forces which will lead our nation ahead again. She, the German mother, is the sole bearer of the German national idea. *The idea of "mother" will always be the same as "being German."* What could unite us more strongly than the idea of honoring the mother?

As untrue as these sentences are, economically and socially speaking, they are correct with regard to human structure. Nationalist feeling is the direct continuation of family attachment and, like the latter, is based on the unconscious, deeply anchored mother fixation. This cannot be explained biologically. For this mother fixation itself is a *social* product. The attachment to the mother would be replaced at puberty by other attachments, for example, by natural sexual relationships, if it were not made permanent by the general suppression of natural love life. Only this socially caused perpetuation makes it the basis for nationalist feeling in the adult and makes it a reactionary social force. The fact that the industrial workers develop nationalist attitudes to a much lesser degree is to be ascribed to the difference in their family situation.

This statement by no means implies a biologizing of sociology. For we do not forget for a moment that the difference in the industrial worker's family situation is itself conditioned by his position in the production process. One must ask oneself why it is that the industrial workers are especially accessible to internationalism while the lower middle class tends equally strongly to nationalism. Only the inclusion of the specific family situation in its dependence on the economic process explains this. The Marxist theorists display a peculiar aversion to considering the family situation as a factor which is *equally* as important as the economic factors in the formation of structure; more than that, it is the *decisive* factor for the anchoring of the social system in the psychic structure. This aversion is caused by their own family attachments. The fact that the family fixation is the most intensive and most highly emotionally charged cannot be overestimated.[7]

The basic identity of familial and of nationalist ideology goes further. The families are set against each other precisely as are the nations. In either case, the ultimate basis lies in economic motives. The lower middle-class family is always under the pressure of economic worries. The economic tendency to expansion on the part of the lower middle-class family with many children thus reproduces the imperialist ideology of the "Lebensraum" of the nation. This is why the lower middle class individual is so easily accessible to imperialist ideology. He tends to identify himself fully with a personified nation. In this way, state imperialism reproduces itself in family imperialism. In this connection, it is interesting to see what Goebbels writes (in DIE VERFLUCHTEN HAKENKREUZLER) in answer to the question whether the Jews are humans:

> If somebody hits your mother in the face with a whip, are you going to say, thank you? Is he human? He is not human, he is a beast! How many worse things has the Jew done to *our mother Germany* [italics mine, W.K.] and is he still doing! He has spoiled our race, he has undermined our morality and has sapped our strength ... The Jew is the personified demon of decay ... he begins his criminal butchery of the nations.

One cannot properly judge the effect of such sentences on the unconscious emotional life of the mass reader unless one knows the significance of the idea of castration as punishment for sexual wishes; the sex-psychological background of the phantasies of ritual murders and of antisemitism in general; and the magnitude of the sexual guilt feelings and the sexual anxiety of the reactionary individual. Here are the psychological roots of National Socialist antisemitism. Could this be called "just obfuscation of the masses"? True, it is obfuscation also. But the fact should not be overlooked that fascism, ideologically, is the revolt of a deathly sick society, sick sexually as well as economically. It is the revolt against the painful and forceful tendencies of revolutionary thinking in the direction of sexual as well as economic freedom. The very thought of this freedom makes the reactionary individual tremble with fear. The establishment of economic freedom of the working people goes hand in hand with the dissolution of the old institutions, especially the sexual ones, a process of which the reactionary individual is afraid. Specifically, the fear of "sexual freedom"—which in reactionary thinking is represented as "sexual chaos"—checks the longing for freedom from economic exploitation. This will be so as long, but only as long, as this idea of the sexual chaos prevails. It can continue to prevail only as long as these decisive problems remain unclarified in the masses. This is why sex-economy belongs in the center of any endeavor to regulate social conditions in general. The more extensive and the deeper the reactionary structure formation of the masses, the more decisive is the sex-economic work on the education of the masses in social responsibility.

In this interplay between economic and structural facts, the authoritarian family stands out as the most important place where reactionary thinking of any kind is reproduced: it is the factory of reactionary ideology and structure. The "preservation of the family," that is, of the reactionary family with many children, is therefore the primordial cultural tenet of reactionary politics. This is what hides behind the slogan of the "protection of the state, of culture and of civilization."

In a proclamation before the Presidential election in 1932 (Adolf Hitler: *Mein Programm*) we read the following:

> Woman, by nature and by fate, is the life companion of man. They are not only life companions but also work companions. Just as the economic development over thousands of years changed the fields of work for the man, so it did for the woman. But higher than the compulsion of working together is the duty to preserve the race. In this, the most noble mission of the sexes, lie their individual and unalterable differences which Providence in its eternal wisdom gave them. The highest task, therefore, is that of making possible for the two life and work companions the *founding of a family*. The *final destruction of the family would mean the end of any higher form of humanity*. No matter how far the woman's field of activity may be extended, *the*

> *ultimate goal of a truly organic and logical development must always be the formation of the family*. It is the smallest *but most valuable unit in the whole structure of the state*. Work honors the woman as it does the man. But the child raises the woman to nobility.

In the same proclamation, under the heading, "Preservation of the peasantry means preservation of the German nation," Hitler stated:

> In the preservation and maintenance of a healthy peasantry I see the best protection against social ills as well as against the racial degeneration of our nation.

In this connection, one has to remember the traditional family fixation among the peasantry. Hitler goes on to say:

> I believe that a nation, in order to increase its resistance, should not live according to principles of reason alone. It also needs a spiritual and religious hold. The poisoning and disintegration of the national body by our Kulturbolschewismus are almost more disastrous even than the effect of political and economic Communism.

Since, like Italian fascism, the National Socialist party took its origin from the interests of the large landowners, it had to win over the masses of small farmers as a mass basis for its movement. Naturally, it could not emphasize the interests of the large landowners in its propaganda, but had to appeal to the structure of the peasants, a structure as it develops from the identity of economic and familial existence. Only in this stratum of the lower middle classes is it true that man and wife are work companions. It is not true among the industrial workers. Even with the peasants it is true only in a formal sense, for in reality the peasant woman is the domestic servant of the peasant. The fascist ideology of the hierarchic structure of the state is preformed in reality in the hierarchic structure of the farm family. The farm family is a nation in miniature and every member of the farm is identified with this miniature nation. The soil for the acceptance of the imperialist ideology, then, is given in the peasantry and wherever in the lower middle classes economic unit and family are identical. We are struck by the idealization of motherhood. What is the connection between this idealization and reactionary sexual politics?

Nationalistic Self-confidence

In the mass-psychological structure of the lower middle class individual, national and family fixation are identical. This fixation is intensified by another process. The Nationalist Führer means, to the masses, the personification of the nation. A personal fixation on him develops only to the extent to which he actually personifies the nation in terms of the nationalistic feeling of the masses. If he knows how to arouse the familial fixation in the mass individual he also becomes an authoritarian father figure. He becomes the object of all the emotional attitudes which the mass individual, as a child, had toward the protecting and—in the child's thinking—representative father. In discussing the untenability of the contradictory program of the NSDAP with National Socialist followers, one heard again and again the argument that Hitler knew all these things much better, that "he would do it all." Here we see clearly the infantile leaning on paternal protection. It is this attitude of blind trust and of seeking protection on the part of the masses which gives the dictators the power to "do it all." This attitude is at variance with social self-determination, with rational independence and cooperation. No genuine democracy should try to build on this.

Even more important, however, is the *identification* of the mass individual with the "Führer." The more helpless the individual was made by his upbringing, the more strongly does he identify himself with the Führer, the more does the infantile helplessness take the form of the feeling-one-with-the-Führer. This tendency to identification is the psychological basis of *national narcissism*, that is, of a self-confidence based on identification with the "greatness of the nation." The reactionary middle-class individual believes he discovers *himself* in the Führer, in the authoritarian state. On the basis of this identification, he feels himself the defender of "the nation," even though, on the basis of this very identification, he despises "the masses" toward whom he has an individualistic attitude. His economic and sexual misery is drowned out by the exalting idea of "Herrentum" and of the genius of the Führer; it makes him forget to what extent he has become an insignificant, uncritical follower.

In contrast, the *professionally conscious worker* identifies himself with his work instead of the Führer, with the international totality of working individuals and not with the national homeland. *He feels himself a leader*, not on the basis of an identification but on the basis of doing vital, socially necessary work.

It is not difficult to see what causes this difference. The *emotions* in this opposite mass-psychological type are the same as in the nationalist. But the *content* is different. The need for identification is the same, but its object is the fellow worker instead of the Führer, the work instead of the illusion, the working individuals of the earth instead of the family. It is a matter of international professional consciousness versus mysticism and nationalism. The self-confidence of the worker is not based on his identification with illusory concepts but on his identification with his work.

The past fifteen years have confronted us with a fact which is difficult to understand: Economically, society is sharply divided into various social strata and professions. According to economistic concepts, social ideology derives from the respective social position. If that were so, the ideological strata would always correspond to the socio-economic strata; the industrial workers as a whole would develop more collectivism, the small tradespeople more individualism. The employees of large concerns would have a collective feeling similar to that of the industrial workers. As we have already seen, structure and social position are rarely concordant. We distinguish the professionally conscious, responsible worker from the nationalistically mystical reactionary subject. *Both* types are seen in *any* social or professional group. There are millions of reactionary industrial workers, and there are as many work-conscious revolutionary teachers and physicians. In other words, there is no such thing as a mechanistic relationship between social position and character structure.

The social position is no more than the external factor in the determination of the ideological process in the mass individual. What remains to be investigated is the *emotional force* which causes the various social factors to attain *exclusive* dominance in the psychological structure. It certainly is not hunger, otherwise the economic world crisis of 1929 to 1933 would have led to international revolution. As much as this finding conflicts with well-established economistic concepts, it cannot be doubted.

When sociologically limited psychologists explain the social revolution by the "infantile rebellion against the father" they are thinking of revolutionaries in intellectual circles. In them, this is indeed the decisive motive. But the same is not true of the industrial workers. The suppression of the children by the fathers is no less pronounced among the workers; it is often even more brutal. This is not the difference. The difference lies in their different attitude toward sexuality. True, the parents among the industrial workers also suppress infantile sexuality. But among the lower middle classes, there is *only* suppression of sexuality. Among the industrial workers, things are different. They show, along with their moralistic ideology, their own sexual attitudes which are strictly opposed to the moralistic ones. The difference in housing and the collective work life of the factory are further factors which tend to counteract a moralistic sexual ideology.

The average industrial worker differs from the average middle-class individual by his open and matter-of-fact attitude toward sexuality. He is incomparably more accessible to sex-economic concepts than the typical middle-class individual. What makes him more accessible is the absence of precisely those attitudes which play a central role in the ideology of National Socialism and of the church: the identification with the authoritarian state power, the "supreme Führer," the nation. This is further proof that the basic elements of National Socialist ideology have a sex-economic origin.

The peasantry, due to its individualistic economy and marked familial isolation, is very accessible to reactionary political ideology. This is the reason for the divergence between its social position and its ideology. In spite of strictest patriarchy and the corresponding morality, the peasantry develops a natural—though distorted—sexuality. As among the industrial workers, its youth starts having sexual intercourse at an early age, but as a result of the strict patriarchal education sexuality is disturbed or brutal; the sex life is clandestine; frigidity among the girls is the rule; sex murders, brutal jealousy and subjugation of the woman are typical phenomena among the peasantry. Hysteria is nowhere as prevalent as out in the country. Peasant economy makes patriarchal marriage the ultimate goal of education.

Among the industrial workers, an ideological process has been taking place during the past few decades which one can observe in pure culture in the workers' aristocracy but which did not spare the average industrial worker. The industrial workers of the 20th century are no longer the proletariat of the 19th century of which Marx speaks. They have essentially taken over the forms of living and the attitudes of the middle class. True, formal democracy has not eliminated economic class distinctions any more than race prejudices. But the social endeavors which took place within its framework obliterated the structural and ideological boundaries between the various social strata. The industrial workers of England, America, Scandinavia, and Germany took on more and more a middle-class character. In order to understand the manner in which fascism penetrates the workers' stratum one has to follow this process in its various stages from formal democracy to openly fascist dictatorship.

The Middle-Class Adaptation of the Industrial Workers

Fascism penetrates the stratum of the industrial workers from two sides: the so-called "Lumpenproletariat" (a revolting expression) by means of direct economic corruption, and the so-called "worker's aristocracy" by means of material corruption as well as by ideological influence. German fascism unscrupulously promised everything to everybody. Dr. Jarmer, in an article entitled "Kapitalismus" (*Angriff*, Sept. 24, 1931) wrote the following:

> On the German National party day in Stettin, Hugenberg took an admirably clear stand against international capitalism. But at the same time he emphasized the necessity of a national capitalism.
>
> In doing so, he made again clear what separates the German Nationals from the National Socialists; for the latter clearly realize that the capitalist order which is in a state of collapse all over the world must be replaced by a different order, because even in national capitalism there can be no justice.

This sounds almost Communistic. Here, the fascist propagandist appealed to the revolutionary feeling of the industrial worker, consciously and with fraudulent intent. The question was why the National Socialist industrial workers did not see that fascism promised everything to everybody. It was well known that Hitler negotiated with the captains of industry, received financial support from them and promised them anti-strike legislation. Obviously, there was something in the structure of the average worker which made him overlook such contradictions, in spite of the intensive propaganda of revolutionary organizations. In talking with the American journalist Knickerbocker, Hitler said with regard to the recognition of private debts to foreign countries:

> I am convinced that the international bankers will soon realize that Germany under National Socialism is a safe place for investment, that an interest rate of about three per cent will be readily granted.
>
> ("Deutschland so oder so," p. 211)

If the task of revolutionary propaganda was that of "defogging the proletariat," this could not be done merely by appealing to its "class consciousness," nor by keeping the subjective economic and political situation constantly before their eyes, nor simply by unmasking the fraud that was being perpetrated on them. The primordial task of revolutionary propaganda should have been that of comprehending the *inner contradictions in the worker*, the fact not that the worker had a clear-cut revolutionary will which may have been covered up or "befogged," but, rather, that the revolutionary element in his psychic structure was partly underdeveloped, partly counteracted by opposite reactionary elements in his structure. The crystallizing out of the revolutionary elements in the masses is the prime task in the process of liberating their social responsibility.

In times of "quiet" formal democracy, the industrial worker has, in principle, two possibilities open to him: identification with the middle class above him, or identification with his own social position which gives birth to forms of living of its own which are contrary to the reactionary forms. The first means envying and imitating the reactionary and—given the economic opportunities—completely adopting his way of living. The second means refuting the ideologies and forms of living of the reactionary and emphasizing one's own. Due to the simultaneous influence of both the social and the class living, there is an equally strong pull in either direction. The revolutionary movement also underestimated the significance of the seemingly unimportant small habits of everyday living; more than that, it made the wrong use of it. The middle-class bedroom which the "proletarian" acquires at the first opportunity even though he may be Communist; the suppression of the woman which goes with it; "decent" clothes on a Sunday; stilted forms of dancing; these and thousands of other little things, in their everyday repetition, have an incomparably more powerful reactionary influence than can be counteracted by thousands of revolutionary meetings and pamphlets. The impact of a narrow reactionary life is continuous and fills every cranny of everyday living; the factory work and the pamphlet have an effect only for hours. To try to "reach the masses" by arranging festivities was, therefore, a miscalculation, because it appealed to the conservative tendencies in the workers. In such methods, reactionary fascism was far more successful. The budding revolutionary forms of living were not being developed. The "evening dress" which a worker's wife put on for such a "festivity" contained more truth about the reactionary structure of the worker than hundreds of learned articles. The evening dress and the family beer parties are, after all, only the external manifestations of a structural process in the worker, a sign that the soil was already prepared for the acceptance of National Socialist propaganda. When the Fascist then promised "abolition of the proletariat" and was successful in such propaganda, his success, in ninety out of a hundred cases, was due not to his economic platform but to the "evening dress." These aspects of everyday living deserve much more attention. It is they that form, in a *concrete* manner, the social process, be it progress or reaction, and not the political slogans which create only a fleeting enthusiasm. Here waits a field for fruitful and important work. The revolutionary mass propaganda in Germany was restricted almost exclusively to the propaganda "against hunger." As important as this argument is, it proved too narrow. The youthful worker, for example, has innumerable worries of a sexual and cultural nature as soon as he has stilled his hunger to a degree. True, the fight against hunger is of primary importance, but the backstage processes of human life must also be ruthlessly placed in the spotlight of the comedy in which we are both spectators and actors.

If that were done the working people would show themselves infinitely creative in their attempt to develop their own concepts and their own natural forms of living. No matter how infested they might be with reactionary attitudes, social comprehension of their everyday life would give them an invincible impetus. Detailed and concrete work on this problem is imperative; it will safeguard the victory of the revolution. To object that such a proposition is an illusion means failure to grasp the problem. This fight for the development of work-democratic living means a militant turning away from what is reactionary and the development of a mass culture which alone will guarantee lasting peace. As long as social irresponsibility outweighs social responsibility in the worker he will hardly learn revolutionary, that is, rational behavior. This mass-psychological work, furthermore, is indispensable for still another reason.

The debasement of manual work—which makes the manual worker ape the reactionary white-collar worker—is the mass-psychological strength of fascism when it tries to reach the workers. Fascism promises the abolition of classes, that is, doing away with one's being a proletarian; in this manner, it appeals to the social inferiority feeling of the manual worker. Workers which have only recently migrated from the country to the city still have the family ideology of the peasant, which, as we have shown, is one of the most fertile soils for imperialistic nationalist ideology. There is, in addition, an ideological process which thus far has been neglected in judging the chances of the revolutionary movement in countries with a high industrial development on the one hand and those with a low industrial development on the other.

Kautsky (Soziale Revolution, 2. Aufl, pp. 59–60) found that the worker in highly industrialized England was politically backward compared with the worker in industrially little developed Russia. The political events of the past thirty years the world over leave no doubt that revolutionary movements develop more readily in countries with a low industrial development as is shown, e.g., by a comparison of China, Mexico, and India on the one hand and England, America, and Germany on the other. This in spite of an older, better trained and organized labor movement in the last mentioned countries. Leaving out of consideration the bureaucratization of the labor movement—which in itself is a pathological symptom—one must ask oneself what is the reason for the extraordinary anchoring of conservatism in the Social Democracy and the trade unions of the Western countries. *The mass-psychological basis of Social Democracy is the conservative structure of its followers.* As in fascism, the problem is not so much one of the politics of the party leadership as one of the mass-psychological basis in the workers. I shall point out only a few significant facts:

In early capitalism, there was not only a sharp cleavage line between bourgeoisie and proletariat but an equally sharp ideological, in particular, structural demarcation. The lack of any social politics, the exhausting workday of sixteen or eighteen hours, the generally low living standard of the industrial workers (as classically described by Engels in his *Lage der arbeitenden Klasse in England*)—all these things prevented a structural adaptation of the proletariat to the bourgeoisie. The structure of the proletarian of the 19th century was characterized by humble submission to his fate. The mass-psychological characteristic of this proletariat, the peasantry included, was indolence. Middle-class thinking was absent. This indolence did not prevent revolutionary feelings, on appropriate occasions, from breaking into the open with unexpected intensity and determination.

In late capitalism, however, things became different. The workers' movement had made certain gains such as shorter hours, the right to vote, social security, etc. This meant, on the one hand, a strengthening of the working class. At the same time it had an opposite effect: the raising of the living standard led to a structural adaptation to the middle classes. In times of prosperity this middle-class adaptation was intensified; in ensuing economic crises, it acted as an inhibition of a further development of revolutionary feeling.

The strength of the Social Democracies during the years of the crises—which cannot be explained on political grounds—was the expression of this conservative infestation of the workers. This has two main reasons: the Führer fixation, that is, the unshakeable belief in the infallibility of the political leader[8]; and the sex-moralistic adaptation to the conservative lower middle class. The upper middle class helped this adaptation along as best it could. While in its beginning it had literally used the stick, it now held it in reserve in the countries which were not yet fascist and used it only against the revolutionary worker. For the mass of the Social-Democratic workers, however, it had a far more dangerous weapon: the use of conservative ideology.

When the Social-Democratic worker found himself in the economic crisis which degraded him to a coolie, the development of his revolutionary feelings was inhibited by the conservative structure which had been cultivated in him for decades. Either he remained in the Social-Democratic party, in spite of all his criticism and rebellion. Or, oscillating between his revolutionary and his conservative feelings, and disillusioned by Social-Democratic leadership, he followed the path of least resistance and switched to the NSDAP, hoping to find better leadership there. In this situation, it depended on the correct or incorrect mass leadership of the revolutionary party whether or not the worker would give up his conservative tendency and would develop the full consciousness of his responsibility in the production process, that is, his revolutionary consciousness. The Communist contention that it was Social-Democratic politics which had helped fascism come to power was—mass-psychologically—correct. *Disillusionment in Social Democracy must, in the presence of a conflict between pauperization and conservative thinking, lead into the fascist camp* if there are no effective revolutionary organizations. Thus there was, for example, a fascization of the workers in England after the fiasco of the Labor party in 1930–31; in the elections of 1931, the workers, instead of swinging to Communism, shifted to the right. Democratic Scandinavia, also, was threatened by such a development.[9]

Rosa Luxemburg contended that a revolutionary struggle with "coolies" was not possible. The question is which kind of coolie is meant: the coolie *before* he has acquired a conservative structure, or *afterwards*. Before this alteration of structure, there is an indolence which is difficult to break through, but there is also a great capacity for revolutionary action. After the alteration of structure, there is the *disillusioned* coolie. He is much less accessible to the revolution. How long will fascism be able to utilize for its own purposes the disillusionment of the masses in Social Democracy and their "rebellion again the system"? Though this question cannot be answered now, it is certain that the international revolutionary movement will have to take it into consideration if it is not to fail.

Notes

1 *Translator's note*: The quotations from Mein Kampf—with the exception of one, which is so marked—are taken from Mein Kampf, by Adolf Hitler, Translated by Ralph Manheim, Houghton Mifflin Company, Boston, 1943. Permission to use these quotations was kindly granted by the Houghton Mifflin Company and is hereby gratefully acknowledged.—T.P.W.

2 After the seizure of power, in March and April, there was a mass attack on the department stores to which the NSDAP soon put a stop.

3 This is true of Europe. In America, the middle-class character of the industrial workers obliterates this distinction.

4 Particularly instructive in showing these connections is a book by the National Socialist, Ernst Mann, Die Moral Der Kraft.

5 *Editors' note*: Reich is referring here to Chapter VII of his own book, from which the current chapter is excerpted.

6 The "Oedipus complex" discovered by Freud, then, is not so much the cause as the result of the social inhibition of infantile sexuality. The parents, however, quite unconsciously execute the intentions of society.

7 He who has not overcome his fixation on family and mother, or is not able at least to exclude it from his judgment, should not engage in the study of ideology formation. Brushing these facts aside by calling them "Freudian" betrays scientific cretinism. Talking without knowing the facts is not scientific argumentation. Freud discovered the Oedipus complex. Without this discovery there could be no revolutionary family politics. But Freud is as far from a sociological interpretation of the family fixation as the mechanistic economist from a comprehension of sexuality as a social factor. To deny facts which every worker knew even before Freud discovered the Oedipus complex, instead of pointing out a possible erroneous application of natural science, is inadmissible. Fascism cannot be overcome with slogans but only with knowledge. Errors occur and can be corrected, but scientific narrow-mindedness is reactionary.

8 In the summer of 1932, after a meeting in Leipzig, I talked with Social-Democratic workers who had attended it, about the political crisis. They agreed with all the arguments brought forth against the Social-Democratic propaganda on the "way to Socialism," but otherwise did not differ from Communist workers. I asked one of them why they did not draw the consequences and separate from their leaders. The answer amazed me: "*Our leaders know what they are doing*." Here was the conflict of the Social-Democratic worker in a tangible form: the fixation on the Führer, which kept the worker from translating his criticism—which he did not lack—into action. It was a mistake, then, to try to win the Social-Democratic worker by attacking his leaders. As he was identified with them, such attacks would only repulse him. The inner rottenness of German Social Democracy showed itself when, shortly before Hitler's seizure of power, a few armed men arrested Severing, the Social-Democratic Minister of the Interior. There were twelve million Social Democrats, but they did not prevent it.

9 The collapse of Norway in 1940 was in no small part due to the same effect of Social-Democratic conservatism. The Social-Democratic government had, for example, prohibited the parading of military organizations. But in 1939 the Norwegian Fascists were the only ones who still marched through the streets and held training exercises. Quisling's betrayal was greatly helped by such "liberalism."

Chapter 10

Capitalism Without Capitalism

Fascism According to Žižek

Alberto Toscano

Reasons for Inclusion

Toscano's essay is a concise and focused summary of Žižek's important contributions to the psychoanalytic study of fascism. Žižek uses his powerful theoretical perspective to advance the Marxist theory of fascism as a response to the crises of capitalism, grounding his theorization in a Lacanian framework that relates trauma and perversion to capitalism and radical right political ideology. Žižek's theory, however, is not presented concisely or in one location in his writings. While Toscano is, in his own right, an important critical theorist of fascism in its relation to racial capitalism and the "politics of crisis" (see Toscano, 2023), his contribution here is to collate and synthesize Žižek's distinctive account and to present it in a single paper. The essay is included for these reasons, and because it makes the crucial link between capitalist crisis and fascism that other psychoanalytic studies of the fascist "state of mind" tend to either reject or ignore.

***

If capitalist ideology may be suitably defined as socially necessary false consciousness, how is philosophy to respond to a proliferating surplus of social illusions and to their coalescence into politically efficacious movements or organisations? The emergence of interwar fascisms has constituted a kind of generative impasse, or even trauma, for Marxism and critical theory—the realisation that, notwithstanding the instrumentality of this revolution without a revolution[1] for the reproduction of relations of exploitation amid organic crisis, *why* and especially *how* the socio-political contradictions of capitalism issue into the particular ideological *form* of fascism is something that an orthodox historical materialism found itself unable properly to account for. In the twentieth century, fascism thus became the *locus classicus* for thinking the disjunction of the economic and the political, the asynchrony of base and superstructure, but also the rifts and asynchronies between the material and the psychic.

The symptomatology of interwar fascisms (especially their articulation with the experience of the war front, their distorted mimesis of socialist and communist mass movements, and their particular figures of leadership) make for

DOI: 10.4324/9781003742876-15

striking dis-analogies with the present, and yet both the content of contemporary planetary reaction (fantasies of law and order, mythologies of racial superiority, desires for rebirth) and aspects of its form—its irreducibility to socio-economic causation, but also many leitmotifs of its discourse and affective disposition—means that talk of fascism is not, *pace* the liberal mainstream, simply misplaced or, worse, hysterical. Elsewhere, I have tried to capture our ideological conjuncture through the notion of *late fascism*—a concept constructed both by resonances with and dis-analogies from some of the fundamental tenets that make up the legacy of critical theories of fascism. Unlike "classical" fascism, this late fascism is not inhabited by the non-contemporaneity or non-synchronicity that, according to Ernst Bloch, characterised the psycho-social bases of Nazism; if anything, it is nostalgic for the contemporaneity or synchronicity of industrial modernity (a kind of "white" Fordism). Contrary to Georges Bataille's pioneering analyses of the psychological structure of fascism, contemporary reaction is not pervaded by reference to a heterogeneous, "sovereign" surplus that would be required to bolster the homogeneity of state and capital. And, against images of the totalitarian or even the "ethical" state, late fascism, moulded by the capillary influence of neoliberalism, is driven by a desire for the state but also by a hatred of government. Though it often fantasizes opposition to a fantastical red threat, in a kind of anti-communism without communists, late fascism reacts against what is already a (neo)liberal reaction to the revolutionary upsurges of the short twentieth century. In other words, late fascism is not primarily counter-revolutionary—and in that sense even less "necessary" or "instrumental" for a capital whose threat is principally endogenous. As I have put it elsewhere, late fascism is not consolidated by a ruling class effort to use the autonomy of the political to deal with an external limit of capital but one of the offshoots of an endogenous protracted crisis of legitimacy of capital, in which the political is autonomous more at the level of fantasy than function; it is "a symptom of the toxic obsolescence of the modern figure of the political, namely a 'national and social state' in which citizenship is organised across axes of ethno-racial and gender identity, and articulated to labour" (Toscano, 2017).

For about four decades, the theorisation of fascism (and Nazism) has played a prominent part in Žižek's work, often taking the guise of efforts to distinguish it from Stalinism, thus troubling or undermining the very category of "totalitarianism". In this article, I want to explore some of the theses and insights that emerge from this sustained concern on Žižek's part with fascist ideology, in view of evaluating the extent to which his thinking can contribute to the *aggiornamento* of critical theories of fascism in these "late fascist" times. As I hope to further detail below, the pertinence of Žižek's thoughts on fascism for our own ideological interregnum originates at least in part from the specificity of the conjuncture in which his theorising developed, namely the Slovenia of the early 1980s. Theories of fascism (and Nazism), in their contrastive articulation with accounts of Stalinism, and within the broader purview of disputes about "totalitarianism", emerged in the *sui generis* really-existing socialism of what would be the final decade of Yugoslav self-management. The uses of theories of fascism, but also of fascist symbols (as in the proposals and provocations of the *Neue Slowenische Kunst* and Laibach, to which I'll return), along with the possible lineaments of anti-fascism, are here articulated in a complex critical parallelogram: no longer the face-off between fascism and communism, or the shifting triangle of fascism, communism and liberalism, but the shifting fourfold of fascism (or Nazism)/Stalinism (or communism)/(capitalist) liberalism/"Really-existing Socialism" (Slovenia/Yugoslavia). It is from the "semi-peripheral" angle of vision of an outlier in the ambit of the "Second World" of postwar socialism, and in a decade marked by a profound ideological and social crisis (an uneven transition to liberal capitalism that would traverse the massacres of the civil wars, from which Slovenia itself was spared), that Žižek (alongside his philosophical comrade Mladen Dolar) would develop his characteristic claims regarding the need to supplement and shift the nostrums of the critique of political economy through Lacanian psychoanalysis.

Žižek's inaugural conviction, which he shares with the arc of critical Marxisms from Horkheimer to Postone, is that fascism is fundamentally defined by its violent disavowal of its own continuity (or better, intensification) of the capitalist *status quo ante*. In an interview looking back at Laibach's practical and aesthetic re-articulation of fascism, Žižek presents an admirably concise summary of the link between, on the one hand, the thesis that fascism is an intra-capitalist simulacrum of revolution and, on the other, the methodological imperative to draw on psychoanalysis in the theory of fascism, while also differentiating among fascisms—a task that remains crucial today. This takes place in four steps.

First, the *Verneinung* of capitalism:

> Fascisms are of different sorts. What unites them is a basic reflex: capitalism without capitalism. Fascism wants to preserve the basic relations of capitalism, but simultaneously to take away capitalism's ideological and economic features, which bring individualism, disequilibrium, and so forth. The ideal of fascism is to have capitalism, in the sense of private ownership and relations of capital and labor, but capitalism that is liberated from all of its excesses: no class struggle, but rather cooperation between classes; no spiritless money, but rather patriarchal relations in which the capitalist is not a spiritless exploiter, but one who looks after the workers in a patriarchal and fatherly manner.
>
> (Žižek, 1997, p. 60)

Second, the wrenching contradictions latent in this disavowal, manifest in the wretched travesty of a third way between capitalism and socialism, and generating the indispensable mechanism of racial scapegoating:

> Fascism's goal is organic cooperation. Because this goal is impossible to reach, it is necessary to posit an enemy, onto whom the reason for the difficulty can be projected. Fascism is fond of corporeal metaphors for labor and capital, like "head" and "hand"; it likes to speak of society as an organism in which one social stratum is the head and another is the hand. Because fascism does not work and because the reason for its difficulties cannot lie in the antagonistic relations between head and hand, between capital and labor, the cause of the social disequilibrium is projected onto some cancerous formation, some external enemy. These are the Jews or another foreign people.[2]
>
> (Žižek, 1997, p. 60)

Third, the plurality (and ultimately *duality*) of fascisms, opening up a controversial contiguity with really-existing socialism:[3]

> As analyses indicate, we have two types of fascism. The first type is a savage, self-annihilating fascism that cannot find an equilibrium and, at a certain point, goes crazy and has to destroy itself, burning itself up in self-annihilating wars (Hitler, Mussolini after 1940). The second type is a patriarchically peaceful, principled Catholic fascism (Dollfuss, Pétain in France, Mussolini through 1940) that lacks a self-annihilating dynamic and can peacefully persist to the end of time, as long as it is not buried by economic or other circumstances. Salazar was the longest ruling European dictator and president. Not only is this light fascism still rooted generally in Slovene consciousness, but Slovene self-management has also appropriated it for itself. In its struggle against the evil spirit of statist, evil, totalitarian socialism, self-managing socialism refers to and even reactivates a series of motives that are exceptionally close to light fascism.
>
> (Žižek, 1997, pp. 62–63)

Fourth, the necessity of a psychoanalytic framework to excavate, traverse and inhibit the fascist fantasy:

> The slogan of fascism is "enough of enjoyment, enough of debauchery: a victim is necessary". The whole trick of fascism is certainly in an excess enjoyment, which itself produces the renunciation of enjoyment, the gesture of sacrifice. The Left was never ready to really confront this trauma. From this comes the Left's persistent traumatization, how to kill fascism, and the persistent impotence of its abstractly enlightenment arguments against

> fascism, which simply do not function. The Left emphasizes as its great ascertainment that fascist ideology is irrationally authoritarian. Fascism tells you to obey, but it does not give reasons to obey. Obedience like this, however, has a meaning. Fascism knows everything about this. The tragedy of the Left is that the more it criticizes those who are caught in fascism, the more it gives them arguments to be fascist.

This grounding insight into the psychic rationality of the irrational is at the heart of Žižek's stress on the "impotence of the Left to confront what is, in psychoanalytic terms, the libidinal economy of fascism" (Žižek, 1997, p. 63)[4]—a statement that echoes a dissident strand of theorising about fascism, beginning in the interwar period with Wilhelm Reich, Erich Fromm, and Georges Bataille and reaching all the way to the 1970s and 1980s with the writings of Deleuze & Guattari or Klaus Theweleit. It is no accident, in this regard, that Žižek has defined the theoretical specificity of Lacanian psychoanalysis precisely by the way in which it distinguishes itself from the most sophisticated effort hitherto to combine—in a disjunctive synthesis or parallax as it were—the critique of political economy with the teachings of Freud, namely critical theory in its Adornian guise. The theory of fascism is both where Adorno's appropriation of Freud's theses on mass psychology shows its greatest promise and where it meets its ultimate "deadlock". Žižek recognises and celebrates the superiority of Adorno's work to all the impasses of an undialectical "Freudo-Marxism" incapable of grasping the negativity of the unconscious, or the operative antinomy of repression and sublimation. But he discerns in the German philosopher's writing a tendency, in tension with his own critique of a normative bourgeois individuality, first, to draw from Freud's theory a lesson about the need to strengthen and defend the *ego*, and, second, a correlated conception of fascism as fundamentally a matter of *manipulation*. A tendency to treat the manipulating subject of fascism as instrumental and its manipulated subject-object as a demolished ego prey to mass narcissism, results in a misprision regarding the very status of fascist ideology. For Žižek, this is encapsulated in the "pseudo-concept" of repressive desublimation (as opposed to Freud's repressive *sublimation*), whereby the Id triumphs over the Ego in the same process by which society thoroughly subsumes, or indeed crushes, the individual. While repressive desublimation does foreground real processes and contradictions at work in "post-liberal" societies, the idea that behind fascist irrationality and the "de-psychologised" masses lies a kind of selfish calculation misses the specificity of fascism. The result, as Žižek notes, is that

> Adorno refuses to treat fascism as an ideology in the proper sense of the term—that is, as a "rational legitimation of the existing order". The so-called "fascist ideology" no longer possesses the coherence of a rational construct that calls for conceptual analysis and ideologico-critical

> refutation. "Fascist ideology" is not taken seriously even by its promoters; its status is purely instrumental, and ultimately relies on external coercion. Fascism no longer functions as a "lie necessarily experienced as truth"—the sign of recognition of a true ideology.
>
> (Žižek, 1996, p. 19)

The superiority of Lacanianism as ideology-critique to Adorno's Freud-inspired theory of fascism lies then in the former's capacity, based on the radical disjunction between ego-psychological categories and a concept of the unconscious grounded in a theory of the signifier, to move beyond "psychology" *stricto sensu*. What is at stake, therefore, is a different concept of "de-psychologization": not the loss of the centrality and interiority of the ego analysed and mourned by Adorno, but the operation of a superegoic Law that stands in a signifying relation of exteriority to the subject. As Žižek observes,

> the superego is a Law in so far as it is not integrated into the subject's symbolic universe, in so far as it functions as an incomprehensible, nonsensical, traumatic injunction, incommensurable with the psychological wealth of the subject's affective attitudes, bearing witness to a kind of "malevolent neutrality" directed towards the subject, indifferent to his empathies and fears. At this precise point, as the subject confront the "agency of the letter" in its original and radical *exteriority*, the signifier's nonsense at its purest, he encounters the superego command "Enjoy!" which addresses the most *intimate* kernel of his being.
>
> (Žižek, 1996, p. 20)

This "extimate" working of fascism (to adapt a Lacanian notion), in which the social Law operates as a superego injunction, is for Žižek what repressive desublimation both gestures towards and misses. Lacan's linguistic turn towards the "agency of the letter", and to what Žižek pointedly calls "the strictly *non-psychological* character of the unconscious" is what allows the French psychoanalyst's theory to capture the materiality of fascist discourse in a manner that critical theories of fascist manipulation do not. Similarly, the "distance" that a fascist subject may bear to his discourse is not a kind of instrumental mask—as Adorno's notions of "simulation" or phony fanaticism may suggest—but an integral, and deeply troubling, dimension of fascist ideology itself. As Žižek notes, *contra* the very idea of ideology as manipulation:

> "madness" does not turn on effectively believing in the Jewish plot, in the charisma of the Leader, and so on—such beliefs (in so far as they are repressed, that is, the unacknowledged fantasy-support of our universe of signification) form a constituent part of our ideological "normality". "Madness", however, emerges in the *absence* of such engaging beliefs, in the

> fact that "in the depth of their hearts, people *do not* believe that the Jews are the devil". In short: madness emerges through the subject's "simulation" and "external imitation" of such beliefs; it thrives in that "inner distance" maintained towards the ideological discourse which constitutes the subject's social-symbolic network.[5]
>
> (Žižek, 1996, pp. 21–22)

It is around this question of an inner distance that Žižek's Lacanian theory of fascist ideology turns. Distance pertains to the functioning of social Law under fascist conditions; it is determined by the non-ideological kernel sustaining every fascist ideology; it allows us to identify the capture and colonisation of "popular" energies and desires by fascism; and, lastly, it is the target of that *sui generis* practical critique of fascist fantasy that Žižek, in his several writings on Laibach and the *Neue Slowenische Kunst*, terms *over-identification*. Let us consider these dimensions of distance in turn.

As Žižek details in his brief essay, "Why are Laibach and the *Neue Slowenische Kunst* not Fascists?", the social Law—which, as we've already seen, hinges on the superego injunction and the agency of the letter—cannot be considered as a homogeneous and complete whole. The Law, Žižek argues, is necessarily split, by virtue of its incompleteness, its being "not-all", into "the written public Law and its underside, the «unwritten», obscene secret code". This means that explicit, public rules do not suffice, so they must be supplemented by a clandestine, 'unwritten' code ... The field of Law is thus split into Law *qua* 'Ego-Ideal', i.e., a symbolic order that regulates social life and maintains harmony, and its obscene, superegoic inverse. (Žižek, 2007, pp. 63–64). It is in the obscene inverse of the written order, then, that any "rule of law" is supplemented (but also subverted) by a communal bond, whose substance is transgression:

> What most deeply "holds together" a community is not so much identification with the Law that regulates the community's "normal" everyday rhythms, but rather *identification with a specific form of transgression of the Law, of the Law's suspension* (in psychoanalytic terms, with a specific form of enjoyment). [...] The Nazi community relied on the same solidarity-in-guilt adduced by participation in a common transgression: it ostracized those who were not ready to assume the dark side of the idyllic *Volksgemeinschaft*, the night pogroms, the beatings of political opponents—in short, all that "everybody knew, yet did not want to speak about aloud".
>
> (Žižek, 2007, p. 64)

It is worth noting here the shifts or hesitations in Žižek's own accounts of the play of Law and distance in fascist ideology. In passages like the one above, it seems that fascism (in its Nazi guise), still operates across the two registers of public law and common transgression. Elsewhere, fascism seems to be marked by a peculiar implosion of this distance, and the "fundamental trait of the totalitarian social link" is defined as "the loss of distance between the fantasy that gives the indicators of the enjoyment of the subject and the formal-universal Law that governs social exchange" (Žižek, 2007, p. 102). Indeed, loss of distance is here the differentiating factor between the "two" fascisms (nihilist-accelerationist fascism or "pure totalitarianism", on the one hand, and "light fascism", on the other), which we already encountered above:

> The fantasy is "socialized" in an immediate way insofar as the social Law coincides with the injunction, "Enjoy!" It begins to function as a superego imperative. In other words, in totalitarianism, it is really the fantasy that is in power and this is what distinguishes totalitarianism *stricto sensu* (Germany in 1938–45, the Soviet Union in 1934–51, Italy in 1943–45) from the patriarchal-authoritarian regimes of law-and-order (Salazar, Franco, Dollfuss, Mussolini until 1943) or from "normalized" socialism. Such pure totalitarianism is necessarily self-destructive; it cannot be stabilized; it cannot arrive at a minimal homeostasis that would allow it to reproduce in a circuit of equilibrium. It is constantly shaken by convulsions.
>
> (Žižek, 2007, p. 91)

Though Žižek does elsewhere go against the grain of the liberal-vindicationist theory of totalitarianism, here the dialectic of Law and fantasy, together with the collapse of distance, is seen to provide a theoretical definition of totalitarianism itself as the social order where, although there is no law (no positive legality with universal validity, established in an explicit form), all that we do can at any moment pass for an illegal and forbidden thing. Positive legislation does not exist (or if it does, it has a totally arbitrary and non-obligatory character), but despite this we can at any moment find ourselves in the position of the infractor of an unknown and non-existent Law. (Žižek, 2007, p. 91).

While maintaining an ambivalence about the workings of distance between Law and its underside in fascist ideology and fantasy, Žižek does identify another dimension of distance that provides an insight into the libidinal integument of fascist ideology, namely the distance between ideology and the non-ideological. Contrary to the (liberal) idea that Nazism or totalitarianism is defined by the integral politicisation of life, for Žižek the binding power of fascist ideology lies precisely in the specific way it mobilises a general feature of ideology's efficacy, namely the idea that we can always maintain a distance from it, that beneath ideology there is something (human, natural, spiritual) that exceeds it, an irreducible *quid*. Commenting upon one of Hitler's speeches, as well as the *Führer*'s preference for Wagner's *Tristan und Isolde* over the composer's more explicitly mytho-political operas *Die Meistersinger* or *Lohengrin*,[6] Žižek advances the following thesis about ideology in general and fascist ideology in particular:

> in every ideological edifice, there is a kind of "trans-ideological" kernel, since, if an ideology is to become operative and effectively "seize" individuals, it has to batten on and manipulate some kind of "trans-ideological" vision which cannot be reduced to a simple instrument of legitimizing pretensions to power (notions and sentiments of solidarity, justice, belonging to a community, etc). […] The point is thus not that there is no ideology without a trans-ideological "authentic" kernel but rather, *that it is only the reference to such a trans-ideological kernel which makes an ideology "workable"*… So, paradoxically, the dangerous ingredient of Nazism is not its "utter politicization" of the whole of social life but, on the contrary, the suspension of the political through the reference to an extra-ideological kernel, much stronger than in a "normal" democratic political order.
>
> (Žižek, 2008b, pp. 27–29)

This realisation also prepares an understanding of the third dimension of distance that Žižek identifies in the workings of Fascist ideology, namely its relationship to "utopian" possibilities. Following the path already traced by Bloch in *The Heritage of Our Times* and other texts, Žižek repeatedly counters the false liberal wisdom according to which all desires for community, collectivity or authenticity are tainted by their association with fascism. The underdetermined character of the non-ideological kernel accounts for why "ruling ideas are never directly the ideas of the ruling class" (Žižek, 1999, p. 186),[7] making the domain of fantasy a field of political and ideological struggle:

> Of course Fascist ideology "manipulates" authentic popular longing for a true community and social solidarity against fierce competition and exploitation; of course it "distorts" the expression of this longing in order to legitimize the continuation of the relations of social domination and exploitation. In order to be able to achieve this effect, however, it none the less had to incorporate authentic popular longing.
>
> (Žižek, 1999, pp. 184–185)

That is why "the non-ideological Utopian character of this longing is to be fully asserted" (Žižek, 1999, pp. 184–185). In other words, the non-ideological is both indispensable for the functioning of (fascist) ideology, and the prize of its practical critique. Žižek, who repudiates the very category of the "proto-fascist" (Žižek, 1999, p. 139),[8] takes this to be the case not just for the longing for community, bodily discipline or the political aesthetics of the masses, but also, in the philosophical domain itself, for *decision*. This is the crux of his intervention into the debate over Heidegger and Nazism, where he presents the "second" decisionist Heidegger (the first being identified with the analytic of Dasein, the third with the *Kehre* and a depoliticising *Gelassenheit*) as both the one who threw his cards in with Nazism *and* the one who was closest to a true grasp of political subjectivity. Against a Habermasian criticism of Heidegger which treats the decisionist dimension of *Being and Time*'s account of the historicity of Dasein as proto-Nazi, Žižek regards it as simply a condition of the political that cannot be conceded to the right. Whence his assessment of the philosophical-political regression that Heidegger's famous "turn" represented:

> what Heidegger later dismissed as the remainder of the subjectivity transcendental approach in *Being and Time* is what he should have stuck to. Heidegger's ultimate failure is not that he remained stuck in the horizon of transcendental subjectivity, but that he abandoned this horizon all too quickly, before thinking out all its inherent possibilities. Nazism was not a political expression of the "nihilist, demoniac potential of modern subjectivity" but, rather, its exact opposite: a desperate attempt to avoid this potential.
>
> (Žižek, 1999, p. 21)

We can see here once again the model of fascism or Nazism as a revolution without, or rather *against* revolution, a violent flight forward and away from true philosophical and political radicality, ultimately undergirded by the murderous displacement of class antagonism onto genocidal racial hatred.[9]

Now, if ideology's inner distance (from its non-ideological kernel) is both a condition of possibility for its efficacy and a site of political conflict (over the articulation of popular fantasy, so to speak), it is also the locus for the operations of ideology-critique. But if the rationalist-Marxist unmasking of fascist manipulations and the effort to restore the bourgeois individualist ego-ideal are doomed, what options remain open. In the particular ideological observatory and laboratory that was 1980s Slovenia, Žižek found this opening in the performances and interventions of Laibach and the *Neue Slowenische Kunst*, capturing them under the heading of *over-identification*. I am not so interested here in Žižek's spirited defense of Laibach's signifying strategies—which goes as far as ascribing to them a counter-intuitive anti-fascist valence[10]—but in what it further reveals regarding the nexus of ideological "distance" and our relation to fascism. For Žižek, Laibach provides a model for acting upon (but also *with*) fascism not at the level of its instrumental intentionality, but of fantasy and enjoyment, welding Brechtian traditions of estrangement with an aesthetic-performative equivalent of the function of the Lacanian analyst. The "historical meaning" of the Slovenian group, according to Žižek, lies in

> providing a model of that which in Lacanian terminology would be said to go beyond the fantasm. Laibach confronted us with a fantasmic logic, with fascist enjoyment, and simultaneously, they presented this in such a way as to defamiliarize it and enable us to keep our distance from it.
>
> (Žižek, 1997, p. 63)

But perhaps "keeping one's distance" is still a misleadingly Enlightenmental, liberal formulation? For over-identification truly to operate it surely cannot simply amount to a vanishing mediator towards a position of enlightened lucidity; fantasies must be assumed and traversed, not merely named or performed "at a distance". Here, we need to attend to the way in which over-identification is precisely pitted against "ironic" distance as a variant of that inner distance that according to Žižek, as we saw, defines the very efficacy of ideology. Reflecting on Laibach, Žižek asks us to explore whether variants of ideological distance do not in the end define *both* fascism as the supposed *ne plus ultra* of ideological fanaticism *and* a contemporary "post-ideological" condition defined by ironic or cynical distance towards publicly affirmed values.

> What if this distance, far from posing any threat to the system, designates the supreme form of conformism, since the normal function of the system requires cynical distance? In this sense, the strategy of Laibach appears in a new light: it "frustrates" the system (the ruling ideology) precisely insofar as it is not its ironic imitation, but represents an over-identification with it—by bringing to light the obscene superego underside of the system, over-identification suspends its efficiency.
>
> (Žižek, 1983b, p. 65)

This suspension, however, is not an unmasking, but works rather by analogy with how a Lacanian analyst frustrates transference, making possible the irruptive realisation that the Big Other does not exist. This is the sense in which Laibach's over-identification with the fascist kernel of enjoyment underlying the ruling ideology (in their case, "really-existing socialism", i.e. an ideology grounded on official anti-fascism), "*does not function as an answer but a question*", compelling us "to take up our own position and decide upon our desire"—in what may ultimately be regarded as a Lacanian return to a Kantian definition of Enlightenment as emergence from (or at least interruption of) our self-incurred immaturity (Žižek, in Badovinac, Čufer & Gardner, 2015, p. 65).[11]

By way of conclusion, we can ask whether our current predicament gives the strategy of over-identification any real promise or efficacy. One of the most evident, and commented upon, features of our late fascism (in its "alt-light" and "alt-right" avatars) is the blurring, so to speak, of irony and fanaticism, the germination of something like fanaticism in the guise of irony—an operation on the inner distance of ideology that does not fully chime with Žižek's "classical" typological distinction between "light fascism" and totalitarianism. Further investigation of the way in which Lacanian theory can shed light onto the workings of late fascism would require thinking of the latter not just in terms of its disanalogies from various instances of fascism in power but perhaps also in its ideological kinship with fascism as an ideological movement that had yet to fuse with the state and the social Law. This is the fascism that Mussolini in 1921 presented as a "super-relativist" movement, in keeping with the modern supremacy, including and especially in the sciences, of relativity over objectivism. As he declared, with florid bombast:

> For those who boast of always being the same as themselves, nothing is more relativistic than the fascist mentality and fascist action. If relativism and universal movementism (*mobilismo*) are equivalent, we fascists, who have always manifested our unscrupulous arrogance (*strafottenza*) towards the nominalisms to which the sanctimonious bigots of other parties nail themselves, like bats to rafters; we, who've had the courage of breaking into smithereens all the traditional political categories and calling ourselves, depending on the moment, aristocrats and democrats, revolutionaries and reactionaries, proletarian and anti-proletarian, pacifists and anti-pacifists, we are really the relativists par excellence and our action resonates directly with the most current movements of the European spirit.
>
> (Mussolini, 1921, p. 1)

To borrow from Hans Vaihinger, the post-Kantian philosopher whose reading of Nietzsche Mussolini leans on in this same article, this is a fascism of the *as if*, a fascism, so to speak, of the enjoyment of the very distance that makes ideology function. To the extent that shades of this reactionary relativism are a (more or less conscious) *leitmotiv* in the twenty-first century far right, they will test the capacities of both the Lacanian theory of fascism advanced by Žižek, and of the strategy of over-identification that accompanies it.

Notes

1 Contrary to its rhetoric of intransigent radicality, fascism may be regarded as the paradigmatic "pseudo-event" in the field of the political (and the ideological),

> a spectacular turmoil destined to conceal the fact that, on the most fundamental level (that of the relations of production), *nothing really changes*. The Fascist Revolution is thus the answer to the question: what do we have to change so that, ultimately, nothing will really change?
>
> (Žižek, 1999, p. 200)

2 Elsewhere, Žižek terms this "the fundamental wager of fascism", explaining it as the urge to preserve

> the fundamental relation of capitalism (between Capital and labour), [so that] fascism wants to abolish its organic, anonymous and savage character; that is to say, to make of it an organic relation of patriarchal domination between the 'hand' and the 'head', between the leader and his escort, and replace the anonymous 'invisible hand' by the will of the master. Now, insofar as we remain within the fundamental framework of capitalism, this operation does not work. There is always a surplus of the «invisible hand» that contradicts the design of the master.
> (Žižek, 2007, p. 85)

3 This distinction is also explored in terms of the broader thematics of social fantasy in "The Fetish of the Party", p. 91. The article largely reproduces Žižek's much earlier French article, "Le stalinisme: un savoir décapitonné" (1983a, pp. 57–83). The same volume also contains Mladen Dolar's related "Prolégomènes à une théorie du discours fasciste" (1983a, pp. 39–54).

4 Consider also the observation in "The Fetish of the Party" (Žižek, 2007), according to which Marx

> underestimated the importance of *fantasy* in the historical process, and the importance of inertia that does not dissolve due to its dialectization and whose exemplary intrusion would be what is called the 'negative behaviour of the masses', who appear to be acting against their best interests and let themselves get entangled in diverse forms of the 'conservative revolution'.

5 In an early piece on Laibach and NSK, Žižek instead briefly criticises Adorno's notion of fascist manipulation, for not capturing the coexistence of manipulation with integral, fanatical belief: "in spite of all his professed manipulation [as described in *Mein Kampf*], Hitler actually *completely believes his own views*" (Žižek, 1983b, p. 103). For a lengthy discussion of Adorno's work on fascism, which complements Žižek's account with a deeper exploration of the differences between *The Authoritarian Personality* and the 1951 essay on "Freudian Theory and the Pattern of Fascist Propaganda", as well as a Lacanian reframing of Freud's mass psychology, see, in the same volume, Mladen Dolar's "Fascism through Psychoanalysis" (1982, pp. 50–65).

6 Though I cannot explore it in any depth here, the non-ideological kernel peculiar to fascism and Nazism is also associated, via Lacanian theory, to the distinction between gaze and voice, on the one hand, and writing and the matheme, on the other. As Žižek observes:

> the Fascist discourse's medium par excellence is the living speech that hypnotizes by its very performative strength, without taking into account its signified content. To cite Hitler himself: 'All great events that have shaken the world have been provoked by speech and not writing'. By contrast, the medium par excellence of Stalinist discourse is writing. The Stalinist is almost obliged to read his very discourses in a monotonous voice, clearly attesting the fact that we are dealing with the reproduction of a prior writing. [...] In Lacanian theory, the Real has two principal sides. One is the Real as a reminder that is impossible to symbolize, a scrap, the refuse of the symbolic, a hole in the Other (in other words, the Real aspect of *objet a*, the voice, the gaze...; the other is the Real as writing, construct, number and matheme. These two sides perfectly correspond to the opposition fascism/Stalinism. The hypnotic power of Fascist discourse is supported by the 'gaze' and especially the 'voice' of the leader. The support of Stalinist discourse is, in turn, the writing.
> (Žižek, 2007, pp. 80–81; cf. Dolar, 1983, p. 42)

7 This resonates with Étienne Balibar's argument, according to which the dominant ideology is "a specific universalization of the imaginary of the dominated" (1993, p. 13).

8 Cf. also Žižek (2008a, p. 138), as well as the whole of Chapter 3, on Heidegger's philosophical commitment to National Socialism.

9 [T]he 'Jew', in playing the role of the disruptive element and introducing 'from outside' the surplus of class struggle, is really the positive repudiation of class struggle and of the notion 'there is no class relation'. It is for this reason that fascism, as distinct from socialism, is not a *sui generis* discourse, a global social contract, determining the whole social edifice. We could say that fascism, with its ideology of corporativism, of returning to the prebourgeois master, causes in some way an interference with Capitalist discourse without changing its fundamental nature—the proof being precisely the figure of the Jew as enemy.

(Žižek, 1999, p. 84)

Elsewhere, Žižek notes how Nazism displaces class struggle on to racial struggle and thereby obfuscates its true site. What changes in the passage from Communism to Nazism is the *form*, and it is in this change of the form that the Nazi ideological mystification resides: political struggle is naturalized into racial conflict, the (class) antagonism inherent to the social edifice is reduced to an invasion by a foreign (Jewish) body which disturbs the harmony of the Aryan community. The difference between fascism and Communism is thus "'formal-ontological', not simply ontic" (cf. Žižek, 2007, p. 127). For an elucidation for how this displacement of class onto race is analysed by Žižek through the framework provided by Lacan's theory of the four discourses (Master, University, Hysteric, Analyst)—as well as how this theory allows for a critical discrimination between Nazism and Stalinism, c.f. Dean (2006, ch. 2).

10 Cf. especially his "Letter from Afar" (1987), in *NSK—from Kapital to Capital.*

11 Parenthetically, it may be noted that Žižek's own interventions into the ideological field have been far more fruitful when he has functioned as a question than when, in the stance of the "public intellectual", he has been tempted to provide answers.

References

Balibar, E. (1993) The Non-Contemporaneity of Althusser. In A. Kaplan & M. Sprinkler (eds.) *The Althusserian Legacy*. New York, Verso.

Dean, J. (2006) *Zizek's Politics*. London, Routledge.

Dolar, M. (1982) Fascism through Psychoanalysis. In Z. Badovinac, E. Čufer and A. Gardner (eds.) *NSK—from Kapital to Capital: Neue Slowenische Kunst—an Event of the Final Decade of Yugoslavia*. Cambridge, MA, The MIT Press.

Dolar, M. (1983) Prolégomènes à une théorie du discours fasciste. *Analytica, 33*, pp. 39–54.

Mussolini, B. (1921) Relativismo e fascismo. *Il Popolo d'Italia*, 22 November, p. 1.

Toscano, A. (2017) *Notes on Late Fascism*. Available at: https://www.historicalmaterialism.org/notes-on-late-fascism/

Toscano, A. (2023) *Late Fascism: Race, Capitalism and the Politics of Crisis*. London, Verso.

Žižek, S. (1983a) Le stalinisme: un savoir décapitonné. *Analytica, 33*, pp. 57–83.

Žižek, S. (1983b) Ideology, Cynicism, Punk. In Z. Badovinac, E. Čufer and A. Gardner (eds.) *NSK -from Kapital to Capital: Neue Slowenische Kunst-an Event of the Final Decade of Yugoslavia*. Cambridge, MA, The MIT Press.

Žižek, S. (1987) Letter from Afar. In Z. Badovinac, E. Čufer and A. Gardner (eds.) *NSK—from Kapital to Capital: Neue Slowenische Kunst—an Event of the Final Decade of Yugoslavia*. Cambridge, MA, The MIT Press.
Žižek, S. (1996) *The Metastases of Enjoyment: Six Essays on Woman and Causality*. London, Verso.
Žižek, S. (1997) "Everything Provokes Fascism" (interview with Andrew Herscher). *Assemblage*, *33*, pp. 58–75.
Žižek, S. (1999) *The Ticklish Subject: The Absent Centre of Political Ontology*. London, Verso.
Žižek, S. (2007) *The Universal Exception* (2nd ed.) London, Continuum.
Žižek, S. (2008a) *In Defense of Lost Causes*. London, Verso.
Žižek, S. (2008b) *The Plague of Fantasies* (2nd ed.) London, Verso.

Chapter 11

Studies in Prejudice

Theorizing Anti-Semitism in the Wake of the Nazi Holocaust

Stephen Frosh

Reasons for Inclusion

Building on his pioneering writings about psychoanalysis and psychosocial studies, Nazi Germany, anti-Semitism and racism (see Frosh, 2005, 2023), in this essay Stephen Frosh presents a characteristically lucid review of critical attempts to theorise anti-Semitism in the wake of the Nazi Holocaust. Drawing on a range of relevant theorists, from Adorno and Horkheimer, to Otto Fenichel, Ernst Simmel and Slavoj Žižek, he carefully delineates a series of psychosocial responses to the prevailing psychoanalytic literature, resisting the pull towards 'psychologism' in favour of a more fully realised account of 'the structure of personal life as inextricably bound up with social forces' (this reader, p. 220). Frosh is an immensely important theorist within psychoanalytic studies, continuously reminding psychoanalysis of its critical limitations and shortcomings (e.g. in relation to its colonial assumptions), while drawing on its intellectual sophistication as a key impetus to the emerging transdisciplinary paradigm within psychosocial studies. The forms of racism and anti-Semitism which Frosh describes here are fundamental to the psychodynamics and social structure of historical and resurgent forms of fascism across the West, and, in the context of the present reader, Frosh's work is also notable for consistently highlighting the Jewishness of psychoanalysis as a site of ongoing remembering and working-through (see Frosh, 2005, 2013, 2019).

***

Asking Questions About Hatred: The Mission of *Studies in Prejudice*

In the period immediately after the Second World War, the question of how the murder of millions of people mainly on racial grounds could have come about in the centre of Europe fuelled interest in both the sociology and the psychology of authoritarianism, fascism and prejudice.[1] The topic of anti-Semitism was one focal point for this, understandably because of the specific fate of the Jews under Nazism but also because anti-Semitism could be seen as a prototype of, or perhaps a core element in, all racial hatred. Comprehending what

DOI: 10.4324/9781003742876-16

had happened and how to prevent it recurring was a crucial moral and political endeavour, and it also may have seemed to many people that without a conscious effort the lessons of the immediately preceding period might be lost before they had even been learnt. This was certainly the view of the editors of the American Jewish Committee-backed series *Studies in Prejudice*, produced by adherents of the Institute of Social Research, the 'Frankfurt School'. In their Foreword to the series, Max Horkheimer and Samuel Flowerman famously asserted (1950, p. v), 'Today the world scarcely remembers the mechanized persecution and extermination of millions of human beings only a short span of years away in what was once regarded as the citadel of Western civilization.' The claim that forgetfulness was already happening, that the memory of what had not yet come to be called the Holocaust was being lost, is explicit here and was to become an orthodox point of view amongst many historians in subsequent years. The argument ran that immediately after the war this forgetfulness was motivated by an emotional inability to face the facts of what had happened, a need to focus on personal and social reconstruction, fears provoked by the Cold War and possibly by a triumphalist discourse necessary for the foundation of the State of Israel. In governmental circles, the perceived dangers of communism had overtaken the actual experience of Nazi barbarism, in a shift that had all the hallmarks of the psychoanalytic process of denial writ large. This version of things has now been put severely in doubt, not just by ideologues such as Norman Finkelstein (2000) who have traced the explosion of more recent interest in the Holocaust to the efforts of American Jews and Zionists to create a favourable climate for themselves. More careful scholarship has also revealed a substantial amount of writing and activity around 'remembering' the Holocaust that started immediately at the war's end (and even before it in some cases) and never really ceased, even if it did not come together until towards the end of the 1950s. In his Introduction to the edited collection *After the Holocaust: Challenging the Myth of Silence* (Cesarani and Sundquist, 2012, p. 2), for instance, David Cesarani comments:

> The purpose of this essay collection is to present evidence that in the wake of the Second World War the Jewish survivors of Nazi persecution and mass murder were not 'silent' and that, over the ensuing fifteen years, the world was gifted a plenitude of information about the horrors that had so recently occurred in Europe.

The evidence the collection presents is indeed compelling on this, but it also offers some explanations as to why people who it might be assumed wrote in good faith about the 'silence' could have thought it had existed. One reason was language: much personal testimony written in the early years was in Yiddish or Polish and was not translated; in addition, it was very difficult to sustain networks of international collaboration and memorializing once the post-war East–West divisions were fully in place. This all means that the situation was much more complex than Horkheimer and Flowerman's statement about 'scarcely remembering' suggests: there was plenty of activity, even if keeping track of it and institutionalizing it was hard.

Of course, Horkheimer and Flowerman were not naïve. On the one hand, the warning about forgetting was an important factor in setting the work of the authors of *Studies in Prejudice* and that of the American Jewish Committee in a strongly moral and therapeutic framework—their role was to remind the world of the horror that it had just witnessed and was in the process of denying. But Horkheimer and Flowerman were also aware that the forgetting was nowhere near absolute: they continued by suggesting that the trend they identified towards denial had not fully silenced the troubling questions posed by Nazism; and that these have something to do with the fragility of the structure of civilization within which supposedly advanced cultures live.

> Yet the conscience of many men was aroused. How could it be, they asked each other, that in a culture of law, order and reason, there should have remained the irrational remnants of ancient racial and religious hatreds? How could they explain the willingness of great masses of people to tolerate the mass extermination of their fellow citizens? What tissues in the life of our modern society remain cancerous, and despite our assumed enlightenment show the incongruous atavism of ancient peoples? And what within the individual organism responds to certain stimuli in our culture with attitudes and acts of destructive aggression?
>
> (Horkheimer and Flowerman, 1950, p. v)

This sets up the work very clearly as an attempt to understand *irrationality* and mass psychology. What is articulated here is a polarization of the 'culture of law, order and reason', which one might assume to be the enlightenment project, against 'irrational' forces that are left over as 'remnants of ancient racial and religious hatreds' and which are visible in the willingness of people to tolerate violent destructiveness. 'Irrationality' here is a kind of vestigial but still active process; the account is reminiscent of Freud's (1927, p. 48) seemingly despairing response to the continued hold of religion over people who should know better: 'surely infantilism is destined to be surmounted'.

The way Horkheimer and Flowerman articulate this similarly draws on the idea of a developmentally 'primitive' state that puzzlingly sustains itself and breaks into the mature organism to do damage. The dominant images are colonial and bodily, running together the idea that there is a primitive stain in civilization ('atavism') with the equally familiar one of an apparently healthy body politic that is subjected to a spreading illness. The shock of Nazism was that it could appear as an 'irrational remnant' in a 'culture of law, order and reason'—as if psychoanalysis had not already told the world that such 'culture' is built on shaky foundations, that irrationality is not just something it contests, but is its permanent underside. The 'incongruous atavism of ancient peoples' breaks through, damaging 'our assumed enlightenment' and in this formulation echoing Freud's own colonial imagery of the 'primitive' and the 'savage' (Freud, 1913). Switching from this language of primitivity and 'ancientness', Horkheimer and Flowerman also attribute the going-astray of Western civilization to the attack on it by a bodily pathology: 'What tissues in the life of our modern society remain cancerous?' they ask. The key point, softened by their use of 'assumed' in 'assumed enlightenment', is that there is something left over or extraneous that is damaging contemporary culture, and it is this we need to understand—rather than that it is the culture itself that is wrong. That is to say, they do not prefigure the later suggestion, for example from Zygmunt Bauman (1989), that the Holocaust was not an aberration, but an *expression*, of modernity; rather, they maintain the simplification that there is a fundamental opposition between civilization and barbarism, between the cultured and the primitive, between the healthy organism and that which invades it to make it ill. This is a view not consistently held by Freud himself, despite his push to oppose the civilized European by the other as 'primitive'. Indeed, that the seeds of destruction might be *intrinsic* to 'a culture of law, order and reason' is suggested by his own account of how culture originates in acts of violence (the murder of the father in *Totem and Taboo* and in *Moses and Monotheism*—Freud, [1913], 1939) as well as by the broader psychoanalytic proposal that each human subject, however 'cultured' she or he may be, is inhabited and preoccupied by irrational, unconscious urges that may even take the form of a drive towards death.

Still, Horkheimer and Flowerman ask excellent questions.

> How could they [i.e. "many men"] explain the willingness of great masses of people to tolerate the mass extermination of their fellow citizens? ... And what within the individual organism responds to certain stimuli in our culture with attitudes and acts of destructive aggression?

These questions remain timely: how can it be that such things can (be allowed to) take place? In the full glare and gaze of the populace, with everyone's knowledge, in full daylight—because this is what happened and happens, even if there were shadows too, in which much of the detail was hidden—something bursts through that excites some people into destructive action and terrorizes others into silence, and brutalizes everyone until they hardly see it for what it is. And asking such questions was no trivial matter in the immediate postwar period, even if the claim is heavily overstated that there was little discussion of the Holocaust. As details of the concentration camps seeped into public awareness; as people started to rebuild their lives and particularly as the Jews who had escaped began to trace what had happened to those who had been left behind, the force of these questions was sometimes too much for people to take in and silence was at least sometimes the preferred response (e.g. Roseman, 2001). In articulating the issues at all, the authors of *Studies in Prejudice* were very much on the side of those brave enough to risk seeing what was there.

In search of useful answers, Horkheimer and Flowerman draw heavily on psychoanalysis and social psychology. They are in fact alert to the possibility that they will be criticized for their psychological focus, and attend quickly to it; after all, the Frankfurt School was one of the most influential and sophisticated groups of sociologists and social theorists of the twentieth century. Nevertheless, they choose to stay with psychology in regarding the essential intervention that will follow from their studies as one of *education* and through that protection of the individual against the possibility of being led astray again; and for them, such educational interventions are individually and psychologically based. 'Once we understand, for example, how the war experience may in some cases have strengthened personality traits predisposed to group hatred,' they write (Horkheimer and Flowerman, 1950, p. v), 'the educational remedies may follow logically. Similarly, to expose the psychological tricks in the arsenal of the agitator may help to immunize his prospective victims against them.' The model here is pedagogic and therapeutic; the point is to understand 'irrationality' and 'atavism', and indeed susceptibility to 'agitators' advancing extremely prejudiced views. And for them, this is a personal affair: 'education in a strict sense is by its nature personal and psychological', which means that one has to understand just what the personal and psychological element in 'prejudice' might be in order to find ways to 'eradicate' it. This psychological focus both allows for a nuanced and powerful utilization of psychoanalytic theory, and raises questions about what *Studies in Prejudice* might offer for a fully social analysis of what nowadays we might more easily recognize as racist hate. The rest of this chapter takes up these points in relation to the core racialized component of *Studies in Prejudice*, the issue of anti-Semitism, asking about the limits of the approach taken by the Frankfurt School theorists of the time, and also about how it feeds into some later developments, with particular reference to some of the ideas of Slavoj Žižek.

Cultural Nomadism

Given the emphasis on psychology, the persuasive power of authoritarianism and the 'irrationality' of prejudice and hate, it is not surprising that psychoanalysis was one of the conceptual systems drawn on in *Studies in Prejudice*. Its influence can be seen very profoundly in its best-known volume, Adorno, Frenkel-Brunswik, Levinson and Sanford's (1950) *The Authoritarian Personality*. For Adorno and Horkheimer, the lead figures in the Institute for Social Research, the stakes were high. Wiggershaus (1995 [1986], p. 275) describes how, by 1940, Adorno was seeing the Jews as 'the proletariat of the world-historical process of enlightenment, deprived of every vestige of power', so that analysis of the Jewish situation and of anti-Semitism would cut to the heart of the issues of domination and oppression. Adorno developed a vision of the Jews as representing 'nature' (in the form of an attachment to 'nomadism') against the depredations of 'civilized', alienated class society. This provokes envy amongst non-Jews, with the Jew representing a happier, less constrained humanity, in which the forces of rationality and alienated labour are kept at bay.

It has to be said that this seems an unlikely portrait of Jews, who throughout the twentieth century were more characteristically viewed as urban. Indeed, distance from 'nature' was often used in the rhetoric directed against them, in particular through the trope of 'rootless cosmopolitanism' and divorce from the 'land' or 'soil'. On the other hand, Adorno's reference to nomadism is resonant of some of Carl Jung's notorious commentaries in the pre-war era, in which the Jew is seen as parasitical on the more substantial and genuinely creative Aryan consciousness.

> The Jew, who is something of a cultural nomad, has never yet created a cultural form of his own and as far as we can see never will, since all his instincts and talents require a more or less civilized nation to act as host for their development.
>
> (Jung, 1970 [1934], p. 165)

What is apparent here is that the representation of the Jew as nomadic, which is understood by Adorno as a source of anti-Semitic envy, is turned by Jung into an accusation of parasitism. This combines the idea of rootlessness with a more general feeling that has recently become central to some psychoanalytic thinking on racism: that the core racist fantasy is of having something stolen. The others enjoy themselves too much; this is envied—there is so much freedom in it—and the question arises, why do *they* have so much pleasure, and *we* so little? The answer has to be, because our deserved enjoyment for which we have worked and suffered so hard, has been taken away from us by underhand means. The Jew has stolen the money, the black has stolen sexuality: this is what drives much racist fantasy. For Slavoj Žižek, prime exponent of this view of the racist imaginary, such a fantasy is premised on the repression of a different awareness, that what has been 'lost' or stolen in this way was never part of the subject at all:

> What we conceal by imputing to the Other the theft of enjoyment is the traumatic fact that *we never possessed what was allegedly stolen from us*: the lack ('castration') is originary, enjoyment constitutes itself as stolen.
>
> (Žižek, 1993, p. 203)

Be that as it may, there is a direct line of thought from the presentation of anti-Semitism as constituted around the idea of the Jew as parasite to the broader theorizing of racism as a psychic structure organized around fantasies of the theft of enjoyment. The *currency* of Adorno's thinking in current work (Žižek engages with him thoroughly in several places, for example in a discussion of psychoanalysis and political liberation in Žižek, 1994) is very marked in this way, as it is in many others.

The image of the cultural nomad successfully captures a sense of the Jew as standing outside the social order—the Jew as other—that is powerfully engrained in much anti-Semitic thinking. Building on this in their *Dialectic of Enlightenment* (1989 [1944]), Adorno and Horkheimer make a link between Jews and women, understanding the hatred towards them both as deriving from their status as outsiders to the coercive power of domination. The point here is not so much the more conventional psychoanalytic claim that weakness is despised because it reminds the oppressor of her or his own vulnerability, although this notion is present in *The Authoritarian Personality*. It is rather that women and Jews are excluded from the realm of culture, yet they continue to exist; this makes them less alienated (because less acculturated, hence more 'natural') and so produces envy in the 'strong', who are the victims of their own alienation. Where Jews differ from other minorities, according to Adorno and Horkheimer, is in the unusual combination of this association with nature and 'weakness', and the striving of the Jew for something nonmaterial or spiritual—an argument very much akin to Freud's (1939) idea that the key characteristic of Judaism is the belief in an abstract God and that this provokes antagonism from the more regressed, *less* intellectually cultured (Christian) other. The impact of this, somewhat as in Freud's theorizing, is supposedly to elicit envy in those who are subject to what Wiggershaus (1995 [1986], p. 341) calls the 'failed civilization'. It is worth noting that the idea that the oppressed group bears the responsibility for preserving 'nature' is resonant of some later psychoanalytic accounts of the relationship between slavery and anti-black racism (e.g. Kovel, 1995), in which the repressed sexuality of the white is understood to be projected onto the supposedly animalistic body of the black. If it still seems slightly odd to extol Jews for their closeness to nature, it is nevertheless stimulating to consider that anti-Semitism may in this way connect more strongly with the general fantasy structure of racism: the derogated other who is made subject to racism stands in for what is imagined as having been lost or stolen, that thing that would bring the satisfaction which the 'failed civilization' denies.

Purity and Projection

There are a number of shared themes that emerge from work in the *Studies in Prejudice* tradition. One is the location of responsibility for anti-Semitism firmly with the anti-Semite: Adorno *et al.* (1950, p. 301) state 'anti-Semitism is not so much dependent on the nature of the object as upon the subject's own psychological wants and needs'. The search for purity, both pure goodness within and pure evil without, as a key element in the anti-Semite's consciousness is an example of such 'psychological wants and needs', and links this work with later psychoanalytic traditions of thinking on racism, which suggest that it is one of many refusals to deal with doubt and ambivalence (Rustin, 1991). Denial of the multifariousness of social and psychic phenomena forms the basis of what Adorno *et al.* refer to as 'psychological totalitarianism', the impulse to keep everything completely in its place, under the sway of one powerful, paranoid organizing principle. The cost of this is great because the anti-Semite lives in terror of the persecutory universe she or he has created, but the benefit is that at least this universe makes sense, and nominates one single, identifiable source of danger—the Jew. For *The Authoritarian Personality*, it is the violence of this psychic process that characterizes the fascist and anti-Semitic state of mind, closing down anything soft and welcoming, replacing it with a repudiating harshness that damages the subject as well as the hated other, and that reflects (again to use the anachronistic mode of expression) a kind of enjoyment that masks an inner emptiness.

> It is as if the anti-Semite could not sleep quietly until he has transformed the whole world into the very same paranoid system by which he is beset: the Nazis went far beyond their official anti-Semitic programme ... The extreme anti-Semite silences the remnant of his own conscience by the extremeness of his attitude. He seems to terrorize himself while he terrorizes others.
>
> (Adorno *et al.*, 1950, pp. 324–5)

This compellingly captures both the extremity of the anti-Semitic state of mind and its perversity, a point followed up in other work including Klaus Theweleit's (1987 [1977]) exploration of what he references as the 'monumentalism' of fascism, the way it acts to preserve psychological and social boundaries in the most rigid way, setting them up as a bulwark against fluidity. 'Terrorizing' anti-Semitism is seen by Adorno *et al.* as a kind of addiction demanding increasingly intense satisfaction if it is to leave the subject satisfied, yet with every 'fix' there is something more that is needed, and something more that is lost. Any 'difference' becomes a threat and has to be wiped out, but the more tightly the boundaries around what is acceptable and 'same' are drawn, the more likely it is that difference of one form or another will be encountered. So it is that the capacity of the self to tolerate anything 'outside' is continuously reduced, and the intensity of hatred of all that is other is exponentially increased. This account offers a relatively simple yet quite durable model for understanding anti-Semitism in a psychosocial framework: the Jew is a figure chosen initially for its cultural congruence as a hate object, but is then excessively invested in as a carrier of all this otherness; conspiracy is to be found everywhere. This produces a spiralling of paranoia and hatred, as the Jew serves both to contain and to exaggerate the projected impulses of the anti-Semite. Psychosis is in the air, kept at bay only by endlessly increasing rigidity and escalating anti-Semitic hate. The Jew is a safety valve for destructive impulses, but this use of the Jew has a profound personal and social cost.

This material indicates the weight placed on psychological interpretation of anti-Semitic phenomena, a characteristic shared by many studies of Nazism in the preceding years, as Daniel Pick (2012) has recently shown. That is, like Nazism, anti-Semitism is viewed as a kind of madness that might be responsive to the vocabulary of psychology (prejudice) and psychoanalysis (repression and projection); this also holds the psychopolitical hope that comprehending it in these terms might offer a route towards the 'treatment' or therapy of society. 'The educational remedies may follow logically', state Horkheimer and Flowerman (1950, p. vii), buying into the Freudian and enlightenment idea that knowledge transforms the uncontrollably irrational into the amenably rational. Given the circumstances, one might wonder whether this is an instance of failing to learn from immediately preceding history, in which the rationalistic model implying the inevitability of enlightened progression to mental and political balance so conspicuously failed. On the other hand, it is perhaps ironic to think that there might be a link to ego psychology, the dominant form of psychoanalysis in the USA after the war, which was so despised by some of the Frankfurter theorists, notably Marcuse (1972 [1955]). The usual criticism is that ego psychology, which emphasizes the role of the ego in mediating between unconscious impulses and the requirements of 'external reality', turns too readily into a conformist psychology stressing adaptation to social norms. However, considering what the psychoanalysts who developed it (who were mostly forced emigrants from Nazi Europe, many of them Jewish) had been through, perhaps one should not be too single-minded about pillorying ego psychology's attempt to reinstate rationality as a moral force. The wish to restore some semblance of rationality as an ideal could seem like a genuinely therapeutic and civilized response to the explosion of irrationality so recently endured.

The Frankfurt School theorists were very alert to the potential limitations of their psychological reading of anti-Semitism and balanced it by linking it closely to social and economic analysis. For example, according to Bronner and Kellner (1989, p. 7), Horkheimer's (1989 [1939]) essay 'The Jews and Europe' 'basically interprets anti-Semitism in terms of its usefulness for monopoly capitalism'. Even in this article and with this caveat, however, Horkheimer manages to convey the energy and intensity of Nazi anti-Semitism as 'intimidat[ing] the populace by showing that the system will stop at nothing', but also serving psychic needs.

> People can secretly appreciate the cruelty by which they are so outraged. In continents from whose produce all of humanity could live, every beggar fears that the Jewish émigré might deprive him of his living. Reserve armies

> of the unemployed and the petty bourgeoisie love Hitler all over the world for his anti-Semitism, and the core of the ruling class agrees with that love. By increasing cruelty to the level of absurdity, its horror is mollified … Pity is really the last sin.
>
> (Horkheimer, 1989 [1932], p. 92)

At this time, Horkheimer was generally scathing about the uses of psychological theories applied to social phenomena, but his analysis here is already pointing to the emotional hold that terroristic forms of anti-Semitism might have, even over those who ostensibly oppose them. It also shows the ambiguities that this psychic arrangement produced: 'pity is the last sin', not only pity for the other, but also the pity mobilized by recognition of the actual emotional needs of the hate-filled self.

If the fault lies not with the Jews, then why are the Jews so consistently chosen as the recipients of this particular form of racialized violence? The simple answer is that in the history of Western civilization—specifically its Christian history but, as the Nazis had shown, underpinned by a good dose of paganism—the figure of the Jew constitutes a ready-made container for the destructive urges of the anti-Semite. That is, the psychological formulation provided by psychoanalysis is made *psychosocial* through the thesis of a socially and historically legitimized mode of expression of these psychological forces. For Adorno *et al.*, Jews are suitable 'substitute objects' because of the work that has been done on them historically in the culture, producing a fantasy that is compelling, rigid, and exhaustive. This produces the Jew as a perfect '"object" of unconscious destructiveness', fitting all the necessary requirements to fulfil that role:

> It must be tangible enough; and yet not *too* tangible, lest it be exploded by its own realism. It must have a sufficient historical backing and appear as an indisputable element of tradition. It must be defined in rigid and well-known stereotypes. Finally, the object must possess features, or at least be capable of being perceived and interpreted in terms of features, which harmonize with the destructive tendencies of the prejudiced subject.
>
> (Adorno *et al.*, 1950, p. 300)

According to Adorno *et al.*, the Jew is the ideal, prepared-for hated other for the disturbed individual, who latches onto this escape route in order to preserve psychic integrity when faced with internal destructiveness and an oppressive social order. In addition, the system of domination works to confuse the prejudiced person, creating a sense of being alienated from society, of not understanding how it works or what are the sources of its actual impact. Politically unsophisticated, the anti-Semite seeks respite from a mystifying reality in the reassuring story of the single enemy, a rigid narrative of existence strong enough, and widely-shared enough, to seem to make sense, and one supported by a social order that ensures opposition is directed against an externalized other rather than against itself. The Jew's 'alienness' serves as shorthand for the alien nature of society itself, but the materiality of Jews makes them accessible as an object of hate in the way that society in general is not.

> Charging the Jews with all existing evils seems to penetrate the darkness of reality like a searchlight and to allow for quick and all-comprising orientation. The less anti-Jewish imagery is related to actual experience and the more it is kept 'pure', as it were, from contamination with reality, the less it seems to be exposed to disturbance by the dialectics of experience, which it keeps away through its own rigidity.
>
> (Adorno *et al.*, 1950, p. 310)

It is interesting to note that this theme of the irrelevance of Jews to anti-Semitism—the way anti-Semitism perpetuates itself even, or perhaps especially, in the absence of Jews—is one that continues to thrive in the literature, and has been taken up for example by Žižek. He tracks the ways in which the very unreality of the denigrated other sustains it in the face of violence, making an escalating phenomenon of hatred: 'This paradox, which has already emerged apropos the Jews in Nazi Germany … the more they were ruthlessly exterminated, the more horrifying were the dimensions acquired by those who remained' (Žižek, 1994, p. 78). Being unreal, being fantastic, the hated other cannot actually be eradicated; in a sense, the perfect enemy is the one who does not exist.

In one of Otto Fenichel's last pieces (Fenichel, 1946), written for Ernst Simmel's *Anti-Semitism: A Social Disease*, the situation is still starker and more psychoanalytically specific. He takes up the position also found in *The Authoritarian Personality* that anti-Semitism arises in periods of socially induced misery: the anti-Semite, immersed in confusion and led astray by ideological forces, 'sees in the Jew everything which brings him misery—not only his social oppressor but also his own unconscious instincts, which have gained a bloody, dirty, dreadful character from their socially induced repression' (Fenichel, p. 29). Jews are the ideal object for projection of these unconscious urges 'because of the actual peculiarities of Jewish life, the strangeness of their mental culture, their bodily (black) and religious (God of the oppressed peoples) peculiarities, and their old customs' (Fenichel, p. 29), which remind the anti-Semite of 'old primeval powers' that non-Jews have given up (Fenichel, p. 18). Jews seem uncanny because of these peculiarities, adding to the sense of threat and disgust they provoke. However, the most significant element leading to the intensity of anti-Semitic hate is the way the Jew is the recipient of the anti-Semite's own destructive feelings and also of the fantasized retaliation against them, induced by the individual's own superego. That is, both the repressed impulses and the punitive internal response to these urges are projected outwards, onto the Jew. Linked to this is a more profound identification between the Jew as foreign and uncanny, and the site of foreignness within: 'It can be expressed in one sentence' writes Fenichel (1946, p. 20): 'one's own unconscious is also foreign. Foreignness is the quality which the Jews and one's own instincts have in common.' The Jew as foreigner and preserver of archaic customs can be the object of projection of what is feared and hated within oneself, the 'foreign' unconscious; they thus carry the sense of destruction and desire, of 'what is murderous, dirty and debauched' (p. 19), and racist hate is magnified by the anti-Semite's terror of these inner urges. Again this theme can be found exemplified in some of Žižek's writings, but here turned not into a fundamental psychic structure, but one that is socially overdetermined, the structure of capitalism.

> Is capitalism's hatred of the Jew not the hatred of its own innermost, essential feature? For this reason, it is not sufficient to point out how the racist's Other presents a threat to our own identity. We should rather invert this proposition: the fascinating image of the Other gives a body to our own innermost split, to what is 'in us more than ourselves' and thus prevents us achieving full identity with ourselves.
>
> (Žižek, 1993, p. 206)

Against the implication that it is the inner state of the subject that is primary in seeking out an external cause, Žižek (1997, p. 76) also gives us a more elaborated version of anti-Semitism in which it is produced by the structure of capitalism itself: 'social antagonism comes first, and the "Jew" merely gives body to this obstacle'. Culture's investment in this figure of the 'Jew' produces it as an element in the unconscious, and with it arises the widespreadness of anti-Semitism itself.

Ernst Simmel (1946), writing in the volume of essays that he edited out of a symposium on anti-Semitism organized by the San Francisco Psychoanalytic Society in 1944, draws a familiar parallel here, using the discourses both of Marxism and of anti-Semitism-as-illness and making the connection between modernity ('civilization') and the canker that destroys it.

> Applying our method of psychoanalytic-dialectic thinking, we must infer not that anti-Semitism annihilates the achievements of civilization, but that the process of civilization itself *produces* anti-Semitism as a pathological symptom-formation, which in turn tends to destroy the soil from which it has grown. Anti-Semitism is a malignant growth on the body of civilization.
>
> (Simmel, 1946, p. 34)

For Simmel, thinking back on the Nazi phenomenon, anti-Semitism is both a cancer and a mass psychosis, a 'social disease', despite the individuals concerned not being psychotic; or rather, it is the existence of this mass psychosis that *protects* anti-Semites from becoming psychotic themselves. Although it is the case that there may be various neurotic processes at work within individual anti-Semites, the individual anti-Semite is 'normal'. However, when this person joins a group the crowd dynamic takes over, distinguished particularly by 'unrestricted aggressive destructiveness under the spell of a delusion' (Simmel, 1946, p. 39)—exactly the characteristic of psychosis. This is also the epitome of the splitting process: 'he can split in two the re-externalized parental power: into the leader whom he loves and into the Jew whom he hates' (Simmel, 1946, p. 50). All this further clarifies the comfortable way in which the anti-Semite can live with irrational beliefs:

> The anti-Semite believes in his false accusations against the Jews not in spite of, but *because* of their irrationality. For the ideational content of these accusations is a product of the primary process in his own unconscious and is conveyed to his conscious mind through the mediation of the mass-leader's suggestions.
>
> (Simmel, 1946, pp. 51–52)

The lie at the heart of racism, as Rustin (1991) describes it, comes out in full force here as a mode of psychic truth—not in the sense of an ethical truth, which it clearly is not, but rather as a symptomatic statement and a mode of containment-by-excess. The anti-Semite is attracted to 'irrational' beliefs precisely because they express the turmoil of a mind at war with itself and with the world, yet one that is structurally and socially weak, and needs the prop of its containing madness to keep itself sane. And at the root of this turmoil, according to Simmel, is 'the process of civilization itself', taking us back to the original theme that has at times been hard to preserve: that anti-Semitism is not something grafted onto modernity as an external force that disturbs what would otherwise be 'a culture of law, order and reason'; rather, as in Bauman's (1989) articulation, it is expressive of the irrationality that lies within modernity itself, and is generated by it.

Conclusion

It can be seen that despite the sophistication of the social theory on which these post-war writers drew, there is quite a simple psychosocial argument about anti-Semitism being posited. Society is anti-Semitic in its construction of the Jew as a hate object; and this construction allows individual anti-Semites to project their unconscious disturbances into that hate object. This simplicity is part of the reason both why the argument remains accessible and influential, and why it is also important to see how it is developed and deepened in later work. One question is, is it possible to go further than this essentially static presentation of the individual–social divide when considering anti-Semitism and other forms of social hatred? For example, might one build more fully on Simmel's argument that the contradictions in society are not simply accompaniments of, or accidental parallels to, the contradictions of the unconscious, but that they actively *produce* them, through all the micro- and macrosocial processes (parental interactions and anxieties; socialization practices; familial beliefs; gendered and 'racialized' institutional practices, etc.) out of which each person is made? Part of the point of the links made here with some later psychoanalytically-imbued sociological writing is to suggest that the ideas developed by the *Studies in Prejudice* authors prefigure a possibly more nuanced understanding of how the dynamics of racism and anti-Semitism are intrinsic to modernity and of the mechanisms through which this works to make them both 'personal' (in Horkheimer and Flowerman's sense) and fundamentally social, produced by 'the process of civilization'. For example, Slavoj Žižek, who has appeared frequently in this chapter, often turns to the exposure of anti-Semitism as a key topic, and even goes so far as to see anti-Semitism as paradigmatic for an understanding of racism itself. In this regard he writes that today, '"normal", nonexceptional, non-anti-Semitic racism is no longer possible' (Žižek, 1994, p. 74). His suggestion is not only that some basic psychic mechanisms are at work, but also that the fantasy structure of anti-Semitism is central to that of racism in general. For Žižek this turns on the idea of enjoyment and its theft, on how deprivation is clung to by the anti-Semite and on how the Jew is constructed, we might say, as the one who 'gets away with it', who can always turn the law to advantage. It should be noted that Žižek is often criticized for the way in which he approaches this material, for his own apparent 'enjoyment' of the anti-Semitic discourses that he describes (Frosh, 2011). Nevertheless, the detailed examination of the fantasy structure of anti-Semitism and racism that he uses can be seen to lean on the work of the critical theorists of the Frankfurt School, but also to radicalize it through its articulation of the *social* imaginary as the source of, and arena for, psychoanalytic exploration.

In all this, the figure of the Jew is a particularly powerful instance of the figure of the 'other' in general. Through its historically-derived cultural pervasiveness it is perpetuated as a representation of that which is needed yet despised, that which holds in place the otherwise potentially intolerable destructiveness of a social system founded on inequality and alienation. Such systems *create* their own psychic structures and psychological disturbances; thus, given the organization of Western society, anti-Semitism is as much an element in the unconscious of every subject as is any other psychosocial state—love, loneliness or loss, for example. The Jew is a constitutive feature of Western consciousness, primed by centuries of Christian anti-Semitism; and it is therefore one element out of which subjectivity is made. However, there are plenty of others, as postcolonial theory and feminism respectively have shown around racism and sexism, so anti-Semitism is by no means unique. One additional question that this gives rise to is over the extent to which the very specific and urgent focus on anti-Semitism that dominated in *Studies in Prejudice* limits or facilitates the application of its thinking to other modes of racist activity. Is it the case that European anti-Semitism's roots in the history of Christianity mean that what is theorized about the cultural function of the Jew as other is too specific to have lessons for, say, American anti-black racism? Or, as psychoanalysts have tended to assume, are we dealing with universal psychic mechanisms called into play under certain social conditions (extreme economic insecurity, for example) that then seek out whatever category of denigrated othering might be made available by the particular history of that culture? Whilst to the psychoanalytically attuned ear this seems a plausible assumption, the work still remains to be done, as some of the debates around the appropriateness of using psychoanalytic meta-categories in postcolonial theory have shown (Khanna, 2003) and as criticisms of psychoanalysis' own colonial and at times racist assumptions have also made clear (Brickman, 2003).

The post-Second World War effort to trace the psychodynamics of 'prejudice' was understandably focused on the recent experience of fascism and Nazism and concern over the danger of their resurgence; but it was also highly productive. These texts embody a principled attempt to construct a sophisticated psychosocial theory in the sense of one that understands the structure of personal life as inextricably bound up with social forces. However, the pull back to psychologism in this work inhibits the full development of such an account, effectively polarising the theory so that the social becomes either the true cause of anti-Semitism, or the 'container' for individual pathology. This makes sense within the prevalent discourse of Nazi 'madness', but perhaps is not so persuasive when one considers the durability of anti-Semitism and racism across time and space.

Note

1 Some material in this chapter was used in Stephen Frosh (2005), *Hate and the Jewish Science*. London: Palgrave.

References

Adorno, T. and Horkheimer, M. (1989 [1944]) *Dialectic of Enlightenment*. London: Verso.
Adorno, T., Frenkel-Brunswik, E., Levinson, D.J. and Sanford, R.N. (1950) *The Authoritarian Personality*. New York: Harper & Brothers.
Bauman, Z. (1989) *Modernity and the Holocaust*. Ithaca, NY: Cornell University Press.
Brickman, C. (2003) *Aboriginal Populations in the Mind*. New York: Columbia University Press.
Bronner, S. and Kellner, D., eds. (1989) *Critical Theory and Society: A Reader*. London: Routledge.
Cesarani, D. and Sundquist, E., eds. (2012) *After the Holocaust: Challenging the Myth of Silence*. London: Routledge.

Fenichel, O. (1946) 'Elements of a Psychoanalytic Theory of Anti-Semitism'. In Simmel, E., ed. *Anti-Semitism: A Social Disease.* New York, NY: International Universities Press: 11–32.
Finkelstein, N. (2000) *The Holocaust Industry: Reflections on the Exploitation of Jewish Suffering*. London: Verso
Freud, S. (1913) *Totem and Taboo. SE*, vol. XIII: vii–162. London: Hogarth Press.
Freud, S. (1927) *The Future of an Illusion. SE*, vol. XXI: 1–56. London: Hogarth Press.
Freud, S. (1939) *Moses and Monotheism. SE*, vol. XXIII: 1–138. London: Hogarth Press.
Frosh, S. (2005) *Hate and the Jewish Science: Anti-Semitism, Nazism and Psychoanalysis.* London: Palgrave.
Frosh, S. (2011) 'Psychoanalysis, Anti-Semitism and the Miser'. *New Formations* 72: 94–106.
Frosh, S. (2013) *Hauntings: Psychoanalysis and Ghostly Transmissions.* New York, NY, Palgrave Macmillan.
Frosh, S. (2019) *Those Who Come After: Postmemory, Acknowledgment and Forgiveness.* Palgrave Macmillan.
Frosh, S. (2023) *Antisemitism and Racism: Ethical Challenges for Psychoanalysis.* London: Bloomsbury Academic.
Horkheimer, M. (1989 [1939]) 'The Jews and Europe'. In S. Bronner, and Kellner, D., eds. *Critical Theory and Society: A Reader*. London: Routledge: 77–94.
Horkheimer, M. and Flowerman, S. (1950) 'Foreword to Studies in Prejudice'. http://www.ajcarchives.org/AJC_DATA/Files/AP1.pdf
Jung, C. (1970 [1934]) 'The State of Psychotherapy Today'. In Jung, C.G. *Collected Works*. London: Routledge, vol. 10: 157–173.
Khanna, Ranjana (2003) *Dark Continents: Psychoanalysis and Colonialism.* Durham, NC: Duke University Press.
Kovel, J. (1995) 'On Racism and Psychoanalysis'. In Elliott, A. and Frosh, S., eds. *Psychoanalysis in Contexts*. London: Routledge.
Marcuse, H. (1972 [1955]) *Eros and Civilization*. London: Sphere.
Pick, D. (2012) *The Pursuit of the Nazi Mind: Hitler, Hess, and the Analysts*. Oxford: Oxford University Press
Roseman, M. (2001) *The Past in Hiding*. Harmondsworth: Penguin.
Rustin, M.J. (1991) *The Good Society and the Inner World.* London: Verso.
Simmel, E. (1946) 'Anti-Semitism and Mass Psychopathology'. In Simmel, E. (ed.) *Anti-Semitism: A Social Disease*. New York: International Universities Press.
Theweleit, K. (1987 [1977]) *Male Fantasies*, vol. 1. Cambridge: Polity.
Wiggershaus, R. (1995 [1986]) *The Frankfurt School*. Cambridge: Polity.
Žižek, S. (1993) *Tarrying with the Negative: Kant, Hegel and the Critique of Ideology*. Durham, NC: Duke University Press.
Žižek, S. (1994) *The Metastases of Enjoyment*. London: Verso
Žižek, S. (1997) *The Plague of Fantasies*. London: Verso.

Part V

Afterword

Chapter 12

"Don't You See I'm Burning?"

Fascism Amnesia and the Failure of Witnessing

Jill Salberg

Reasons for Inclusion

Salberg's article provides a fascinating psychoanalytic perspective on memory, transgenerational trauma, and the re-emergence of fascism in contemporary politics. Focusing on the United States and the incipient fascism of Trump's Republican party, Salberg argues that the collective failure to countenance the terror and trauma of fascism in the past has contributed to its return in the present. The erasure of history, Salberg suggests, guarantees its repetition. Salberg's article concludes with an impassioned plea for adequate social processes of mourning, describing the work done by the Abuelas de Plaza de Mayo in Argentina. By linking the psychoanalysis of fascism to work on mourning and melancholia from Freud to Abraham and Torok, and to work the transgenerational transmission of trauma, Salberg highlights an important, understudied element of the fascist mind. Her work also suggests a path for a psychoanalytically informed anti-fascism—a kind of non-fascist mindstate, which relies on our capacity to accept loss and experience grief.

***

Conversations like the following were happening more frequently: "Where could we go? Where will they let us in and let us work? Is it safer to try someplace nearby or best to go further away?" Or this,

> Three generations of my family have lived in the same house in the same town. All of a sudden, we are told to leave and walk out with a single suitcase. I remember the night of the packing very well. Things went in the suitcase; things were taken out of the suitcase. In the end my mother filled it with food and warm clothing and bedding. Plus we took a watch, some earrings, a wedding ring with us to exchange for food. The next day my father was forced to hand over his remaining money to a delegation at the town hall
>
> (Weiss, as told to Connolly, 2015)

DOI: 10.4324/9781003742876-18

Listen to this excerpt from *The Atlantic*, December 2022, by Gal Beckerman titled, "What It Feels Like When Fascism Starts." He writes:

> Among the many Holocaust anecdotes I heard again and again as a child … none was more common than the tale of the brother who stayed and the brother who left. One brother couldn't bear to abandon his parents or homeland, while another brother packed a suitcase at the first inkling of danger and set off. The more impetuous one lives. The takeaway: When the social and political barometric pressure begins to drop, when you can feel that tingling: Leave.

Can you tell what year any of these are from? Is it the 1930s in Germany? Or is it 1970s in Argentina, 2014 in Venezuela? Or 2017/2025 in the United States? I raise this because—in many ways, in many places in the world—"we" have been here before, and we certainly know how things can turn out. Although I was born in the U.S., post-WW II, many historical residues flood me. I am aware of how endangered many are feeling and there is a foreboding in me, barely contained, just beneath the surface.

In the U.S. since 2020, early in the COVID pandemic, we have imploding racism, increased anti-Semitism, increasingly weekly incidences of gun violence and mass killings (in the U.S. we have more guns owned than people[1]), the banning of books, the overturning of the legal right of women to choose to end a pregnancy, and hatred of immigrants. These are all examples of reemerging, deeply oppressive forces and the ways that regimes of power exert control over minorities, their most vulnerable citizens.

We can consider all of this with the push to restrict what can be taught to children, the Florida anti-WOKE, "Don't Say Gay" laws, and extreme abortion bans and violence toward transgender people. In Texas, there is a move to remove any books in schools or libraries that make parents feel uncomfortable, books that relate to subjects such as slavery, 'critical race theory,' or gender and sexual diversities. When you ban teaching history and attack the news, memory is foreclosed. Amnesia becomes instilled.

In 2023, a *New York Times* article predicted Donald Trump's plan if he was restored to the presidency.[2] Even then, according to the article, Trump and Project 2025 intended to "centralize more power in the Oval Office" by "increasing the president's authority over every part of the federal government" (Richardson, 2023). The *New York Times* reporters envisioned a "president" who could not be checked by the Congress or the courts. At that time, I didn't know which would be more terrifying: the blatant plan to seize and centralize power, or the public posting of this intention. In the aftermath of the election, this has now come to fruition with many signed executive orders that place us on the brink of a Constitutional crisis. We are now facing—with the attacks on journalists, newspapers and lawsuits against lawyers who represented any cases against Trump—the kind of repressiveness toward controversy or criticism of Trump, including a denial of historical facts. This tips us toward autocracy and fascism.

Who were the many, nearly half the country, who have returned this authoritarian menace to the White House? As with prior dictators in the world, his sense of injury over being criticized and challenged takes forefront in his ongoing lawsuits and calls for impeachment of judges who rule against him. And further, the refusal to address the growing climate emergency, undoing all EPA rulings and promising to drill for more oil or gas. In January 2025, we all had to watch Los Angeles in flames, devastated by the worst wildfires that, despite all efforts, could not be contained for weeks. With the focus on autocratic power and not the health, safety, and well-being of all citizens my terror is continuing to climb.

Judith Herman (1992) coined the term episodic amnesia to describe how the field of psychology (and I would add psychoanalysis) briefly considers trauma and then looks away, episodically remembering and then forgetting completely. The events of the world over the past few years suggests a broader understanding of this amnesic process. I view it as a kind of refusal to allow memory that is filled with terror, with pain and great loss, into awareness. It is a negation of the anguished process that is necessary for true transformative healing to take hold. Empathy exhaustion takes over and too often we all look away. I know *I* can dissociate, forget, believing it won't happen or doubting that the reality I am seeing can possibly be true.

There is growing consensus that the global political universe has shifted away from democracy and is leaning toward illiberal autocratic governments with increased social repression, greater levels of openly expressed hatred and violence, embracing dictatorial strongman rulers. These moves toward fascism suggest a further disavowal of how far from a humane world we have moved, a kind of amnesia surrounding the trauma history in the United States and the world. The currents I am pointing to—of hatred, violence, and suppression of diverse points of view or historical facts—are, I believe, the reawakening of a fascism that never went away. The dissemination of what was once considered fascistic propaganda has now found the light of day in the term, 'alternative facts,' or real news being called 'fake news.' Conspiracy theories have enormous currency.

How do we awaken ourselves from the amnesic response to the traumatized burden of history? How do we live with a sense of terror and yet mobilize? I believe these political movements are heading directly toward negating truth and erasing history—a violent obliteration of any memory of a nation's trauma past. How many steps away is fascism? This is a clear sign of what I want to call '*fascism amnesia*.' One side of this fascism is not forgotten but in fact wished for and planned for. I imagine that the ultra-right wing of political movements have, what Ferenczi first termed, an identification with the aggressor. No matter what their personal history may have been with the fascistic past, these individuals have identified with the power of the leader and the movement.

Their hungering is for restoration of a power that orders and defines who is deserving of benefits and who is not, and is often based on traditional values of White male Christianity, patriarchy, and heteronormativity.

The alternate side are groups of people who feel these are just the wild rantings of the fringe, that we live in a democracy, with the rule of law, and something more ominous cannot happen here in a democracy. Yet again. (McCarthyism was a type of fascism.) There is denial and nonrecognition that there have been years of clear planning with millions of dollars put toward these goals. The people who cannot see what is happening believe that we must keep working to take care of ourselves and families, believing things will get better, i.e., the "moral arc bends toward justice." I wish, if only.

Davoine and Gaudilliere (2004) have written about the psychic consequences of negation regarding World War II. Working in Paris, they found, in their patients' psychosis, a response to this scotoma, this blindness or failure to register the trauma of the war. Is the current amnesia regarding fascism and its insidiousness in our political lives a kind of psychotic social-political scotoma? There are treacherous movements to erase history by not teaching a full historical record, by limiting books and discussions, and by rewriting historical events. The newly inaugurated President Trump insists, and wants recorded into our history, that January 6, 2021 was not an insurrection that he helped plan and fuel. Instead, he persists with his lie of the election having been stolen and that January 6 was a peaceful "day of love." He has now pardoned all those who were convicted of crimes in that insurrection. Are the scales tipping and the social/political barometric pressure dropping drastically enough? Is there 'tingling'?[3]

While my focus is not on the proto-fascist leader but on the group's susceptibility to these leaders and populist movements, I realize this to be a near-impossibility; they are so intertwined and codependent. Hamburger (2018) has written, "social trauma is executed in a societal context, thus involving the surrounding society in the traumatic process, printing the cliché of victim and perpetrator on the whole group" (p. 110). The Kleinian paranoid maneuver of splitting the world into 'good and bad' is forcefully perpetrated on us all in this scenario. Disappeared memory and history erased remains its best weapon. In the world as it exists, the proto-fascist leader purports omnipotence, forcing helplessness and weakness into the minority group to be victimized. Which part of the split would any of us need to inhabit to stay sane, in the world?

This simultaneous diffusing of victim/perpetrator processes into the collective rests upon, I argue, a failure of witnessing, an aborted mourning process of the atrocities of prior generations. Now you may respond that this is categorically wrong: Look at the Holocaust testimony projects that Dori Laub and others created, the Truth and Reconciliation Commission in South Africa, or the Genocide Studies graduate program at Yale, which take testimonies from Rwanda, Cambodia and elsewhere in the world, or the vast data from the legacies of the world wars? And now the war in Ukraine, where they are fighting on some of the same battlefields as WW II with Putin's propaganda declaring they are 'purging more Nazis' while Ukrainians are relentlessly fighting for their lives and freedom. We must ask, why has this documenting, reporting, and disseminating findings not impacted the outcomes? How did the cry of *never again* become yet again? Where is our horror and grief? Where is our action?

Mourning was first brilliantly compared by Freud (1917) to melancholia using the former to inform the latter. He wondered why often the work of mourning was accomplished, and melancholia persisted. Freud believed that the work of mourning would follow and be accomplished from a summoning up and then relinquishing of memories, a decathexis of libidinal attachment to the lost loved object. Eventually this is finished, and now you move on to a new object. While it remains one of my favorite papers of Freud, I have never been comfortable or in agreement with his assertion. This has always struck me as a romanticized version of mourning, not the gut-wrenching depth of loss that is felt when a parent or a spouse/life partner dies or that parents feel when a child dies. Or the sadness of our patients, when they have suffered loss.

Slochower (2011) suggests that we tend to pathologize when patients repetitively remember and talk about their losses, seeing it as evidence of trauma or unresolved conflicts. She writes, "We valorize, indeed idealize, 'moving on' and 'letting go'" (p. 677). I agree with her sensibility and it helps clarify for me my disagreement with Freud. He argues that the normal state of mourning is one that passes before too long, and unlike melancholia, which takes up residence in someone, it—the state of mourning—ends. This feels too simplistic. My sense is that the agonizing early stages of grief change but the feeling of loss of a loved one and mourning that loss never completely leaves. We don't actually fully surrender the loss and move on to a new object, although we may re-partner when we've lost that kind of significant other. And what of the loss of country, of a moral world, of a code of living that values all human life and protects truth and freedom?

These kinds of losses alter and shape us. What needs to be relinquished, according to Freud, is the longing for the restoration of the loved one. I would argue that in giving up longing, in acceptance of a loss, we learn to live with the loss and with the *ongoingness* of mourning. It continues as a tribute to the love we felt and/or received and have lost; it is our internal candle of remembrance that continues. The loss of a moral world order, however, may be too hard to bear in this way and may become a choice between dissociative amnesic-like forgetting or anguished despair. Mourning becomes aborted because it feels impossible or overwhelming to do in the absence of others' recognition and external validation. We are left adrift, unanchored.

Fascistic leaders opportunistically capitalize on our internal unsettledness, our unexpressed grievances, losses, and longings. Vamik Volkan (2017) has written extensively about how large group identity can be manipulated to cohere around what he has termed "chosen traumas." These are often events from a historical past and transfer psychically transgenerationally. Volkan's work is part of psychoanalytic transgenerational transmission literature that argues when traumas are insufficiently mourned, the result can be—as in the work of Abraham and Török's (1994) encrypted phantom—ghostly hauntings affecting the minds of many generations.

Chosen traumas, however, call upon succeeding generations for restitution, repair, and/or revenge, or what Apprey (1999, 2014) has termed *errands*. These chosen traumas or errands become urgent in subsequent generations and yet impossible. They can be neither ignored nor fulfilled since the trauma is not of the current generations' lived experience. Faimberg ([1988] 2005) termed these trauma transmissions "a telescoping of generations." She conceptualized the parent's narcissistic appropriation of the child's identity as a co-opting by the parent of the child's mind. In this way the proto-fascist leader has also drafted the minds of the collective, stoking the flames of past grievances, past traumas, but without any recourse toward grieving, mourning, or metabolizing the trauma. It is to be reenacted anew in the world linked to the past without benefit of witnessing or reconciliation and healing.

The witnessing we have accomplished has been very important. But have we gone far enough? Or have we failed to witness fully the evil and destruction and meet it with profound grief and with what Watkins (2018) coined, "deserved shame"? Can we respond to our shame and be more moved toward reparative social justice, as Grand (2018) has urged? Has it remained too much on the surface level in the academy? Where is our communal obligation to each other and how inexorably linked our lives are now and to the prior generations? And I even wonder, have we begun a collective amnesia process about the COVID pandemic and all the deaths—to date 1.2 million in the U.S., 11 million worldwide? And the denial and chaotic mishandling of the public health crisis by President Trump in his last term?

I want to offer an example of what a deeper and fuller witnessing has been. In 1977, amidst the Argentinian state terror unleashed during the dictatorship years, a group of grieving women were trying to find the whereabouts of their arrested daughters and the daughters' babies, some of whom were born in captivity. In writing about the effects of Argentinian social and political life on psychoanalysis, Volnovich writes

> Just as Argentines were scarred forever by state terror, so were we all shaken by the presence of the Mothers and Grandmothers of Plaza de Mayo (Abuelas de Plaza de Mayo). They opened a space, a gap, a crevice through which the ability to think could flow. They put a desire, a boundary opposite to overwhelming totalitarian power.
>
> (Volnovich, 2017, p. 14)

Here is a quote from the Abuelas website:

> The Armed Forces that carried out a coup d'état in our country on March 24, 1976, consolidated a regime of terror and persecution that resulted in the disappearance of 30,000 people of all ages and social classes for political reasons. Among them were hundreds of pregnant women who gave birth in captivity and children kidnapped along with their mothers and/or fathers.
>
> The victims' families scoured courts, police stations, hospitals, churches, and public agencies in search of information, only to be met with complicit silence. Little by little, we began to group together to share information and give each other strength. By April 1977, the Mothers of Plaza de Mayo had already transformed the police order to "move around" into "the Thursday rounds," and they wore, to identify each other, a white scarf tied around their heads, symbolizing the cloth diapers worn by their children. Six months later, a mother who was also a grandmother stepped aside from the crowd and asked, "Who is looking for their grandchild, or has their daughter or daughter-in-law pregnant?" At that moment, twelve of us women realized we had to organize to search for the children of our children kidnapped by the dictatorship. The following Saturday, October 22, 1977, we met for the first time and began a collective struggle that continues to this day ... The Grandmothers will continue to transmit the collective memory to build the legacy of the struggle and ensure that this terrible violation of human rights is never repeated.
>
> (Grandmothers of the Plaza de Mayo, n.d.)

Their relentless search embodies an impossible feat; mourning a loss that is not confirmed but felt in the silence. The Abuelas insisted a crime, kidnapping, and possible death had occurred, and they held on to memory despite loss. At the International Psychoanalytic Association (IPA) congress in 2017 held in Buenos Aires, I had the opportunity to go to the Plaza de Mayo on a Thursday when the Abuelas and others who join them continue to demonstrate. They march with pictures of their children and loved ones; in their continuing insistence they chant and sing, "We will not forget you."

Their persistence over these many years has been remarkable. Not just because it started during the military takeover and threatened their own lives, not just because they sought out every legal avenue they could and, when thwarted, went to the international level. This was not just because with the technology of science and gene mapping they could now find matches from their DNA to their grandchildren, and not just because they have found and/or reunited over 136 grandchildren (from an estimated 500 who were taken or born in captivity) with their biological families. In their insistence of the longevity of memory and mourning they were standing up to the autocratic military regime who refused accountability for its crimes.

While witnessing lies at the heart of the work on trauma, the continuing mentalizing process successive generations inherit is integral to the work on intergenerational transmission of trauma and its repair. The urgency of restoring attachment and repairing damaging ruptures is crucial to both. Witnessing needs to be in the service of defying and refusing fascistic amnesia. Every episode of mass violence is enabled by willful obliviousness and collective denial. The urgency of restoring attachment and repairing damaging ruptures is crucial. It is my belief that when "wounds touch," that is, whether in our clinical work when a patient's wound stirs our own or in our reaction to what is happening in the world, a deeply profound, enlivened, and embodied form of witnessing needs to occur. In the aftermath of atrocity, cultures rarely offer survivors a reflective, recognizing container for their Big History trauma. Actions can derive from love or from hate, from reparative wishes or destructive ones. Without working-through processes for the social, political, racialized, or sexualized traumas that entail fully remembering with recognition, we cannot expect fascism to remain in the past.

I end with a dream fragment found in Freud's (1900) *Interpretation of Dreams*.

> A father had been watching beside his child's sick-bed for days and nights on end. After the child had died, [an old man had been] engaged to keep watch over the body murmuring prayers. After a few hours' sleep, the father had a dream that his child was standing beside his bed, caught him by the arm and whispered to him reproachfully: "Father, don't you see I'm burning?"
>
> (Freud, 1900, p. 509)

Freud's interpretation of this dream rested upon his wish fulfilment theory. He suggested that the father was keeping the son alive a few more minutes in the dream. While he did not identify the old man hired to sit with the son's body saying prayers, I want to make this the dream focus. This is a very old Jewish tradition of *shimrah* which requires the deceased not be left alone prior to burial. The rationale for this ritual is that the *nehsamah*, the soul, should not be alone until the burial when this divine spark returns to God. For me this dream represents twofold, our witnessing that our world in fact may be on fire and we should not forget or fail to take notice, to witness the prior fires and the ones now ignited and burning. As the Abuelas have done, we must take up this cause of remembering, not repeating prior relinquishing of our responsibility, and renewing our protests against fascism. Lastly, we must treat our democracy as the soul of our country. It too needs watching and safeguarding.

Disclosure Statement

No potential conflict of interest was reported by the author.

Notes

1 See Ingraham (2018, June 19). *The Washington Post*.
2 See Swan et al. (2023, July 17). *The New York Times*. Also, see Richardson (2023) for additional commentary
3 See Beckerman (2022), *The Atlantic*, referenced above: "When the social and political barometric pressure begins to drop, when you can feel that tingling: Leave."

References

Abraham, N., & Török, M. (1994). *The shell and the kernel: Renewals of psychoanalysis* (N. Rand, ed. & trans.). University of Chicago Press.

Apprey, M. (1999). Reinventing the self in the face of received transgenerational hatred in the African American community. *Journal of Applied Psychoanalytic Studies*, 1(2), 131–143.

Apprey, M. (2014). A pluperfect errand: A turbulent return to beginnings in the transgenerational transmission of destructive aggression. *Free Associations: Psychoanalysis and Culture, Media, Groups, Politics*, *66*, 15–28.

Beckerman, G. (2022). What it feels like when fascism starts. *The Atlantic*, December 19. https://www.theatlantic.com/books/archive/2022/12/the-oppermanns-book-holocaust-nazi-fascism/672505/

Connolly, K. (2015). Tales from Auschwitz: Survivor stories. *The Guardian*. https://www.theguardian.com/world/2015/jan/26/tales-from-auschwitz-survivor-stories

Davoine, F. G. & Gaudilliere, J.-M. (2004). *History beyond trauma*. Other Press.

Faimberg, H. (2005). *The telescoping of generations: Listening to the narcissistic links between generations*. Routledge.

Freud, S. (1900). The interpretation of dreams. In J. Strachey (Ed.), *The standard edition of the complete works of Sigmund Freud* (Vol IV, p. 627). Hogarth Press.

Freud, S. (1917). Mourning and melancholia. In J. Strachey (Ed.), *The Standard edition of the complete works of Sigmund Freud* (Vol. XIV, pp. 237–258). Hogarth Press.

Grand, S. (2018). The other within: White racial shame and the Native American genocide. *Contemporary Psychoanalysis*, *54*(1), 84–102. https://doi.org/10.1080/00107530.2017.1415106

Grandmothers of the Plaza de Mayo. n.d. https://www.abuelas.org.ar/las-abuelas

Hamburger, A. (2018). After Babel: Teaching psychoanalysis on a former battlefield-experiences in an international research network. *International Forum of Psychoanalysis*, *27*(2), 105–113. https://doi.org/10.1080/0803706X.2017.1390252

Herman, J. L. (1992). *Trauma and recovery: The aftermath of violence from domestic abuse to political terror*. Basic Books.

Ingraham, C. (2018). There are more guns than people in the United States, according to a new study of global firearm ownership. *The Washington Post*, June 19. https://www.washingtonpost.com/news/wonk/wp/2018/06/19/there-are-more-guns-than-people-in-the-united-states-according-to-a-new-study-of-global-firearm-ownership/

Richardson, H. C. (2023). Letters from an American. *Substack*, July 17. https://heathercoxrichardson.substack.com/p/july-17-2023

Slochower, J. (2011). Out of the analytic shadow: On the dynamics of commemorative ritual. *Psychoanalytic Dialogues*, *21*(6), 676–690. https://doi.org/10.1080/10481885.2011.629565

Swan, J., Savage, C., Haberman, M. (2023). Trump and allies forge plans to increase presidential power in 2025. *The New York Times*, July 17. https://www.nytimes.com/2023/07/17/us/politics/trump-plans-2025.html

Volkan, V. (2017). Large-group identity and massive trauma. In J. Alpert & E. Goren (Eds.), *Psychoanalysis, trauma and community: History and contemporary reappraisals*. Routledge.

Volnovich, J. (2017). Trauma and contemporary forms of subjectivity: Contributions of Argentine psychoanalysis. *American Journal of Psychoanalysis*, *77*(1), 7–22. https://doi.org/10.1057/s11231-016-9083-0

Watkins, M. (2018). The social and political life of shame in the U.S. presidential election. *Psychoanalytic Perspectives*, *15*(1), 25–37. https://doi.org/10.1080/1551806X.2018.1396125

Conclusion

Fascism Terminable and Interminable

Alasdair Cannon and Tom Fielder

It is March 2026 at the time of writing, and the nightmare of fascism continues to encroach on the exploding horizons of contemporary psychopolitics. As we complete this conclusion, bombs rain down upon Iran and Lebanon. Antifa protesters in the US are convicted of terrorism offences for the first time (Office of Public Affairs, 2026). And leading researchers of democracy publish a report that states, "The speed with which American democracy is currently dismantled is unprecedented in modern history" (Varieties of Democracy Institute, 2026, p. 5). We read the papers collected in this volume, these sophisticated and bold attempts to theorise the fascist individual and state's vociferous appetites for destruction and terror, and yet their deeply resonant arguments hardly register as real against the absurd violence of our world today. What purchase can a psychoanalytic theory of perverse and sadistic cruelty possibly have on the world when the US Secretary of War, his skin inked with the symbols of extremist Christian nationalism, tells reporters that his country "literally never targets civilians" after his military murders over 100 Iranian schoolgirls (Amnesty International, 2026; Wilson, 2024)? When Israel's Secretary of Defence openly signals genocidal intent in Lebanon, dropping leaflets over Beirut that read, "In light of the remarkable success in Gaza, the newspaper 'The New Reality' arrives in Lebanon. Where is your country heading?" (Ward, 2026). Or when the Iranian government allegedly murders more than 30,000 people who protest their "clerofascist" regime, then publicly executes young people for their defiance (Armin, 2026; Armstrong, 2026; Žižek, 2026)? To speak of the "unconscious", "fantasy", "psychopolitics", and "late fascism" as we witness this parade of atrocities reminds us only of how quixotic—how worldless—our dreams of resistance have become. As news breaks about new illegal wars and human rights violations, about "free" countries who now seek to define antifascism as a terrorist ideology—allegedly characterised by "adherence to radical gender ideology, anti-Americanism, anti-capitalism, or anti-Christianity" and "hostility towards traditional views on family, religion and morality" (see Office of the Attorney General, 2025)—it can feel as if fascism is returning from historical memory into present reality.[1] As if fascism,

DOI: 10.4324/9781003742876-19

like a symptom that surges and recedes but never disappears, is both "terminable" and "interminable" (Freud, [1937] 2024).

Psychoanalytic theorists present fascism as a recalcitrant and undying threat, issuing forth from both the individual unconscious and the social and economic order at large. Reading the psychoanalytic studies of fascism collected in this reader, it can sometimes feel as though the authors have collectively plundered the extensive archive of pathological constructs within psychoanalysis, turning the full range of its diagnostic arsenal against the deadly allure of fascism, while ineluctably falling short in their critical reckonings with its "mental pandemonium which also had a strict inner logic" (Rose, this reader, p.112). At one level, the authors each seek to describe the psychodynamics of fascism—its strict inner logic—in lucid psychoanalytic terms. Yet at another level, this need for conceptual precision is possessed by the excessive urgency and bewilderment—the pandemonium—of the thing itself, plagued by the insistent fear that we cannot, in fact, find the right words for this menace. Across this body of work, fascism emerges not as a stable object of psychoanalytic diagnosis, but as an uncanny zone of conceptual proliferation which generates an unsettled field of heterogenous pathological categories. From Bollas's and Diamond's "fascist states of mind," through McAfee's Kleinian paranoid–schizoid politics, Kernberg's compound category of "malignant narcissism", and Grand's "web of perversion", to Rose's account of "total belief" as cultural delirium, fascism is repeatedly redescribed through overlapping, hybridised diagnostic frames which resist mutual reconciliation within a synthetic critical schema. Classical distinctions—between neurosis and psychosis, narcissism and paranoia, individual pathology and group regression—are strained to breaking point, producing ever more sophisticated formulations of psychoanalytic reason, ranging from characterological diagnoses (authoritarian character), to group-psychological processes (large-group regression), to structural accounts of ideology (ideological fantasy), and trauma-inflected notions of cultural dissociation (fascism amnesia), that seek, and somehow fail, to stabilise the phenomenon. The result is not smooth theoretical coherence as such, but a kind of disciplined, white-knuckled excess: psychoanalysis, confronted with fascism's historical and libidinal intensity, and the limits of its own power, appears "maddened" beyond the bounds of its own classificatory system into a restless multiplication of categories that both registers and displaces its own difficulty in thinking the object, the (re)emerging nightmare of our times.

In *The Interpretation of Dreams*, Freud ([1900a] 2024, p. 99) famously observed that in every dream, there is "at least one spot … at which it is unplumbable—a navel, as it were, that is its point of contact with the unknown". As the recurring nightmare—or transgressive dream—of liberal modernity, fascism similarly confronts us with an "unplumbable" depth, even as its depthless evil "can lay waste to the entire world like a fungus growing rampant on the surface" (Arendt, [1964] 2017, p. 209). The irascible violence and degradations of fascist fantasy, which represents a negative extreme of politics and relationality, provokes psychoanalysis to deploy all its intellectual resources to understand, contain and control its power—to castrate the fascists, as it were. But drawn into this yearning for mastery, resolved to interpret, diagnose, and theorise the inner logics of fascism, psychoanalysis soon discovers its own impotence. For all our efforts, the fascist terror continues unabated. Much like a psychoanalyst, confounded by symptoms and dreams that persist after interpretation, a confrontation with fascism undoes our illusions of intellectual mastery and delivers us to the very limits of political and psychoanalytic thought, where we glimpse something finally incomprehensible. In fascism as in dreams, we confront signifiers whose meaning is overdetermined, which, like "a mushroom out of its mycelium", emerge from a "tangle of thoughts" and branch through the whole "intricate network of the world of thought" that has no "definite ending" (Freud, [1900b] 2024, pp. 469–470). The particular knot of signifiers that organise our fantasies draw their vitality and power from the drives that operate across the "frontier between the mental and the somatic" (Freud, [1915] 2024, p. 107), both animating and exceeding conscious experience in their insistent (unconscious) striving for expression. The analysis of fascism thus pits us against the real and senseless force of human urges and the labyrinth of language—against the incomprehensibility of nightmares as such. Psychoanalysing fascism thereby returns us to the aporetic task that makes the project of psychoanalysis both so deeply alluring and simultaneously impossible: the mind's analysis of the unconscious that, by definition, always already exceeds it. In the psychoanalysis of fascism, psychoanalysis discovers its own constitutive madness—the madness of the conscious mind discovering and resisting the weakness of its own agency within the totality of the psychic and social (dis)order of which it is a part.

At the end of his life, Freud expressed a profound pessimism about the efficacy of psychoanalysis in the face of the violent, sadomasochistic drives characteristic of fascist politics. "No stronger impression", he writes, "arises from the resistances during the work of analysis than of there being a force which is defending itself by every possible means against recovery and which is absolutely resolved to hold on to illness and suffering." "These phenomena", Freud continues, "are unmistakable indications of the presence of a power in mental life which we call the instinct of aggression or of destruction according to its aims, and which we trace back to the original death instinct of living matter" (Freud, [1937] 2024, p. 219). Fascism presents itself as an ecstatic and profoundly unsettling "alloy" (Freud, [1930] 2024, p. 107) of aggressive and erotic impulses. Garbed and disguised in the symbolic idealism of nation and race, "the instinct of aggression or destruction" is allowed full expression, first driving but ultimately overwhelming fascistic bids for domination and self-edification in the pursuit of its final, unconscious aim—total destruction. Though psychoanalytic and political theory can help us to understand the social, historic, and psychic processes that result in the fascistic alloying of the death drive, they are impotent if we hope to grasp the fully metaphysical dimensions of this nightmare. They cannot help us finally understand *why* fascism, destructiveness, and death, strive towards expression in a world of living matter: "Why this has to happen", just as Freud wrote of the erotic drives' activities, "we do not know" ([1930] 2024, p. 109). The interminability of fascism finally escapes us.

What, then, of the analysis of fascism? Knowing the weakness of our powers against the nightmare that so troubles us, do we continue in our analysis indefinitely? Do we work for another century to identify its unconscious mechanisms, to voice the pleasures and terrors that secure its power in psychic and political life? Or do we instead terminate the analysis of fascism? Do we dispense with further theoretical elaboration so that we might open a space of possibility where something else might emerge—the *sui generis* lineaments of the Trumpian conjuncture and some other, currently unthought form of non-fascist life? Or will abandoning our analytic efforts allow fascism to return and surge forward without resistance, leading to the violence that we desired beyond all else to avoid? These are properly ethical questions that all those who hope for an end to fascism must ask. And perhaps it is in this *doubt* which comes by asking necessary and impossible questions, by pursuing these queries that have no definite answers but which excite the full range of our imaginative and mnemic faculties, that we might discover a future for anti-fascism.

In his paper included in this collection, Bollas argues that doubt is antithetical to ideological extremism and "the fascist state of mind". "Doubt, uncertainty, self-interrogation, are equivalent to weakness", he writes, "and must be expelled from the mind to maintain ideological certainty" (p. 24). Elsewhere, Salberg argues in her paper that fascism's resurgence today demands a level of amnesia. The fascism of our times occurs in the wake of fascisms past, and thus requires either a conscious desire for violence, or an unconscious refusal to recognise that violence: for Salberg, the "moves toward fascism suggest a further disavowal of how far from a humane world we have moved, a kind of amnesia surrounding the trauma history in the United States and the world" (p. 227). Taken together, these statements suggest that fascism's certainty, its unimpeachable righteousness, is secured by a refusal of questioning and memory—indeed, by a rejection of the questions those memories raise for one's own investments in fascistic political movements today. Fascism, in other words, is not strong enough to endure the "weakness" of doubt. Strangely, then, the doubt that our analytic failure elicits is anti-fascist: the failure to master fascism in ourselves, in our theoretical systems, and in our world, forces us to embody the position of weakness, vulnerability and metaphysical brokenness that fascism cannot avow.

Beyond any specific theory of fascist psychopolitics, the psychoanalysis of fascism illuminates a certain ethic of anti-fascism—a kind of strong weakness, as it were, more forceful than the brittle power of fascism. Psychoanalysis invites hesitation and forwards an "ethic of honesty (Rieff [1959] (1979))" which may be more softly spoken than fascism, but is ultimately more radical and subversive.

Psychoanalysis can help us to find what Philip Rieff ([1959] 1979, p. 306) called the "analytic attitude", to construct "little communions of counterbelief", and to continue the "remembering, repeating, and working-through" (Freud, 1914a) which might strip fascism of its compulsive, deadly allure. In its own small way, the psychoanalysis of fascism can allow us to share this subject position and praxis with others—including, perhaps, the fascist agitators themselves who perversely threaten and plague our world with catastrophic violence. At the very least, psychoanalysis can prepare us to pick up the pieces, for the "wake work" that follows in the paths of destruction, even after the agents of ruin have exhausted themselves (Sharpe, 2016; Frosh, 2023, pp. 165–182).

At the risk, then, of simply expanding the list of names used to attack fascism, the curses impotently circling around the hated object, and with full understanding of the weakness and acute vulnerability of our theorising, we conclude this reader by presenting our own "psychosocial" theory of fascism. This theory embraces a series of key contributions to both psychoanalysis and political theory without claiming to present a coherent or settled image of fascism, or to resolve the integral aporia of anti-fascism. Nonetheless, we hope that our own take on fascism today might help to better signpost this ongoing debate within psychoanalysis.

Towards a Psychosocial Theory of Fascism?

In his essay included in this reader, Adorno writes that "Psychological dispositions do not actually cause fascism; rather, fascism defines a psychological area which can be successfully exploited by the forces which promote it for entirely nonpsychological reasons of self-interest" (p. 86). Distinguishing between psychological "dispositions" and a psychological "area", Adorno suggests that fascism does not arise as an aggregation of individual psychopathologies or destructive mental states, but politically *defines* and gives shape to psychological experience by harnessing socially produced insecurities to the strategic, political-economic interests of a particular individual or class, a self-interested agency who finds something usable in the "psychological area" which fascism defines. Stephen Frosh celebrates Adorno in this reader for attempting to construct "a sophisticated psychosocial theory" of anti-Semitism, which "understands the structure of personal life as inextricably bound up with social forces" (p. 220). But he also observes a "pull back to psychologism" which "inhibits the full development of such an account, effectively polarising the theory so that the social becomes either the true cause of anti-Semitism, or the 'container' for individual pathology" (p. 227). This "pull back to psychologism" is evident in appeals to a "fascist state of mind" within certain psychoanalytic texts (cf. Bollas, this reader; see also "Directions for Future Research and Further Readings"), which tend to replicate this polarisation of theory by positing fascism as the authentic political "container" for a particular state of mind.

Following Frosh and others, and recognising these shortcomings of some psychoanalytic writings on fascism, we argue that fascism must not be understood as a purely psychological, sociological, or political phenomenon. Instead, we believe it should be theorised as a "psychosocial" phenomenon (Frosh & Baraitser, 2008). Psychosocial theorists argue that neither the psyche nor the social can be understood as discrete entities, locked in an uncomprehending, binary relationship of domination and subordination. Rejecting the reductionism of psychology and sociology, the psychosocial project involves understanding psychic and social processes "as always implicated in each other, as mutually constitutive, co-produced, or abstracted levels of a single dialectical process" (Frosh, 2018). For psychosocial theorists, the psyche is political and the political is psychic; they are inseparable and neither term has ontological priority over its other. From this perspective, "fascism"—but also liberalism, communism, and any other conceivable political movement or ideology—is a kind of "transitional" phenomenon, generated within the space between the mind and the world where subjective fantasy and objective reality intertwine (Winnicott, 2005). Political ideology both constitutes and is constituted by the mind, material reality, and social relationality in the area where they intermingle. But rather than supporting the freedom of the mind to "play with" the world and to be affected by its difference and objectivity, fascism overwrites the reality of the world with fantasy, delirium, and total belief: Rose, 2027 (the paper in this reader) the mind is "played with" to the extent that it is itself destroyed together with the world through which it is inseparably constituted (Yates, 2015).

Rather than describing the psychic dimension of fascist politics in terms of a fascist "state of mind", we aim to present a more fully *psychosocial* version of fascist psychopolitics. To do so, we propose instead the notion of fascist "states of fantasy", substituting "mind" for "fantasy", and pluralising "state", to more accurately represent the delirious, dreamlike psychic and social pandemonium of fascist movements. We derive this notion from Jacqueline Rose's seminal *States of Fantasy*, which seeks to resituate the psychoanalytic account of fantasy, alongside the historical "states" to which it is intimately related, "at the heart of our political vocabulary", proposing a "theoretical turn" which we wish to commend to psychoanalytic theorists of fascism (Rose, 1996, p. 10). For Max Weber, as Rose notes, the modern state relies on the "inner meaning it holds for its subjects" (1996, p. 8) to secure rationally purposive actions, and Rose in fact compares Weber's theorisation of the modern state with the form of the Freudian superego, "binding its subjects to a violence which … is pure *means* without end" (1996, p. 10). But these "inner" factors, as Rose writes, "precisely because of their intangible, speculative component, cannot be held to reason", threatening political composure—and the body politic—with all the "tortuous vagaries of the inner life", running into the arms "of all the other 'borderline' factors which Weber lays out as most recalcitrant to sociological explanation", such as mystical experience, ends which defy the intellect, hidden "motives" and "repressions" (1996, p. 8). "It is because fantasy arrogates an authority which properly belongs to the ego alone", Rose writes, which "threatens the ego's supremacy, and forces it to step down, that … it could be described as a 'State within a State'" (1996, p. 7). Describing the incredible potency of "the unconscious dreams of nations" (1996, p. 3) in the political field, Rose borrows the phrase "State within a State" from Freud's account of pathological phenomena in *Moses and Monotheism*: "an inaccessible party, with which co-operation is impossible, but which may succeed in overcoming what is known as the normal party and forcing it into its service" (1996, quoted on p. 1). For Rose, then, the relationship between fantasy and the state is both integral and profoundly unsettled, sustaining the inner meaning of statehood even as it renders acutely vulnerable the putative reason of any political state. The notion of fascist "states of fantasy" seeks to capture the flight into mental delirium inherent in fascist politics, which channels real political forces and material anxieties, as well as resentments and antagonisms into dreamlike and morbidly rigidified political logics without ever mastering the mobility and intractability of unconscious mental life, or collapsing the vicissitudes of fantasy into a singular "state of mind".

With our notion of fascist "states of fantasy", we aim to suggest that fascism is a psychosocial phenomenon, of which the subjective or imaginary is an essential, dynamic and unpredictable component, determined by both the operations of the unconscious and the social symbolic order. In fascist states of fantasy, causal relations operate dynamically across mutually implicated, co-constitutive and analytically inseparable areas of the continuous psychosocial terrain—intrapsychic, relational, organisational, institutional, governmental, and cultural. These states of fantasy bridge fascism's psychic elements, with its broadly narcissistic, paranoid-schizoid, perverse and psychotic features, and its affectively charged fantasies related to desires for rebirth and vitality and fears of decline and victimhood (see Griffin, 1991; Paxton, 2004, pp. 219–220), with its "social" elements and self-constitution as ideology, group, movement, and state. These intrapsychic factors, we argue with reference to Roger Griffin's notion of the "fascist minimum", are embedded within the ideological programme of "palingenetic ultranationalism": a yearning for national and racial rebirth achieved through emergency political action that transcends the norms, rules, and behaviours of ordinary liberal democracy (Griffin, 1991, 2018). Historically speaking, the state of fantasy defined by "palingenetic ultranationalism", to borrow from historian of fascism Robert O. Paxton, has been "marked by obsessive preoccupation with community decline, humiliation, or victimhood and by compensatory cults of unity, energy, and purity", as well as a sense of unrelenting crisis that must be resolved by some powerful authority. "[A]s a form of political behaviour", Paxton continues, fascism has often operated as "a mass-based party of committed nationalist militants, working in uneasy but effective collaboration with traditional elites" which "abandons democratic liberties and pursues with redemptive violence and without ethical or legal restraints goals of internal cleansing and external expansion" (Paxton, 2004, pp. 218–220).

Our notion of fascist "states of fantasy" seeks to connect these conventional political-theoretical and psychoanalytical explanations, figuring them as different or abstracted aspects of a continuous psychosocial phenomenon. Following Žižek (2006) and other psychoanalytic theorists (e.g., McAfee, 2019; Wieland, 2014; Kernberg, this reader), we also wish to emphasise that fascism appeals especially to individuals and groups living through times of social crisis—specifically, *capitalist* crises. Crises of capitalism, the economic system which generally drives and sustains liberal democracies, frustrate the logics of growth and accumulation and—especially when combined with the mechanisms of state austerity—reveal the exploitation and precarity inherent within those societies. Capitalist crises can be validly described as "ontological crises" (Burleigh, 2000) that shake society at all levels. They rupture the symbolic, imaginary, and material orders of liberal democratic societies and subjectivities and expose people to the "traumatic real" of their socioeconomic systems. Those who cannot bear this encounter, or who seek to perpetuate the existing social order for reasons of material self-interest, their fear of alternatives, or due to their powerful libidinal investments, disavow that the crisis originates from capitalism and the class struggle. Unable or unwilling to recognise the constitutive injustices of their socioeconomic system, and therefore incapable of considering any appropriately radical, or indeed revolutionary alternatives with which to address the crisis, fascist agitators instead project the system's antagonisms outwards onto socially denigrated, othered groups—typically, racialised minorities. In their socioeconomic anxiety, "fear of breakdown" (Winnicott, 1974; McAfee, 2019), and "ontological insecurity" (Laing, [1960] 2010; see also Giddens, 1991), those who experience a given crisis of capitalism are prey to a variety of psychic defences—suicidality, narcissism, melancholia, mania, splitting, psychosis, and so on (Bollas, 2027; McAfee, 2019; Cannon, 2024). A generic set of desires (for revival, restoration, pride, power, and domination) and fears (of disintegration, collapse, contamination, and being dominated) also develop, which typically assert themselves by triggering transgenerational or otherwise "chosen traumas" (Volkan, 2001, 2020). These defences and fantasies chaordically combine and are captured, conducted, and amplified through movements, audiences, and groups corralled and excited by the charismatic power and instinctive genius of messianic demagogues. Ultimately, they are expressed in a phantasmatic political programme that responds to a period of capitalist crisis with a blindly narcissistic project for restoring collective identity and pride, achieved via paranoid-schizoid processes of violent exclusion and persecution, perversely channelling repressed rage, fear, and ecstatic destructiveness through the moral and metaphysical idealism of the superego.

The passionate delirium of "palingenetic ultranationalism" can therefore emerge from crises of capitalism—and, indeed, from other kinds of disruption occurring at the juncture between psyche and society, including the breakdown of identities (white hetero-masculinity), social structures (patriarchal and colonial white supremacy), and state institutions (historic colonial governments and imperial power). In fascism, the psychical, political, and economic desperation caused by social crises are typically used to justify and energise criminal violence against national enemies, the lethal expansion of state capacity at home and abroad, the systematic destruction of worker unions and organised labour, and the violent suppression of political opponents. While industrial leaders are instructed to follow the regime's demands, they often support the regime voluntarily because it is immensely profitable for them to do so: fascism preserves capitalist class relations and private property rights, and corporations are given a free hand to extract maximal value from their workforce and from the planet. The relations between capitalists and fascists are at times relatively harmonious and mutually beneficial, then, proceeding on a shared commitment to the logic of accumulation and the acceleration of production.[2] But as the destructive and delusional elements of fascism increasingly take hold, the fascist state inevitably clashes with capitalism, impeding or destroying the material, relational, institutional, and legal bases of capitalist economic activity through its addictions to spiralling destructiveness, authoritarian domination, and military overreach. Fascism is finally unstable as a psychosocial programme because of this antagonism between its psychical, political, and economic dimensions. Annihilating workers and the means of production while depending on the capitalist logic of accumulation, fascism creates an internal tension that cannot be contained by a single personality or state, eventually degenerating into a kind of generalised madness that erodes and eventually destroys the psychosocial terrain of political life.

Ante-Fascism

By highlighting how fascist "states of fantasy" emerge symptomatically from crises of liberal capitalism and subjectivity, psychoanalytic theorists suggest that a pathological process of psychosocial radicalisation, exploitation, and mass regression links fascism with liberal democratic politics. When we refer to liberalism, we mean especially the narrower version of the liberal tradition which was promulgated by US-based theorists during the Cold War (Moyn, 2023). This Cold War liberalism was epitomised by the "authoritarian liberalism" or neoliberalism of theorists like Hayek and Friedman, who argue for market-based societies that privilege economic "freedom", "property", and "universal rules of justice" over and above substantive democracy and material equality (Brown, 2019, pp. 72 & 103). But we also wish to encompass the much longer history of implication between liberalism and capitalism, with its typical ideals of "liberty, individuality, progress, rationality, the general interest, sociability … and constrained and accountable power" (Freeden, 2025, p. 243)[3] continuously conflicting with its histories of dispossession, private property,[4] extractivism, inequity, imperialism, colonialism, racism, slavery, and genocide. Liberal democracy shares a disturbing number of features with fascism, its supposed opposite. Rather than accepting a strict logic of antagonism between the "universal" and "rational" ideals of liberalism on the one hand and the "national/racial" and "irrational" values of fascism on the other hand, then, we envision a wide space of "ante-fascism" in which liberalism and fascism uneasily coexist: a *multidimensional* and *transitional* space of psychosocial becoming, contradiction, and ideological fluidity, within which liberal selves, groups, and societies move towards and through, or else retreat from and traverse, fascist states of fantasy (see Cannon, 2024; Fielder, 2026). This space of ante-fascism is not a linear space of neatly sequential evolution or development, but a fraught, pathologically confused terrain of multiplying shocks and shifts that render both individuals and whole societies vulnerable to states of fantasy suffused with increasingly blatant, public articulations of fascism. The fascist zones of ante-fascist space are thus connected on all levels to so-called "moderate" and "sane" liberal democratic positions via a submerged or repressed terrain of ideological disorder, ambivalence, and negative "playfulness" that runs between them. With respect to the US today, we suggest periodising the onset of this ante-fascist disorder, this ideological slippage between liberalism and fascism, to the beginning of the millennium: starting with 9/11 and the War on Terror and accelerating after the Global Financial Crisis (GFC), ante-fascism has emerged during the end of the "end of history" where we witness the beginning of something bewilderingly new and strange (cf. Cannon, 2024).

Defining fascism as a multi-dimensional psychosocial phenomenon linked to liberalism across the transitional space of ante-fascism introduces both precision and complexity to psychoanalytic theorising. One of this theory's principal contributions is to introduce a psychoanalytic "readiness to contradictory attitudes" in studies of the relations between liberalism and fascism: in political ideology, as in psychic life more broadly, this theory recognises the "ambivalence" which is "present to a greater or less amount in the innate disposition of everyone" (Freud, [1913] 2024; p. 62; [1914b] 2024, p. 236). Nevertheless, this theory also risks presenting fascism as something measurable or quantifiable, as if we could score (ante-)fascist personalities along a linear spectrum in the manner of Adorno's famous studies of the "authoritarian personality" (Adorno et al., 2019). We aim instead to construe fascism as a ghostly, phantasmatic presence, haunting and episodically asserting itself within liberal subjectivities and societies, donning various official or public masks and playfully—farcically—hybridising itself in order to avoid outright condemnation, while also continuously striving for further expression. Although fascism is defined by its historical enactments, it remains interminable to the extent that it resists historical and intellectual containment. The notion of ante-fascism troubles neat definitions of historical fascism, and recentres the vexed boundary between psyche and society as the site of a ghostly "return": it asserts that fascism is both present and absent in the world today.

The Fascist Transformation

From the aforementioned theorists, we ascertain the fascist zones that saturate one end of the liberal-fascist/ante-fascist continuum, simultaneously haunting the entire psychosocial arena of (neo)liberal politics as a symptomatic social motif and permanent psychic potential. However, we have not yet accounted psychoanalytically for the long period of psychosocial transformation during which fascism emerges as a decisive force in the world, where liberal democratic "normalcy" is transformed into an increasingly lurid enactment of the nightmare. We require more from psychoanalysis, too, to comprehend why fascist ideology is often characterised by an essentially arbitrary set of features—namely, nationalism, statism, authoritarianism, illiberalism, anti-democratism, anti-leftism, the defence of private property, racism, patriarchal misogyny, the hatred of queer individuals and sexual freedom, sexual perversion, religious fundamentalism, imperialism, militarism, and genocidal projects,[5] among other things.

One way of reckoning psychosocially with these questions relies on the relation between psychic defences and social ideals established by Freud's work on narcissism and the construction of the ego. In "Group Psychology and the Analysis of the Ego", Freud writes that "from the very first individual psychology … is at the same time social psychology as well" ([1921] 2024, p. 67). The ego—later described by Freud as a "precipitate of abandoned object cathexes" and identifications with different authority figures (see [1923] 2024, pp. 25 & 29)—is a composite of social ideals related to the "race", "nation", "caste", "profession[s]" and "institution[s]" or "crowd of people" to which we belong (Freud, [1921] 2024, p. 68). Freud's perspective here is foundational to psychosocial studies, establishing an inviolable mutuality between inner and outer worlds, making them "mutually constitutive" levels of a "single dialectical process" (Frosh, 2018). Because the Freudian ego is composed of contingently introjected fragments of the social, collective triumphs and hopes are always also personal, intrapsychic pleasures, fantasies, and desires. Mass defeats and threats, too, are redoubled as shame, guilt, humiliation, anxiety, fear, and vulnerability. The psyche is social and *vice versa*, which means social cohesion and psychic stability cannot be separated—a fact we all learned, perhaps, when COVID-19 disrupted the broad "holding environment" (see Winnicott, 1960) of societies worldwide at the start of 2020. Conversely, social "breakdowns" and crises of capitalism are always also psychic disintegration and narcissistic collapse, motivating defence mechanisms that rupture and redefine psychosocial life (see Winnicott, 1974; McAfee, 2019) and accelerate movement across the space of ante-fascism.

Fascist states of fantasy emerge at the intersection between these psychic defence mechanisms, the aggressive and erotic drives, the introjected or "extimate" ideals and histories, and the social world—that is, at the conjuncture that defines psychosocial phenomena as such. Fascism's specific political form emerges when psychic defences radicalise positive and negative attachments to society's ideals and abjects, while the ideals and abjects themselves channel defensive activity, aggression and sexuality in certain directions. As this implies, fascist states of fantasy are thereby latent as an "interminable" potential within liberal democratic psychosocial space, emerging at the behest of opportunistic political actors when the state fails to provide a good-enough holding environment for its citizens.

Naïve commentators often counterpose the ideals and institutions of liberal capitalist democracies against those common to fascism, reifying the strict ideological antagonism between liberalism and fascism. But much like the way in which the Freudian psychoanalysis of neurosis revealed important aspects of mental "normalcy" repressed and occluded by liberal societies, fascism and fascist states of fantasy illuminate key features of liberal democratic "normalcy". Fascist states of fantasy, in short, are latent within the psychosocial space of all capitalist liberal democracies. Some elements of fascism haunt liberal democracy out of structural necessity. Individual freedom defined as economic liberalism, for example, does not and cannot exist without private property protections. Authoritarianism, illiberalism, statism, policing, and militarism thus underwrite all free-market capitalist systems and liberal-capitalist psychosocial spaces, while the rejection of democratic socialism becomes a necessary condition of continued psychosocial existence in such systems. There is a basic conflict in liberal ideology, too, between individualism and freedom. As economist James M. Buchanan once wrote in *The Limits of Liberty*, "In a strictly personalized sense, any person's ideal situation is one that allows him full freedom of action and inhibits the behavior of others so as to force adherence to his own desires. That is to say, each person seeks mastery over a world of slaves" (Buchanan, 1975). Taken to its limit, individual freedom demands relational and political domination. As Alberto Toscano (2023) argues, there is therefore a "fascist freedom" implied in individual freedom—a fact, as he notes, that Mussolini understood: "Fascism stands for liberty, and for the only liberty worth having, the liberty of the State and of the individual within the State" (cited in Toscano, 2023).[6] Other fascistic ideals, abjects, and fantasies endure within liberal democracies as a result of more contingent historical circumstances. Black slavery and the genocide of Native Americans created the United States as we know it today. The racist exclusion of "socially dead" Black individuals (see Wilderson, 2010, 2020) from the formal processes and institutions of democracy was central to US society until mere decades ago. Similarly, anti-Arab racism came to define Western and US consciousness during the wars in the Middle East after 9/11, the direct and indirect death toll of which may be as high as 4.5 million people (see Savell, 2023). Neither form of racism is necessary in any real sense. Nevertheless, they are utterly definitive for the North American psychosocial space and the fascisms that might emerge from it.

Whatever their source and present status, the "average" liberal democratic and capitalist psychosocial space contains all the ideals privileged in fascist ideology. Fascism emerges *en masse* across this space, we argue, when widespread and shared social crises provoke psychic defences that radicalise attachments to the ideals and abjects common to fascism. Simultaneously activating narcissistic and paranoid-schizoid defences, and inciting fear, aggression, and libidinal passion while provoking shifts in relationality, communication, and group behaviour, these crises collapse the pluralistic ambivalence of liberal democratic norms into fascist extremism. During these crises, an overvaluation of the ideals that allow for prideful identifications and dominating impulses surges forth—Whiteness, nationalism, authority, religious fundamentalism, capital accumulation, the possession of wealth and private property, heteronormative masculinity, sexual purity *and* virility (see Herzog, 2007),[7] imperial power, and violence. Alongside these passionate idealisations grows the denigration and demonisation of their opposites: Blackness and brownness, migrants, "un-American" and unpatriotic people, anarchism, socialism, Islam and Arab people, Judaism and Jews, women, what the FBI has recently defined as "nihilistic violent extremism" (see Klippenstein, 2025), LGBTQIA+ identities and sexualities, pacifism, and so on.[8] Over time, these processes of narcissism, melancholia and paranoid splitting transform psychosocial space. The patterns of relationality and communication once underwritten by shared fantasies of mutual recognition break down, and a collective trembling in grief and rage begins. This uncontrollable trembling shakes the "precipitate" of introjects that defines the "character" and form of egos and superegos (Freud, [1923] (2004), pp. 25 & 29): some parts are broken off and projected outwards, while others are denigrated and turned into abjects, elevated into ideals and authorities, or decathected and discarded as irrelevant. Erotic and aggressive impulses are desublimated, resublimated, and redirected during this creative/destructive process of transformation,[9] negation, and identification (see Freud, [1925] 2024). The final result is a redefinition of the highest ideals and lowest abjects, and a transformation of the dynamics of shame, guilt, and inhibition that determine political behaviour—a transformation, that is, of psychosocial existence.

Notably, this transformation does not occur instantaneously: it occurs through a process of "imaginative labour" where the psyche works to accumulate, elaborate, and consolidate different combinations of signifiers, drives, experiences, and defensive mechanisms in order to stabilise and contain its trembling.[10] In situations of deep and chronic psychosocial crises, defences and fantasies grow in number and intensity for as long as those crises go unresolved. From prolonged and compounding social crises, fascism emerges gradually and anarchically as a thoughtless attempt to master the restive destructiveness of the times. In our new century, defined in US consciousness by 9/11, the wars in Iraq and Afghanistan, the GFC, austerity, the Occupy and

BLM movements, "lone wolf" terrorism, the rise of social media and the "surveillance capitalism" of Big Tech, the COVID-19 crisis, the January 6 riots, Russia and the Israeli state's genocidal wars against Ukraine and the Palestinians, and, of course, Trumpism itself, it is hardly surprising that there has been movement across the transitional space of ante-fascism, from liberal democratic "normalcy" toward far-right radicalism. Most of these events alone each provoke what could be called an "ontological crisis"—a reckoning that shakes liberal democratic societies at all levels and generates profound insecurity (see Burleigh, 2000; Giddens, 1991). The psychosocial disintegration they have produced in concert is certainly enough to provoke the processes of transformation that lead to a mass migration—a desperate search for safety or containment—across the space of ante-fascism.

It is in this process of transformation and "imaginative labour" that fascism's shocking violence and perverse sexuality emerge as a way of mastering and sadomasochistically enjoying negative experience. The valorisation and practice of violence is generally (if hypocritically) condemned by liberal democratic societies. Fascism, however, often positions violence as an essential political tool and elevates it into an admirable and necessary ego-syntonic activity that bestows pride and moral virtue upon its practitioners. "War alone", Mussolini once said, "brings up to their highest tension all human energies and imposes the stamp of nobility upon the peoples who have the courage to make it." For fascists, Umberto Eco writes, "pacifism is trafficking with the enemy" and "life is permanent warfare" (Eco, 1995). Fascist violence cannot be reduced to one factor alone, but emerges from the confluence of different affects, fantasies, and defences generated in the psychosocial processes of transformation across ante-fascist space. During a mass crisis, a variety of fears, desires, and emotions resound and reverberate through the psychosocial terrain, invading political discourse with new memories of a lost "golden age" of power, security—and whiteness. Grief, terror, and fury chaotically combine with historical desires, traumas, and national mythologies, supercharging conscious reason with unconscious dreams and phantasies, as annihilation anxiety and "breakdown" (Winnicott, 1974; McAfee, 2019) begin to flow with increasing abandon through trembling bodies, minds, groups, and masses. Desperate yearnings for escape or change become contagious, as do hopeful dreams and fantasies that some messianic figure or "transformational object" (see Bollas, 1979) will arrive and resolve—or, at least, divert and diminish—the crisis. The apparently unending suffering and corresponding sense of political impotence projects melancholic self-reproaches, hate, anger and rage into the air, generating an ambience of privation, frustration, and shame (Freud, [1917] 2024; Kohut, 1972; Winnicott, 1975, pp. 204–218). These feelings incite vengeful, destructive impulses, which are orchestrated into, and harnessed as, aggressive, obscenely self-interested demands for political power, spreading everywhere now "like a fungus" through the liberal democratic capitalist order.

Across the transitional space of ante-fascism, then, a terrible combination of feelings emerges in response to social crises: the need to flee, banish, or annihilate the cause of fear, to melancholically punish and debase the objects that have been bitterly lost, to exact revenge on whatever thing or group produces anger and shame and pain, or to die by suicide, even, and end the suffering for good. These terrible forms of pain are further fuelled through the innate destructiveness of the death drive: floating freely in the wake of an ontological crisis and after the collapse of its sublimation into superegoic self-restraint, the death drive generates violent fantasies, dreams, and social enactments. Phobic defences proliferate as delusional fears and fantasies of identification with the transformed ideals take hold, generating an urgent need and moralistic justification for violence against an external "phobogenic" object (Fanon, 1986). Fearful, prideful, and hateful fantasies roam through psychosocial space, and the desire to dominate the phobogenic object grows. This phobogenic object, which eventually takes the form of othered individuals and groups blamed for the decline of society, in-group, and self, is positioned as a toxic and dominating enemy force that must be defeated. It becomes the focus of conspiratorial fantasies that rationalise desires for control, torture, and extermination. Violence is thus redefined: because it secures identifications with fascist ideals and promises to eliminate the feared object, masochistic urges reverse into a sadistic destructiveness that reduces fear and generates narcissistic pleasure, satisfying "old wishes for omnipotence" (Freud, [1930] 2024, p. 109). Throughout the process of psychosocial transformation, dominating and eventually murderous impulses therefore become tied to feelings of narcissistic pride and pleasure, the fabrication of ontological security, and the relief of anxiety. Violence thus becomes an enjoyable and morally urgent activity in fascism, creating intense affective attachments to its increasingly barbaric enactment as a political practice.

The sexualities, desires, and pleasures of fascism must be understood in relation to the primary role of real and imagined violence. As with violence, there is no single factor that explains these sexualities and enjoyments: they too emerge from varied combinations of multiple factors and processes that generate, "*arouse and activate*" desire (Grand, this reader, p. 149). On a general level, sexuality involves a complex and ever-shifting entanglement of desiring, identifying, and destructive urges, all mediated by psychic defences, the gendered matrices of sexuality and desire (see Butler, 1997), and the vicissitudes of psychosocial becoming. Ante-fascist space contains a multiplicity of erogenous zones. There is the homoerotic enjoyment that surges among the audiences of rallies, group events, and broadcasts on television and social media, who masochistically submit themselves to a paranoid leader and indulge in a phantasmatic orgy of mutual identification (Freud, [1921] 2024; Adorno, this reader). "Pure" and "good" pleasures result from fantasies and sex acts involving white women identified with traditional family values; these acts generate narcissistic identification with the fascist ideals of racialised masculinity. Perverse oedipal enjoyment is available to those who enact their mothers' repressed desires, identifying with fascist ideals as they dominate racialised minorities in rituals of moralistic sadism. Going further into perversion, the rape of those dominated minorities presents an opportunity for transgressive sexual pleasures and feelings of omnipotence, the strange masochistic enjoyment of identifying with a dominated object, and the redirection of shame and moral self-reproaches after the act into sadistic attacks on the other… in the psychosocial and transitional space of ante-fascism, there are endless opportunities for alloying sexual and violent urges. The intense aggressive, negative cathexis of the denigrated other creates a pathway for erotic cathexes to develop, turning them into an object of desire. Those investments also make that denigrated other important for the subject's narcissistic coherence, transforming them into an ontological support for the self, its pleasures, and its continuity. Fascism's deadly allure derives from the fact that it makes erotised aggression acceptable, necessary, and moral. The true horror is that fascism is interminable because it is enjoyable.

Conclusion

In our view, fascism is a syncretic, inconsistent political ideology which manifests itself in "states of fantasy" beset by internal antagonisms. Fascism is a precipitate of signifiers common to capitalist liberal democracies, anarchically cobbled together during times of crisis both personal and systemic. These crises inspire the affective and imaginary foundations of fascism: the narcissistic and paranoid-schizoid psychic defences, the desires for rebirth, pride, and domination, and the fears of decline, contamination, and being dominated or destroyed. Meanwhile, the precipitate of signifiers generated by these defences defines a set of ideals and abjects, typically but not necessarily polarised along the lines of nation, race, gender, and economy. This set of ideals and abjects interacts with those affects and fantasies to define the political programme of fascism, while the crisis inspires a sense of urgency that calls for its attainment by any means necessary, including the destruction of democracy and the violent domination of others. Fascism gradually emerges from liberal democratic "normalcy", especially during times of crisis: individuals and groups traverse the psychopolitical space of ante-fascism as their desires, fears, and defences are increasingly radicalised by a chronic sense of peril.

When fascism appears in the imaginary *en masse*, it may or may not transform political reality: it may remain buried and repressed or adequately contained, or it may irrupt into a full "state of fantasy" that takes hold of the subjective component of political being to the extent of redefining the body politic of an entire society. Whatever the case, fascism typically undoes itself in the long run. While the inconsistencies and contradictions in its political programme may give it energy originally, inspiring additional psychic defences or acts of violence against critics and opponents (see Bollas, this reader), they eventually cause its decline. Ethnic cleansing, genocide, and war, for example, clash with the dream of nationalistic revival, often powered by the capitalist logic of accumulation which requires an increasing population, rising economic demand, and increasing investment in productive capacity. As an intersubjectively odious political ideology and programme, fascism also invites resistance and essentially demands its own destruction. For these reasons, fascism is a basically suicidal ideology: a political manifestation of the death drive, garbed in the signs and symbols of the capitalist liberal democracies it tears apart, aimed outward at the world only so that it might return, one day, to annihilate the self (following Arendt and Césaire, a kind of "boomerang effect").

As we write, individuals, political parties, and states around the world continue their movements across the transitional space of ante-fascism. The extreme nightmare of fascism, however, is not yet fully realised. It may indeed falter and retreat before it manages to colonise our world. There is, for example, a growing sense that Trump is simply not sufficiently competent or effective to carry out "the second American Revolution" that, as Heritage Foundation Director and key proponent of Project 2025, Kevin Roberts, said, "will remain bloodless if the left allows it to be" (Associated Press, 2024). "The United States", Timothy Snyder writes, has "fascists in positions of authority, and federal institutions carrying out policies of oppression that cannot be reconciled with the rule of law"; nevertheless, Trump "is failing at fascism … The [2026] State of the Union was full of fascist atmospherics. But it was also blowhard exhaustion" (Snyder, 2026). Even the most extreme "Dark Enlightenment" theorists are pessimistic: the "second Trump revolution, like the first, is failing", writes Curtis Yarvin. "It is failing because it deserves to fail" (Yarvin, 2025).

Fascism has not yet fully arrived—it remains ghostly and spectral, a potential in the process of emergence, half-real and half-dream. For now, then, countries like the US are best described as ante-fascist: its leaders, government, institutions, and a large number of its people are not yet entrapped in the extremes of fascism. But equally, many of them are no longer liberal or democratic. They live in ambivalent, contradictory and transitional states of fantasy, but they do not yet exist within the nightmarish real of fascism. And here we should not forget, as Rose writes, "that fantasy's supreme characteristic is that of running ahead of itself". "There is something coerced and coercive", she continues, "but also wild and unpredictable, about it. If fantasy can give us the inner measure of statehood, it might also help to prise open the space in the mind where the worst of modern statehood loses its conviction, falters, and starts to let go" (Rose, 1996, pp. 14–15). We cannot say if today's ante-fascist movements are abortive or "terminable". They may yet prove that they are no more than "wishful phantasies which, like the myth of a Golden Age, have been projected back into the past" (Freud, [1913] 2024). And in the doubt that grows when these phantasies begin to falter and let go, we might discover the possibility of a more radical alternative to the systemic crises that afflict global humanity. The navel of a new dream, perhaps, that emerges from the tangle of thoughts at the centre of our crisis to branch out in more hopeful directions.

"But who can foresee", as Freud ([1930] 2024, p. 131) appended to *Civilization and its Discontents* in 1931, "with what success and with what result?"

Notes

1 Elsewhere in the same Memorandum issued by the US Attorney General on December 4, 2025, we read: "violence against what extremists claim to be fascism is the clarion call of recent domestic terrorism" (Office of the Attorney General, 2025).

2 Fascism and capitalism arguably share a commitment to destruction, too. As Schumpeter famously argued, capitalism is driven by the process of "creative destruction", whereby new wealth is produced by destroying the old. The "process of Creative Destruction is the essential fact about capitalism", he writes. "It incessantly revolutionizes the economic structure from within, incessantly destroying the old one, incessantly creating a new one" (Schumpeter, 2003, p. 83). Capitalism, however, is not solely destructive, as accumulation requires creativity. This is where it conflicts with fascism which, as the Nazi regime illustrates, trends in the extreme towards a suicidal and self-destructive spiral that is ultimately incompatible with wealth creation and accumulation.

3 For Freeden, these are the "seven core concepts" that have "recurring status" in the highly diverse "family of liberalisms". According to Freeden, these concepts are "durable" and "ubiquitous" within theories of liberalism; they also encompass "multiple different conceptions, resulting in inevitable permutations within liberalism" (2025, p. 243).

4 One characteristic of neoliberalism, which it shares with some but not all other versions of liberalism, is its assertion that political freedom and democracy rely upon and cannot exist without economic freedom and private property. "We have progressively abandoned that freedom in economic affairs without which personal and political freedom has never existed in the past", Hayek writes in *The Road to Serfdom*. He continues: "If 'capitalism' means here a competitive system based on free disposal over private property, it is far more important to realise that only within this system is democracy possible." Elsewhere still: "The system of private property is the most important guarantee of freedom, not only for those who own property, but scarcely less for those who do not" (Hayek, [1944] 2001, pp. 13, 73 & 108). Though Freeden does not include private property as one of the seven core concepts of liberalism, it is a privileged element of many liberal ideologies and, in practice, nominally liberal democratic states generally observe and uphold (an often-delimited form of) private property as a key institution.

5 For a discussion of the relationship between fascism and genocide or "eliminationism", see Kallis (2008).

6 See also Dagmar Herzog's *Sex After Fascism* (2007), which argues that the Nazi state promoted a kind of circumscribed sexual freedom for heterosexual Aryan people, while proscribing sexual liberty for others.

7 A recent example of the contradictory purity/virility dynamic Herzog discusses in *Sex After Fascism* comes from Andrew Tate. Tate, who faces criminal charges for rape and sex-trafficking in multiple countries and who is widely known for disseminating his misogynistic ideology of extreme "alpha-male" machismo, tweeted in 2024: "Sex is for making children. Any man who has sex with women because it "feels good" is gay… if you are 40 with less than 5 children you're probably gay" (Tate, 2024). On the one hand, Tate allegedly practises criminal sexual transgression; on the other, he preaches extreme asceticism. (His post raises issues, too, about repressed homosexuality, misogyny, and heteronormativity in fascism.)

8 It is interesting to consider the value attached to the signifier "fascism" in this process. Relentlessly demonised in liberal democratic societies since the Second World War, identifying positively with "fascism" would cause most people to experience feelings of shame, guilt, and embarrassment. As the allure of fascism became more intense, individuals who identified with the signifier would thereby need strategies to deal with these negative affects. These strategies might include denial and disavowal, splitting and projection, cynicism, or ironic identification with the signifier. As "fascism" becomes more normalised, we would expect to see individuals transition from a state of defensive shame to a perverse shamelessness, a triumphant sadistic pride in one's identification with fascism, and a joy in seeing the disgust and anxiety that identification provokes in the other. The final stage involves fascism's banality: a point neither of pride nor of shame, fascism simply becomes part of the ordinary social milieu. Some individuals can now be observed at the penultimate stage. Consider the rise of "vice-signalling", exemplified by the footage of individuals like Andrew Tate and Nick Fuentes who now perform Nazi salutes in nightclubs while singing along to Kanye West's song *Heil Hitler* (CBS Miami, 2026).

9 Wendy Brown connects this process of desublimation to Nietzschean nihilism: when the "highest values hitherto" collapse during a time of crisis, the erotic and aggressive impulses once sublimated in conscience and the adherence to those values are freed, allowing them to find new objects (Brown, 2019, pp. 160–165).

10 We borrow the term "imaginative labour" from Afropessimist theorists Jared Sexton and Frank B. Wilderson III (see Sexton, 2003, p. 247; Wilderson, 2010, pp. 30 & 134–136).

References

Adorno, T.W. ([1951] 2027) 'Freudian Theory and the Pattern of Fascist Propaganda', in A. Cannon and T. Fielder (eds) *Psychoanalysis and Fascism: A Reader*. Routledge, pp. 71–90.

Adorno, T., Frenkel-Brunswik, E., Levinson, D., & Sanford, N. (2019) *The Authoritarian Personality*. Verso.

Amnesty International (2026) *USA/Iran: Those Responsible for Deadly and Unlawful US Strike on School That Killed over 100 Children must be Held Accountable*. Available at: https://www.amnesty.org/en/latest/news/2026/03/usa-iran-those-responsible-for-deadly-and-unlawful-us-strike-on-school-that-killed-over-100-children-must-be-held-accountable/ (Accessed: 27 March 2026).

Arendt, H. [1964] (2017) 'Letter 133', in M. L. Knott (ed.) *The Correspondence of Hannah Arendt and Gershom Scholem*. The University Of Chicago Press, pp. 205–210.

Armin, K. (2026) *Iran Protest Death Toll Could Top 30,000, According to Local Health Officials*. Available at: https://time.com/7357635/more-than-30000-killed-in-iran-say-senior-officials/ (Accessed: 27 March 2026).

Armstrong, K. (2026) *Teenager among First to be Executed over Iran's Anti-Government Protests*. Available at: https://www.bbc.com/news/articles/ce9mzn7k722o (Accessed: 27 March 2026).

Associated Press (2024) *Leader of the Pro-Trump Project 2025 Suggests There will be a New American Revolution*. Available at: https://www.politico.com/news/2024/07/04/leader-of-the-pro-trump-project-2025-suggests-there-will-be-a-new-american-revolution-00166583 (Accessed: 27 March 2026).

Bollas, C. (1979) 'The transformational object', *The International Journal of Psychoanalysis*, 60(1), pp. 97–107.

Bollas, C. (2027) 'The Fascist State of Mind', in A. Cannon and T. Fielder (eds) *Psychoanalysis and Fascism: A Reader*. Routledge, pp. 19–35.
Brown, W. (2019) *In the Ruins of Neoliberalism: The Rise of Antidemocratic Politics in the West*. Columbia University Press.
Buchanan, J. (1975) *The Limits of Liberty*. The University of Chicago Press.
Burleigh, M. (2000) *The Third Reich: A New History*. Macmillan.
Butler, J. (1997) *The Psychic Life of Power: Theories in Subjection*. Stanford University Press.
Cannon, A. (2024) *Infinite Discontent: Writings on the Allure of Fascism*. eidolon ink.
CBS Miami. (2026) *Controversy at South Beach Club as Far-Right Influencers Request Banned Kanye West Song*. Available at: https://www.youtube.com/watch?v=_PRCNVYkaE0 (Accessed: 5 March 2026).
Eco, U. (1995) 'Ur-Fascism', *The New York Review of Books* (22 June). Available at: https://www.nybooks.com/articles/1995/06/22/ur-fascism/ (Accessed: 27 March 2026).
Fanon, F. (1986) *Black Skin, White Masks*. Pluto Press.
Fielder, T. (2026) Infinite Discontent: Writings on the Allure of Fascism. *Psychoanalysis, Culture and Society*, 31, pp. 546–555.
Freeden, M. (2025) 'Liberalism', in G. F. Gaus, F. D'Agostino, & R. Muldoon (eds.) *The Routledge Companion to Social and Political Philosophy* (2nd ed.). Routledge, pp. 237–248.
Freud, S. [1900a] (2024) 'The Interpretation of Dreams', in M. Solms (ed.) *The Revised Standard Edition of the Complete Psychological Works of Sigmund Freud, Volume IV*. Rowman & Littlefield, pp. 1–302.
Freud, S. [1900b] (2024) 'The Interpretation of Dreams', in M. Solms (ed.) *The Revised Standard Edition of the Complete Psychological Works of Sigmund Freud, Volume V*. Rowman & Littlefield, pp. 303–555.
Freud, S. [1913] (2024) 'Totem and Taboo', in M. Solms (ed.) *The Revised Standard Edition of the Complete Psychological Works of Sigmund Freud, Volume XIII*. Rowman & Littlefield, pp. 7–156.
Freud, S. [1914a] (2024) 'Remembering, Repeating, and Working Through: (Further Recommendations on the Technique of Psychoanalysis II)', in M. Solms (ed.) *The Revised Standard Edition of the Complete Psychological Works of Sigmund Freud, Volume XII*. Rowman & Littlefield, pp. 145–158.
Freud, S. [1914b] (2024) 'Some Reflections on Schoolboy Psychology', in M. Solms (ed.) *The Revised Standard Edition of the Complete Psychological Works of Sigmund Freud, Volume XIII*. Rowman & Littlefield, pp. 235–238.
Freud, S. [1915] (2024) 'Drives and their Vicissitudes', in M. Solms (ed.) *The Revised Standard Edition of the Complete Psychological Works of Sigmund Freud, Volume XIV*. Rowman & Littlefield, pp. 103–123.
Freud, S. [1917] (2024) 'Mourning and Melancholia', in M. Solms (ed.) *The Revised Standard Edition of the Complete Psychological Works of Sigmund Freud, Volume XIV*. Rowman & Littlefield, pp. 217–238.
Freud, S. [1921] (2024) 'Group Psychology and the Analysis of the Ego', in M. Solms (ed.) *The Revised Standard Edition of the Complete Psychological Works of Sigmund Freud, Volume XVIII*. Rowman & Littlefield, pp. 67–138.
Freud, S. [1923] (2024) 'The Ego and the Id', in M. Solms (ed.) *The Revised Standard Edition of the Complete Psychological Works of Sigmund Freud, Volume XIX*. Rowman & Littlefield, pp. 10–62.
Freud, S. [1925] (2024) 'Negation', in M. Solms (ed.) *The Revised Edition of the Complete Psychological Works of Sigmund Freud, Volume XIX*. Rowman & Littlefield, pp. 237–248.

Freud, S. [1930] (2024) 'Civilization and its Discontents', in M. Solms (ed.) *The Revised Standard Edition of the Complete Psychological Works of Sigmund Freud, XXI*. Rowman & Littlefield, pp. 59–136.

Freud, S. [1937] (2024) 'Analysis Terminable and Interminable', in M. Solms (ed.) *The Revised Standard Edition of the Complete Psychological Works of Sigmund Freud, Volume XXIII*. Rowman & Littlefield, pp. 195–232.

Frosh, S. (2018) 'Psychosocial Studies and Psychoanalysis', in H. Stam & H. Looren de Jong (eds.) *The SAGE Handbook of Theoretical Psychology*. Sage. Available at: https://doi.org/10.4135/9781526402073.n31 (Accessed: 31 March 2026).

Frosh, S. (2023) *Anti-Semitism and Racism: Ethical Challenges for Psychoanalysis*. London, Palgrave Macmillan.

Frosh, S. (2027) 'Studies in Prejudice: Theorizing Anti-Semitism in the Wake of the Nazi Holocaust', in A. Cannon and T. Fielder (eds) *Psychoanalysis and Fascism: A Reader*. Routledge, pp. 206–221.

Frosh, S., & Baraitser, L. (2008). 'Psychoanalysis and psychosocial studies', *Psychoanalysis, Culture & Society*, 13(4), pp. 346–365. Available at: https://doi.org/10.1057/pcs.2008.8 (Accessed: 28 March 2026).

Giddens, A. (1991) *Modernity and Self-Identity: Self and Society in the Late Modern Age*. Stanford University Press.

Grand, S. (2027) 'Fascism and the Web of Perversion', in A. Cannon and T. Fielder (eds) *Psychoanalysis and Fascism: A Reader*. Routledge, pp. 144–161.

Griffin, R. (1991) *The Nature of Fascism*. Routledge.

Griffin, R. (2018) *Fascism: An Introduction to Comparative Fascist Studies*. Polity Press.

Hayek, F. [1944] (2001) *The Road to Serfdom*. Routledge.

Herzog, D. (2007) *Sex After Fascism: Memory and Morality in Twentieth-Century Germany*. Princeton University Press.

Kallis, A. (2008) *Genocide and Fascism: The Eliminationist Drive in Fascist Europe*. Routledge.

Kernberg, O.F. (2027) 'Malignant Narcissism and Large Group Regression', in A. Cannon and T. Fielder (eds) *Psychoanalysis and Fascism: A Reader*. Routledge, pp. 91–109.

Klippenstein, K. (2025) *What are "Nihilistic Violent Extremists"?* Available at: https://www.kenklippenstein.com/p/what-are-nihilist-violent-extremists (Accessed: 05 March 2026).

Kohut, H. (1972) 'Thoughts on narcissism and narcissistic rage', *The Psychoanalytic Study of the Child*, 27, pp. 360–400. Available at: https://doi.org/10.1080/00797308.1972.11822721 (Accessed: 28 March 2026).

Laing, R. D. [1960] (2010) *The Divided Self*. London, Penguin.

McAfee, N. (2019) *Fear of Breakdown: Politics and Psychoanalysis*. Columbia University Press.

Moyn, S. (2023) *Liberalism Against Itself: Cold War Intellectuals and the Making of Our Times*. Yale University Press.

Office of Public Affairs (2026) *Antifa Cell Members Convicted in Prairieland ICE Detention Center Shooting*. Available at: https://www.justice.gov/opa/pr/antifa-cell-members-convicted-prairieland-ice-detention-center-shooting (Accessed: 27 March 2026).

Office of the Attorney General (2025) *December 4, 2025: Memorandum for All Federal Prosecutors*. Available at: https://www.washingtonpost.com/documents/b610d753-733b-4eee-8a17-5035bc94cd6c.pdf (Accessed: 27 March 2026).

Paxton, R. O. (2004) *The Anatomy of Fascism*. Alfred. A. Knopf.

Rieff, P. [1959] (1979) *Freud: The Mind of the Moralist*. Chicago University Press.

Rose, J. (1996) *States of Fantasy*. Clarendon Press.

Rose, J. (2027) 'Total Belief: Delirium in the West', in A. Cannon and T. Fielder (eds) *Psychoanalysis and Fascism: A Reader*. Routledge, pp. 110–125.
Salberg, J. (2027) '"Don't You See I'm Burning?": Fascism Amnesia and the Failure of Witnessing', in A. Cannon and T. Fielder (eds) *Psychoanalysis and Fascism: A Reader*. Routledge, pp. 225–236.
Savell, S. (2023) *How Death Outlives War: The Reverberating Impact of Post-9/11 Wars on Human Health*. Available at: https://costsofwar.watson.brown.edu/sites/default/files/papers/How-Death-Outlives-War.pdf (Accessed: 28 March 2026).
Schumpeter, J. (2003) *Capitalism, Socialism and Democracy*. Routledge.
Sexton, J. (2003) 'The consequence of race mixture: Racialised barriers and the politics of desire', *Social Identities*, 9(2), pp. 241–275. Available at: http://doi.org/10.1080/1350463032000101588 (Accessed: 28 March 2026).
Sharpe, C. (2016) *In the Wake: On Blackness and Being*. Duke University Press.
Snyder, T. (2026) *Fascist Failure*. Available at: https://snyder.substack.com/p/fascist-failure (Accessed: 27 March 2026).
Tate, A. (2024) *Sex is for making children*. April 24, 2024. Available at: https://x.com/Cobratate/status/1783049915800736108 (Accessed: 05 March 2026).
Toscano, A. (2023) *Late Fascism: Race, Capitalism and the Politics of Crisis*. Verso.
Varieties of Democracy Institute (2026) *Democracy Report 2026: Unraveling the Democratic Era?* Available at: https://www.v-dem.net/documents/75/V-Dem_Institute_Democracy_Report_2026_lowres.pdf (Accessed: 27 March 2026).
Volkan, V. D. (2001) Transgenerational transmissions and chosen traumas: An aspect of large-group identity. *Group Analysis*, 34(1), pp. 79–97. Available at: https://doi.org/10.1177/05333160122077730 (Accessed: 28 March 2026).
Volkan, V. D. (2020) *Large-Group Psychology: Racism, Societal Divisions, Narcissistic Leaders and Who We Are Now*. Karnac.
Ward, E. (2026) *Israeli Leaflets over Beirut Invoke Gaza's Destruction and Stoke Fear*. Available at: https://www.nytimes.com/2026/03/13/world/middleeast/israeli-leaflets-over-beirut-invoke-gazas-destruction-and-stoke-fear.html (Accessed: 27 March 2026).
Wieland, C. (2014) *The Fascist State of Mind and the Manufacturing of Masculinity: A Psychoanalytic Approach*. Routledge.
Wilderson, F. B. (2010) *Red, White & Black: Cinema and the Structure of U.S. Antagonisms*. Duke University Press.
Wilderson, F. B. (2020) *Afropessimism*. New York, Liveright.
Wilson, L. (2024) *Pete Hegseth's Tattoos and the Crusading Obsession of the Far Right*. Available at: https://newlinesmag.com/essays/pete-hegseths-tattoos-and-the-crusading-obsession-of-the-far-right/ (Accessed: 27 March 2026).
Winnicott, D. W. (1960) The Theory of the Parent-Infant Relationship. *The International Journal of Psychoanalysis*, 41, pp. 585–595. Available at: https://pep-web.org/search/document/IJP.041.0585A (Accessed: 28 March 2026).
Winnicott, D. W. (1974) Fear of Breakdown. *The International Review of Psychoanalysis*, 1, pp. 103–107. Available at: https://pep-web.org/search/document/IRP.001.0103A (Accessed: 28 March 2026).
Winnicott, D. W. (1975) *Through Paediatrics to Psycho-Analysis*. Basic Books.
Winnicott, D. W. (2005) *Playing and Reality*. Routledge.
Yarvin, C. (2025) *You Can't Handle the Truth*. Available at: https://graymirror.substack.com/p/you-cant-handle-the-truth (Accessed: 28 March 2026).
Yates, C. (2015) *The Play of Political Culture, Emotion and Identity*. Palgrave Macmillan.
Žižek, S. (2006) 'The Fetish of the Party', in R. Butler & S. Stephens (eds.) *The Universal Exception*. London, Continuum, pp. 67–93.
Žižek, S. (2026) *Iran from Heidegger to Kant*. Available at: https://slavoj.substack.com/p/iran-from-heidegger-to-kant (Accessed: 27 March 2026).

Directions for Future Research and Further Readings

Alasdair Cannon and Tom Fielder

One of our key motivations for publishing this collection was to inspire future research in psychoanalysis and fascism. In this spirit, we close this book by suggesting some directions for research that could be explored by academic researchers or students working at the graduate or even undergraduate level. We have also included a list of papers that readers may wish to explore to gain a deeper understanding of the field.

Much of the research in psychoanalysis and fascism utilises a relatively narrow range of psychoanalytic references to theorise fascism—typically, Freud, Klein, Winnicott, Bion, and Lacan. We note that there has been little use of ideas and concepts from relational and intersubjective psychoanalysis in papers theorising fascism. Applying Jessica Benjamin's works on gender and domination (e.g., Benjamin, 1988) to fascistic politics, we suggest, is a largely unexplored and potentially fruitful avenue for further work (see Cannon, 2024, pp. 124–132; Rabinbach & Benjamin, 1989). Similarly, there has been less application of Lacanian ideas to fascism than one would expect (but see MacCannell, 1993, 2000; Vadolas, 2009; McGowan, 2022). As Alberto Toscano's essay in this reader shows, Žižek provides a highly interesting Lacanian take on fascism at various points in his oeuvre (see e.g. Žižek, 2006, pp. 67–93): future research could extend both his Lacanian articulation of fascism and its application to fascistic political movements and phenomena. Among existing psychoanalytic studies, there is often a tacit reliance on anxiety as a central mechanism of the fascist state of fantasy. To explain fascism, psychoanalysts refer to Reichian sexual anxiety, Winnicottian disintegration anxiety, Lacanian anxiety and perversion, and so on. A comparative study of psychoanalytic perspectives on anxiety and political ideology would, no doubt, be of significant value for theorising fascist states of fantasy. As alumni of Birkbeck College's Department of Psychosocial Studies, the editors also believe that the work of researchers like Stephen Frosh, Jacqueline Rose, Margarita Palacios, and more, could be highly useful for researchers looking to explore how the psyche and the social co-constitute one another within fascist movements—how fascist ideology, psychic phenomena, political groups, media technologies, and the state generate and shape one another simultaneously.

DOI: 10.4324/9781003742876-20

We also believe that both psychoanalytic and political theoretical studies of fascism would be enriched through greater interdisciplinary mutuality. As discussed in the introduction, psychoanalytic studies often portray fascism as a psychopathological condition without specific political or ideological attributes. "Fascism" is thereby flattened into a term essentially coextensive with states of psychopolitical extremism, however opposed these states might be in simple ideological terms. Meanwhile, political theorists tend to generate psychological concepts and implicit theories of mental life in their discussions of the psychic-affective dimensions of fascist politics which, from a psychoanalytic perspective, leave much to be considered and more carefully substantiated. A brief consideration of the work of fascist scholar Roger Griffin is instructive here. None of the papers included in this reader book cite Griffin's seminal definition of fascism as "palingenetic ultranationalism" (Griffin, 1991) despite its great influence in the field of fascist studies. Griffin, however, does not cite any psychoanalysts besides Jung when he theorises the psychological basis of fascism in his work; his conclusion that fascism relies on the "basic" and "ancient psychological mechanisms of mythopoeia and self-transcendence" (1991, p. 192) arguably follows from his neglect of psychoanalytic theory, which would position both phenomena as derivatives of more basic sexual and narcissistic urges. Greater interdisciplinary awareness and exchange, both in this instance and in general, would improve both the political theoretical and psychoanalytic perspectives on fascism as a psychopolitical phenomenon.

As mentioned in this reader's Introduction, there is also a relative dearth of psychoanalytic work on fascism outside its classical European contexts—Germany and Italy—and its rise in the United States today. This reflects a widely Eurocentric/Western bias within psychoanalytic studies of politics, which is only exacerbated by the linguistic barriers researchers face when analysing political movements elsewhere in the world. Putting to one side the political theoretical question of whether the following regimes are fascist in Griffin's (1991) strict sense, the English-language literature on psychoanalysis and fascism has largely neglected Second World War Japan. Other European and Asian movements and governments that some historians have classified as fascist—for example, the earlier years of Franco's Spain, Rhee's South Korea after 1948 (see Yang, 2025), and Suharto's Indonesia of the 1960s, three countries where tens of thousands of people were killed in anti-communist purges—have also been ignored by psychoanalytic scholars. The same goes for South American movements like Peronist populism that, while not precisely fascist, share important "genealogical" and "ideological continuities" with fascism (cf. Finchelstein, 2014). Psychoanalytic scholars have also left fascism in the Middle East untheorised. The Lebanese Phalangist Party or Rashid Ali al-Gaylani's Nazi-aligned regime in Iraq, whose collapse in 1941 led to the Farhud against Baghdad Jews, are both ripe for study. Similarly, there is some potential for psychoanalytic studies of fascism in African contexts. Influential African nationalist Marcus Garvey once claimed that the members of his Universal

Negro Improvement Association were "the first Fascists" (Gilroy, 2000, p. 70). Though the decolonial context of Garvey's pan-Africanism greatly complicates its status as a fascistic movement, there is nonetheless ample scope for psychoanalytic studies of African movements of this kind. The same goes for the relationship between fascism, decolonial movements, and reactionary colonial suppression more broadly—a question given new urgency by Israel's genocidal war against the Palestinians in Gaza.

Psychoanalytic studies of fascism would also benefit from greater engagement with critical race theory, especially by Black writers. In her paper included in this collection, Grand notes that the Nazis were inspired by the US regime of racial segregation and that Paxton (2004) considers the KKK to be the first fascist movement (Grand, this reader, pp. 145 & 152). Psychoanalytic writers mostly neglect the anti-Black elements of fascism, however, meaning there is much scope for further work connecting critical race theory and psychoanalytic studies of fascism. One potential area for further work is in the application of Afropessimism to contemporary fascism—something one of the editors of this collection has explored in an article that uses Afropessimism and psychoanalysis to examine Kanye West's strange Black-liberation Nazism (Cannon, 2025). Afropessimism, Wilderson states, is a critical metatheory of psychoanalysis; it is also a theory of anti-Black racism that regularly deploys psychoanalytic concepts (see Wilderson, 2010, 2020). There is much scope for using Afropessimism and other critical race theories to analyse the libidinal economy of fascist politics and their racist elements. This is especially true for Trump's America, where anti-Black racism is an increasingly explicit feature of the administration's official rhetoric: we recall, with dismay, the video Trump posted depicting Barack and Michelle Obama as apes, and Trump's comment to Homeland Security Advisor, Stephen Miller, that "if we had it your way, everyone would look like you" (see Matza, 2026; Parker, Scherer & Miroff, 2026).

This short section covers only a small selection of possibilities for additional research. We trust it suffices, though, to show that the field of psychoanalytic studies in fascism is wide open for further development.

References

Benjamin, J. (1988) *The Bonds of Love: Psychoanalysis, Feminism, and the Problem of Domination*. Pantheon Books.

Cannon, A. (2024) *Infinite Discontent: Writings on the Allure of Fascism*. London: eidolon ink.

Cannon, A. (2025) 'Kanye's Black Nazism', *Arena Quarterly*, 22. Available at: https://arena.org.au/kanyes-black-nazism/ (Accessed: 28 March 2026).

Fielder, T. (2026) 'Infinite Discontent: Writings on the Allure of Fascism', *Psychoanalysis, Culture and Society*, 31, pp. 546–555.

Finchelstein, F. (2014) *The Ideological Origins of the Dirty War: Fascism, Populism, and Dictatorship in Twentieth Century Argentina*. Oxford Academic.

Gilroy, P. (2000) Black Fascism. *Transition*, 81/82, pp. 70–91. Available at: https://www.jstor.org/stable/3137450 (Accessed: 20 February 2026).

Grand, S. (2027) 'Fascism and the Web of Perversion'. In A. Cannon and T. Fielder (eds) *Psychoanalysis and Fascism: A Reader*. Routledge, pp. 144–161.
Griffin, R. (1991) *The Nature of Fascism*. Routledge.
MacCannell, J. F. (1993) 'Facing Fascism: A Feminine Politics of Jouissance', *Topoi*, 12, pp. 137–151.
MacCannell, J. F. (2000) 'Fascism and the Voice of Conscience', in *The Hysteric's Guide to the Future Female Subject*. University of Minnesota Press, pp. 127–152.
McGowan, T. (2022) *The Racist Fantasy: Unconscious Roots of Hatred*. Bloomsbury Publishing.
Matza, M. (2026) *Obama Addresses Racist Video Shared by Trump Depicting Him as an Ape*. Available at: https://www.bbc.co.uk/news/articles/c74754j7qwgo (Accessed: 26 February 2026).
Parker, A., Scherer, M., & Miroff, N. (2026) 'The Wrath of Stephen Miller', *The Atlantic*, 7 January. Available at: https://www.theatlantic.com/politics/2026/01/stephen-miller-trump-white-house/685516/ (Accessed: 20 February 2026).
Paxton, R. O. (2004) *The Anatomy of Fascism*. Alfred. A. Knopf.
Rabinbach, A., & Benjamin, J. (1989) 'The Emotional Core of Fascism in Its Most Virulent Psychic Manifestations'. In: S. Geroulanos & D. Herzog (eds) *Staging the Third Reich: Essays in Cultural and Intellectual History*. Routledge, pp. 66–82.
Vadolas, A. (2009) *Perversions of Fascism*. Routledge.
Yang, S. (2025) 'The Highest Stage of Nationalism: Postcolonial Fascism in Korea and Breaking Fascism Out of a Eurocentric Frame', *The American Historical Review*, 130(4), pp. 1512–1534. https://doi.org/10.1093/ahr/rhaf476
Žižek, S. (2006) 'The Fetish of the Party', in R. Butler & S. Stephens (eds.) *The Universal Exception*. Continuum, pp. 67–93.

Further Readings

Adorno, T., Frenkel-Brunswik, E., Levinson, D., & Sanford, N. (2019) *The Authoritarian Personality*. Verso.
Barratt, B. B. (2021) 'Reassessing Wilhelm Reich's Mass Psychology: Libidinality, Authoritarianism and the Rise of Fascism', *Philosophy and Global Affairs*, 1(2), pp. 179–208.
Bettelheim, B. (1943) 'Individual and Mass Behavior in Extreme Situations', *The Journal of Abnormal and Social Psychology*, 38(4), pp. 417–452.
Butler, J. (2019) 'Genius or Suicide', *London Review of Books*, 41(20). Available at: https://www.lrb.co.uk/the-paper/v41/n20/judith-butler/genius-or-suicide
Cannon, A. (2024) *Infinite Discontent: Writings on the Allure of Fascism*. eidolon ink.
Caspary, A. (2002) 'The Conformist: Psychoanalytic Perspectives on Fascism', *Canadian Journal of Psychoanalysis*, 10(1), pp. 115–131.
Chasseguet-Smirgel, J. (1990) 'Reflections of a Psychoanalyst Upon the Nazi Biocracy and Genocide', *International Review of Psycho-Analysis*, 17(2), pp. 167–176. https://psycnet.apa.org/record/1990-28120-001
Cooklin, K. (2021) 'Borders of Identity: Abjection, Foreignness and Fascism', in R. Pine & V. Konidari (eds.) *Borders and Borderlands: Explorations in Identity, Exile and Translation*. Cambridge Scholars Publishing, pp. 252–259.
Diamond, M. J. (2023) 'Perverted Containment: Trumpism, Cult Creation, and the Rise of Destructive American Populism', *Psychoanalytic Inquiry*, 43(2), pp. 96–109.
Faramelli, A., & Piper, I. (2022) 'Everybody Wants to be a Fascist Online: Psychoanalysis and the Digital Architecture of Fascism', *CLCWeb: Comparative Literature and Culture*, 24(4). https://doi.org/10.7771/1481-4374.4089
Fenichel, O. (1940) 'Psychoanalysis of Antisemitism', *American Imago*, 1(2), pp. 24–39.

Ffytche, M., & Pick, D. (eds.) (2016) *Psychoanalysis in the Age of Totalitarianism*. Routledge.

Fielder, T. (2026) 'Infinite Discontent: Writings on the Allure of Fascism', *Psychoanalysis, Culture and Society*, 31, pp. 546–555.

Figlio, K. (2006) 'The Absolute State of Mind in Society and the Individual', *Psychoanalysis, Culture & Society*, 11, pp. 119–143

Finchelstein, F. (2007) 'The Anti-Freudian Politics of Argentine Fascism: Anti-Semitism, Catholicism, and the Internal Enemy, 1932–1945', *Hispanic American Historical Review*, 87(1), pp. 77–110.

Finchelstein, F. (2009) 'Fascism Becomes Desire: On Freud, Mussolini and Transnational Politics', in J. Damousi & M. B. Plotkin (eds.) *The Transnational Unconscious: Essays in the History of Psychoanalysis and Transnationalism*. Palgrave Macmillan, pp. 99–123.

Fisher, D. J. (2004) 'Towards a Psychoanalytic Understanding of Fascism and Anti-Semitism: Perceptions from the 1940s', *Psychoanalysis and History*, 6(1), pp. 57–74.

Freud, S. [1921] (2024a) 'Group Psychology and the Analysis of the Ego', in M. Solms (ed.) *The Revised Standard Edition of the Complete Psychological Works of Sigmund Freud, Volume XVIII*. Rowman & Littlefield, pp. 67–138.

Freud, S. [1933] (2024b) 'Why War?', in M. Solms (ed.) *The Revised Standard Edition of the Complete Psychological Works of Sigmund Freud, Volume XXII*. Rowman & Littlefield, pp. 211–230.

Friedrich, V. (1995) 'The Internalization of Nazism and its Effects on German Psychoanalysts and their Patients', *American Imago*, 52(3), pp. 261–279.

Fromm, E. (2001) *The Fear of Freedom* (2nd ed.) Routledge.

Frosh, S. (1999) *The Politics of Psychoanalysis*. Bloomsbury Publishing.

Frosh, S. (2005) *Hate and the "Jewish Science": Anti-Semitism, Nazism and Psychoanalysis*. Palgrave Macmillan.

Frosh, S. (2012) 'The Re-enactment of Denial', in Gülerce, A. (ed.) *Re(con)figuring Psychoanalysis*. Palgrave Macmillan, London.

Frosh, S. (2019) *Those Who Come After: Postmemory, Acknowledgement and Forgiveness*. Palgrave Macmillan.

Frosh, S. (2023) *Antisemitism and Racism: Ethical Challenges for Psychoanalysis*. Bloomsbury Publishing.

Goldblatt, M. J., & Harvey, A. (2026) Fascist States of Mind: Individual Psychology and Group Functioning. *The International Journal of Applied Psychoanalytic Studies*, e70055. https://doi.org/10.1002/aps.70055

Grunberger, B. (1989) *New Essays on Narcissism*. Free Association Books.

Guattari, F. (1984) 'The Micro-Politics of Fascism', in *Molecular Revolution*. Penguin Books, pp. 217–232.

Guattari, F. (2009) 'Everybody Wants to be a Fascist', in S. Lotringer (ed.), *Chaosophy: Texts and Interviews 1972–1977*. Semiotexte, pp. 154–175.

Hartmann, D. D. (1984) 'Anti-Semitism and the Appeal of Nazism', *Political Psychology*, 5(4), pp. 635–642.

Holland, E. W. (2012) 'Schizoanalysis, Nomadology, Fascism', in I. Buchanan & N. Thoburn (eds.) *Deleuze & Politics*. Edinburgh University Press, pp. 74–97.

Hook, D. (2018) 'Racism and Jouissance: Evaluating the "Racism as (The Theft of) Enjoyment" Hypothesis', *Psychoanalysis, Culture & Society*, 23(3), pp. 244–266.

Jacoby, R. (1986) *The Repression of Psychoanalysis: Otto Fenichel and the Political Freudians*. Basic Books.

Kernberg, O. F. (2003a) 'Sanctioned Social Violence: A Psychoanalytic View – Part I', *The International Journal of Psychoanalysis*, 84(3), pp. 683–698.

Kernberg, O. F. (2003b) 'Sanctioned Social Violence: A Psychoanalytic View – Part II', *The International Journal of Psychoanalysis*, 84(4), pp. 953–968.

Kohut, H. (1972) 'Thoughts on Narcissism and Narcissistic Rage', *The Psychoanalytic Study of the Child*, 27, pp. 360–400.
Laub, D. & Auerhahn, N. C. (1989) 'Failed Empathy – A Central Theme in the Survivor's Holocaust Experience', *Psychoanalytic Psychology*, 6(4), pp. 377–400.
Leeb, C. (2018) 'Mystified Consciousness: Rethinking the Rise of the Far Right with Marx and Lacan', *Open Cultural Studies*, 2(1), pp. 236–248.
Levine, H. B. (1982) 'Toward a Psychoanalytic Understanding of Children of Survivors of the Holocaust', *The Psychoanalytic Quarterly*, 51(1), pp. 70–92.
Lifton, R. J. (1986) *The Nazi Doctors: Medical Killing and the Psychology of Genocide*. Basic Books.
Loewenstein, E. A. (2018) 'The Agitator and His Propaganda Machine: Donald Trump and the Road to American Fascism', *Fort Da*, 24(2), pp. 40–55.
Loewenstein, E. A. (2023) 'In Dark Times: Psychoanalytic Praxis as a Form of Resistance to Fascist Propaganda', *Psychoanalytic Inquiry*, 43(2), pp. 130–144.
MacCannell, J. F. (1993) 'Facing Fascism: A Feminine Politics of Jouissance', *Topoi*, 12, pp. 137–151.
MacCannell, J. F. (2000) 'Fascism and the Voice of Conscience', in *The Hysteric's Guide to the Future Female Subject*. University of Minnesota Press, pp. 127–152.
Mandelbaum, B., & Facchinetti, C. (2025) 'Nazism and Psychoanalysis in Brazil: The Institution of Silence in the First Psychoanalytic Societies', in S. Frosh & D. Baum (eds.) *The Routledge International Handbook of Psychoanalysis and Jewish Studies*. Routledge. https://doi.org/10.4324/9781003371311-9.
McAfee, N. (2019a) *Fear of Breakdown: Politics and Psychoanalysis*. Columbia University Press.
McAfee, N. (2019b) 'Politics and the Fear of Breakdown', in Allen, A., O'Connor, B. (eds.) *Transitional Subjects: Critical Theory and Object Relations*. Columbia University Press.
McGowan, T. (2020) 'Citizen Trump', *Continental Thought and Theory*, 3(1). http://doi.org/10.26021/1173
McGowan, T. (2022) *The Racist Fantasy: Unconscious Roots of Hatred*. Bloomsbury Publishing.
McGowan, T., Garberg, N. (2025) 'Psychoanalytic Reflections on America after Trump's Re-election: A Conversation with Todd McGowan', *Psychoanalysis, Culture & Society*. https://doi.org/10.1057/s41282-025-00598-x.
Mitscherlich, A., & Mitscherlich, M. (1984) *The Inability to Mourn: Principles of Collective Behavior*. Grove Press.
Moellenhoff, F. (1942) 'A Projection Returns and Materializes: Some Observations about Nazi Germany', *American Imago*, 3(3), pp. 3–13.
Ostow, M. (1986) 'The Psychodynamics of Apocalyptic: Discussion of Papers on Identification and the Nazi Phenomenon', *International Journal of Psychoanalysis*, 67, pp. 277–285
Pick, D. (2009) '"In Pursuit of the Nazi Mind?" The Deployment of Psychoanalysis in the Allied Struggle Against Germany', *Psychoanalysis and History*, 11(2), pp. 137–157.
Pick, D. (2012) *The Pursuit of the Nazi Mind: Hitler, Hess, and the Analysts*. Oxford University Press.
Prince, R. M. (2023) 'Locating the Fascist Mind', *Psychoanalytic Inquiry*, 43(2), pp. 70–83.
Rabinbach, A., & Benjamin, J. (1989) 'The Emotional Core of Fascism in Its Most Virulent Psychic Manifestations', in S. Geroulanos & D. Herzog (eds.) *Staging the Third Reich: Essays in Cultural and Intellectual History*. Routledge, pp. 66–82.
Rose, J. (1993) 'Margaret Thatcher and Ruth Ellis', in *Why War? – Psychoanalysis, Politics, and the Return to Melanie Klein*. Blackwell, pp. 41–86.
Rose, J. (1996) *States of Fantasy*. Oxford University Press.

Rosenfeld, H. (2022) 'Applying My Theory of Psychosis to the Nazi Phenomenon', in J. Arundale (ed.) *The Omnipotent State of Mind: Psychoanalytic Perspectives*. Routledge. https://doi.org/10.4324/9781003185192-22.
Seymour, R. (2024) *Disaster Nationalism: The Downfall of Liberal Civilization*. Verso.
Shapira, M. (2013) *The War Inside: Psychoanalysis, Total War, and the Making of the Democratic Self in Postwar Britain*. Cambridge University Press.
Sheehi, L., & Sheehi, S. (2022) *Psychoanalysis Under Occupation: Practicing Resistance in Palestine*. Routledge.
Shomron-Atar, E. N. (2017) 'Psychoanalysis Against Fascism: Fascism, Terrorism, and the Fascist and Terrorist Within', *Psychoanalytic Perspectives*, 15(1), pp. 48–63.
Shukla, R. (2021) 'Aspects of Male Sexuality Enmeshing with Rise of Fascism in India: Tentative Psychoanalytical Explorations', *International Journal of Applied Psychoanalytic Studies*, 18(1), pp. 3–17.
Simmel, E. (1946) 'Anti-Semitism and Mass Psychopathology', in E. Simmel (ed.) *Antisemitism: A Social Disease*. International Universities Press, pp. 33–78.
Theweleit, K. (1987) *Male Fantasies, Volume 1: Women, Floods, Bodies, History*. University of Minnesota Press.
Theweleit, K. (1989) *Male Fantasies, Volume 2: Male Bodies: Psychoanalyzing the White Terror*. University of Minneapolis Press.
Toscano, A. (2023) *Late Fascism: Race, Capitalism and the Politics of Crisis*. Verso.
Vadolas, A. (2009) *Perversions of Fascism*. Routledge.
Volkan, V. D. (2001) 'Transgenerational Transmissions and Chosen Traumas: An Aspect of Large-group Identity', *Group Analysis*, 34(1), pp. 79–97.
Volkan, V. D. (2009) 'Large-group Identity, International Relations and Psychoanalysis', *International Forum of Psychoanalysis*, 18(4), pp. 206–213.
Volkan, V. D. (2020) *Large-Group Psychology: Racism, Societal Divisions, Narcissistic Leaders and Who We Are Now*. Karnac.
Weiss, J. M. (2020) 'Understanding Fascism Today: Nationalism, Group Psychology, and the Return of the Old', *Rethinking Marxism*, 32, pp. 496–520.
Wieland, C. (2014) *The Fascist State of Mind and the Manufacturing of Masculinity: A Psychoanalytic Approach*. Routledge.
Wieland, C. (2017) 'The Primitive Container of Fascism: Masculine Anxieties and Defences in Times of Trauma and Uncertainty', in N. Mintchev & R. Hinshelwood (eds.) *The Feeling of Certainty: Psychosocial Perspectives on Identity and Difference*. Palgrave Macmillan, pp. 129–148.
Wilderson, F. B. (2010) *Red, White and Black: Cinema and the Structure of U.S. Antagonisms*. Duke University Press.
Wilderson, F. B. (2020) *Afropessimism*. Liveright.
Winnicott, D. W. (1974) 'Fear of Breakdown', *The International Review of Psychoanalysis*, 1, pp. 103–107.
Yates, C. (2015) *The Play of Political Culture, Emotion and Identity*. Palgrave Macmillan.
Zaretsky, E. (2015) *Political Freud: A History*. Columbia University Press.
Zaretsky, E. (2018) 'The Mass Psychology of Trumpism', *LRB Blog*, 18 September. Available at: https://www.lrb.co.uk/blog/2018/september/the-mass-psychology-of-trumpism
Žižek, S. (2006) 'The Fetish of the Party', in R. Butler & S. Stephens (eds.) *The Universal Exception*. Continuum, pp. 67–93.
Zolkos, M. (2022) 'The Phantasmatic Core of Fascism: Psychoanalytic Theories of Antisemitism and Group Aggression Amongst the "Political Freudians"', *Redescriptions: Political Thought, Conceptual History and Feminist Theory*, 25(1), pp. 49–64.
Wieland, C. (2023) 'Trauma and the Fascist State of Mind: The Emptying of the Self and the Road to Perdition', *Psychoanalytic Inquiry*, 43(2), pp. 84–95.

Index

Note: Pages followed by "n" refer to notes.

For Product Safety Concerns and Information please contact our EU representative GPSR@taylorandfrancis.com
Taylor & Francis Verlag GmbH, Kaufingerstraße 24, 80331 München, Germany

www.ingramcontent.com/pod-product-compliance
Ingram Content Group UK Ltd.
Pitfield, Milton Keynes, MK11 3LW, UK
UKHW022248051026
476334UK00010B/419
9781041246374